The Wounded Breast
Intimate Journeys through Cancer

Evelyne Accad

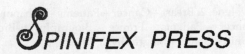
SPINIFEX PRESS

Spinifex Press Pty Ltd
504 Queensberry Street
North Melbourne, Vic. 3051
Australia
women@spinifexpress.com.au
www.spinifexpress.com.au

Published by Spinifex Press, 2001

Edited by Deborah Doyle (Living Proof – Book Editing)
Cover design by Deb Snibson (Modern Art)
Photographs by Eva Enderlein
Back-cover photograph by Paul Vieille
Designed and typeset by Sam Bunny (Fire Ink Press)

Made and printed in Australia by McPherson's Printing Group

National Library of Australia Cataloguing-in-Publication data:
Accad, Evelyne, 1943–

The wounded breast: intimate journeys through cancer.

ISBN 1 876756 12 8.

1. Accad, Evelyne. 2. Breast – Cancer – Patients – Lebanon – Biography. 3.
Breast – Cancer – Patients – France – Biography. 4. Breast – Cancer –
Patients – United States – Biography. I. Title.

362.196994490092

To the memory of my little sister, Séverine, victim of this terrible disease, who struggled against it so courageously

And to all my beautiful friends, survivors like me: Alex, Caryl, Charlotte, Elizabeth, Louise, Nadia, Nina, Paul, Rita, Yolaine-Esmeralda, Yoline and Zohreh

To forget nothing, to efface nothing: that is the obsession of survivors; to plead for the dead, to defend their memory and honor. So much has been said about them. They have been subjected to countless analyses, dissected, exhibited, and made 'presentable' for theological, scientific, political, and commercial purposes. Treated like objects, they have been insulted, belittled, and betrayed. To resist this tide, survivors … have only words, poor, ineffectual words, with which to defend the dead. So some of us weave these words into tales, stories, and pleas. It is all we can do for the dead. And our only wish is to be heard by the living. (Wiesel: 1995)

None of these *[10,940 people who die each year in the United States from environmentally caused cancers]* will die quick, painless deaths. They will be amputated, irradiated, and dosed with chemotherapy. They will expire privately in hospitals and hospices and be buried quietly. Photographs of their bodies will not appear in newspapers. We will not know who most of them are. Their anonymity, however, does not moderate this violence. These deaths are a form of homicide. (Steingraber: 1997)

With all the data we have at our disposal today, burying one's head in the sand constitutes a crime against humanity that will cause more death and suffering than the concentration camps. (Séralini: 1997)

Contents

Acknowledgements

The anguish, sadness and despair!

Bettina: These first three words are very pessimistic! Isn't your message to give hope, because, as you also say, there are survivors, and you are one of them?

Yes, it is! However, I'm first and foremost trying to attract attention to an acute and tragic problem that's often ignored and trivialised.

The barbarism of the twentieth century, and the mutilations and deaths suffered the world over as a result of cancer, are at the core of my writing this book.

In deciding the book's structure and content, I was expressing my commitment to women, men, ecology and peace issues, and the book's tone is coloured by my deep concern about oppression and injustice.

I was freed of my other responsibilities as a result of the institutional support and fellowship given to me through the Program for the Study of Cultural Values and Ethics at the University of Illinois, located in Urbana–Champaign, and I wish to thank the people associated with the program.

I wish to thank all the following wonderful women and men who supported and uplifted me, and through whom I found the courage and energy I needed in order to both overcome the disease and its treatment and write the book: Madeleine and Noureddine Aba, Zahra Belghiti, Amel Ben Aba, Sihem Bensedrine, Marie Claire Boons, Charlotte and David Bruner, Marianne Burkhard, Monique Chajmowiez, Yoline Chandler, Judith Checker, Andrée Chedid, Richard Cogdal, Françoise Collin, Miriam Cooke, Samira Didos, Eva Enderlein, Rachida Ennaifer, Marianne Ferber, Dorothy Figueira, Renate Fisseler-Skandrani, Claire Gebeyli, Hayet

Gribaa, Cynthia Hahn, David Hajjar, Lynn Hajjar, Antje Kolodziej, Youenn Kervenic, Cheris Kramarae, Caryl Lloyd, Diane Long, Monique Loubet, Julie Miesle, Robin Morgan, Elizabeth Moritz, Rod MacLeod, Merri Scheitlin Nordman, Barbara Oehlschlaeger, Ramin Parham, Souad and Pierre Peigné, Sharon Pinkerton, Ann Priesel, John Reuter-Pacy, Nina Rubel, Mary Lee Sargent, Gail Scherba, Yolaine Simha, Louise and Robert Sinclair, Yvette Smith, Alex Sorkin, Beth Stafford, Zohreh Sullivan, Elizabeth Talbot, Mona Takyeddine-Amyuni, Barbara Vieille, Nazik and Ibrahim Yared, Jay Zerbe, and the many members of my family. It would take too long to name each and every person who was present, even if from afar, who brought me hope and comforted me during the dreary and difficult days, weeks and months.

I wish to thank my doctors who were (w)human, listened, were willing to discuss and answer my questions, admitted when they didn't know the answer and weren't taken in by the fads of the day or the promises of profit-making pharmaceutical companies, but who truly prioritised their patients' welfare over their own career and remained aware of the alternatives as well as sensitive to pain and their own limitations. Among them are doctors Aractingi, Belhessen, Espié, Giulivi-Boyer, Heuzé, Karoubi , Kotynek, Martinaud, Mico-Képès, Palazzo, Rowland and Tawil.

I want to especially thank the love of my life, Alban. Without his love, patience, humour, tenderness and encouragement to continue undergoing the treatment and keep writing, I wouldn't have been able to keep my spirits up and my energy flowing, even during the darkest days, when I felt debilitated by the treatment and mutilation my body had to adjust to. Because he has insights into postmodern issues and remains sensitive to the problems of the contemporary world, he has an acute vision of the relationship between the specific and the global. The discussions we continue to have are a source of discovery and understanding of major aspects of these questions – discoveries and understandings I wouldn't have had without his help.

I want to thank my wonderful physical therapist, Bettina Zorayan, whose precise yet gentle lymphatic-drainage massages of my left arm match the pertinent and important comments she was generous enough to make when she was reading the manuscript. Likewise, Jane Kuntz gave me invaluable corrections and comments. Because she has a wide knowledge of American and Tunisian cultures, I was able to understand issues I had either overlooked or incorrectly analysed. I want to thank Cynthia Hahn, who took time from her heavy schedule to re-read and polish the manuscript. I want to thank Dorothy Figueira for finding some of the chapter titles and names and for making me laugh when she thought I was wallowing too much in my misery. I want to thank Antje Kolodziej for making her invaluable comments and corrections. And I want to thank Bjorg Holte, my Norwegian physical therapist in the United States, whose forceful and gentle ways match the life she was able to create for herself: harmonious and peaceful surroundings that are so soothing amid the stress of academia. During the hardest moments of my life, I was often kept going as a result of her massages and lymphatic drainages. I wish to thank the people who most recently read and commented on the text: Deirdre Bucher Heistad, Monique Chajmowiez (Manicha in the text), Françoise Collin, Miriam Cooke and Yolaine Simha: they are so present and stimulating in my life, as well as providers of good and helpful critiques. Madeleine Aba, despite her failing health, was kind enough to both read the manuscript once it was almost complete and make corrections applying the utmost care. Thanks also to Suzanne Jamet, who gave me so many stimulating comments; to Cheryl Toman, for her enthusiasm and willingness to find me a literary agent; and to

Jennifer Solheim, for giving me a boost and wishing to sensitise people to the problems associated with breast cancer.

I also want to thank Lucien Israël: a doctor, an oncologist, a researcher and a writer who is world renowned for being especially encouraging. And Pierre Quet, who gave me judicious editorial advice.

Finally, I owe a special thanks to the wonderful team at Spinifex Press, through whose professional efforts this edition of my book has come up shining. I thank my publishers, Susan Hawthorne and Renate Klein, for having the vision to publish the book in Australia, in English; my editor, Deborah Doyle, for painstakingly working through each section and for giving me a few laughs along the way; the typesetter, Sam Bunny, who gave the book a 'new coat of paint'; the cover designer Deb Snibson for creating such a striking cover; and Spinifex's office manager Maralann Damiano, publicity and promotions manager Johanna de Wever, and overseas marketing and rights manager Laurel Guymer. I've never worked with such a professional and dedicated publishing team.

The book became a collective work. When I was receiving comments, books, articles, tapes or letters from people in general, friends and acquaintances who were concerned about cancer, I thought it was important to incorporate their remarks, experiences and reactions in the text. As I was reading or hearing each story, I was amazed how similar the experiences of dealing with cancer were, for example family members' reactions, doctors' attitudes, social pressures and debilitating treatments. Suddenly, what I was writing acquired a meaning that was more universal.

Evelyne Accad,
Champaign–Urbana, Paris, Tunis and Beirut, 1994–98

Author's note

I have given some people and institutions either a fictional name or two different initials so they cannot be identified. I have given my friends, acquaintances and colleagues either their first name or their full name.

PROLOGUE

THE PRICE OF WASTE AND POLLUTION: AN INSIDIOUS MASSACRE

... a little-known office of the World Health Organization, located in Lyon, France, called the International Agency for Research on Cancer, is charged with the daunting job of monitoring cancer incidence around the world ... The organization concluded that at least 80 percent of all cancer is attributable to environmental influences ... Death from cancer is not randomly distributed in the United States. Shades of red consistently light up the northeast coast, the Great Lakes area, and the mouth of the Mississippi River. For all cancers combined, these are the areas of highest mortality; they are also the areas of the most intense industrial activity ... Investigators found a close overlap between cancer mortality and environmental contamination. Concentrations of industrial toxins were higher in the top-ranked cancer counties than in the rest of the country. (Steingraber: 1997)

And yet if we take no action, we will have to prepare for the worst, not millions of years from now, as some would have us believe, but within the next fifty years. Not at the end of these five decades, but smack in the middle of the mature adult life of today's youngsters. The whole world has always made a swift collapse into history. Those who have lived through history's most profound upheavals know this all too well. (Séralini: 1997)

I decided to keep a journal about my journey through cancer. I needed to do it not only for myself, to exorcise the pain, but for the other women and men who are either suffering through the ordeal now or will suffer through it in the future. I also want to speak out, to shout to the world, about the dangers we are all exposed to: dangers created by the people whose arrogance and ignorance shaped the twentieth century.

It is as if I had somehow been made to pay the price for our so-called standard of living. I am but one of many people who have had to foot the bill for all the pollutants and chemicals ejected into the environment, which affect us through the air we breathe, the water we drink and the sun's rays we absorb, and for all the contaminants dumped into the world's rivers and seas, the pesticides sprayed on fruits and vegetables and the hormones fed to the animals we consume. Our body can stand only so much of this sabotage.

Jane [who first edited the book]: This is the price of affluence: you, Evelyne, are paying for the so-called Western living standard. It is all about a trade-off, a gamble: in exchange for more luxuries, health risks [a higher cancer risk]; in exchange for a youthful body into old age, ERT [Estrogen Replacement Therapy]. This is the hardest thing for us to accept: we will have to give up some of our comforts, our choices, for the good of the planet. People are very reluctant to surrender this so-called freedom.

Alban: But it is important to recognise that this affluence benefits only a small part of humanity, even in the United States. We should be more concerned about changing the needs than about renouncing them. Needs are social constructions; for example, the need for ERT is constructed by the manufacturers of ERT. We could all live richer lives, while consuming differently and less, by effectively shifting our needs: something that should not be as difficult as it sounds. What is harder to change is the capitalist

13

machine itself. If catastrophe is to be avoided, change must occur, and it will occur only when more and more people refuse to carry on living wastefully and destructively, as we are now in the Western world.

I have become the one out of seven women – 14 per cent of all women – who gets breast cancer in her lifetime, according to the 1995 statistics for the United States and Canada. The figures are staggering. All cancers are on the increase: cells gone wild in a world that has reached its limits, reproducing themselves in the human body. However, breast-cancer rate is especially troubling. The breast is body part that is more sensitive, fragile and receptive than any other part to the disruptions to nature and the environment: the font of life transformed into a deadly power.

I did ask, *Why me?* This is the question a woman stricken with the disease typically asks herself. In the United States, an organisation by that name even exists: Y-Me. Yes, I did ask this question. However, one of my friends reversed it to be *Why not me?* Another friend, who had cancer, said, 'If someone had to get it, it had to be me!'

At the time, though, I found it impossible to think this way: only later was I able to ask myself, *What can I learn through this ordeal? What can it teach me?* I was diagnosed as having a lobular carcinoma on 2 March 1994. Nothing had prepared me for the hell I was soon to experience; I never thought it would happen to me. I hadn't been informed in – or rather, I'd ignored – media reports about the subject. Because breast cancer had not stricken one single member of my family, not even a distant relative, I'd thought I was immune: sheltered from the plague, as it were.

I must denounce how ridiculous it is to ask women who have breast cancer about their family history of cancer. It's assumed their answer will be 'Yes: someone in my family has had it,' when we know that breast cancer that includes hereditary factors hits a very small minority of women.

Jane: It is by asking this question that researchers have discovered that so few of today's cancers do, in fact, have a genetic origin. And it will be interesting to see if today's patients with no family history of cancer pass this characteristic on to the next generation; in other words, is there a mutation occurring? It is by studying family histories that this epidemiological information can be made available.

Like most of us, Jane isn't able to see the futility of so common a question. However, cancers of genetic origin have long been drowned in the mass of other cancers: the fact is so obvious it isn't necessary to provide more proof. Also, an epidemiological study can't be undertaken using the vague questions that doctors usually ask their patients.

The tradition of asking about family precedents is based on outdated knowledge and practice, and today it serves as an all too transparent smoke-screen for the medical establishment's ignorance. At the same time, patients are forced to focus on their responsibility and their family history, and the responsibilities of organising collective life are pushed into the background.

This is also the view that Sandra Steingraber expresses in the following quote from her book *Living Downstream: An Ecologist Looks at Cancer and the Environment* (1997: 259), which I've already quoted from to introduce this prologue:

Several obstacles, I believe, prevent us from addressing cancer's environmental roots. An obsession with genes and heredity is one ... Hereditary cancers, however, are the rare exception. Collectively, fewer than 10 percent of all malignancies are thought to involve inherited mutations. Between 1 and 5 percent of colon cancers, for example, are of the hereditary variety, and only about 15 percent exhibit any sort of familial component. The remaining 85 percent of colon cancers are officially classified as 'sporadic,' which, confesses one prominent researcher, is a fancy medical term for 'We don't know what the hell causes it.' Breast cancer also shows little connection to heredity (probably between 5 and 10 percent). Finding 'cancer genes' is not going to prevent the vast majority of cancers that develop. Moreover, even when rare, inherited mutations play a role in the development of a particular cancer, environmental influences are inescapably involved as well. Genetic risks are not exclusive of environmental risks. Indeed, the direct consequence of some of these damaging mutations is that people become even more sensitive to environmental carcinogens.

Apart from the debate about heredity, it is important that report writers emphasise two facts: that cancer is on the increase and that it is striking an ever younger population. It's up to us to promote action, and to promote it loudly and publicly, so we can reverse these nightmarish trends. We must make the facts known to the world so that both today's and tomorrow's generations will know, and so that women who have been hit by the disease won't be forgotten, as so many of their silent sisters have been who've never opened their mouth because they're told to be quiet; or who are never given the chance to speak; or who have their mouth shut as a result of centuries of crushing, sewing up, veiling, masking and closing up.

In the United States, in 1994, more than 165,000 new diagnoses of breast cancer were made, and 46,000 of the women afflicted died of the disease; the numbers continue to increase, year after year. In France, in 1995, 25,000 new diagnoses were made and 9000 women died. In both countries, the figures amount to more fatalities than occur in road accidents. Who will protest about situation, and what's being done? Why are women once again accepting that they are victims?

Cindy: There are organisations speaking out!

Jane: Yes, but is the medical–pharmaceutical complex listening?

The whole world is contaminated, but there is both more contamination and more cancer among the industrialised nations. We in the Western world are paying the price for this so-called *ci-vi-li-sa-tion*, if I may borrow the rhythm of a word used by the Guyanese poet Damas, who visited Urbana when I'd just become employed there as a young professor. Damas's poems are striking in their strength: he expresses revolt by addressing consciousness-raising themes translated into a new language, and inspires his words with the rhythms of African drum beats. The beauty and sensibility of his poems remain with me forever. He was also a rebel who shouted his anger about his people's condition and the injustices of a world that seems doomed to destruction. I have often taught my students his poems, especially the *Pigments* collection.

Steingraber (1997: 268) reinforces my conviction and claim that we have to have a (w)human-rights approach if we are to begin solving the cancer problem through examining its ecological roots, by recognising that:

> the current system of regulating the use, release, and disposal of known and suspected carcinogens – rather than preventing their generation in the first place – is intolerable. So is the decision to allow untested chemicals free access to our bodies, until which time they are finally assessed for carcinogenic properties. Both practices show reckless disregard for human life.

Steingraber is a biologist, poet and cancer survivor. When she was in her twenties, she carefully and scientifically researched and documented the connection between carcinogenic substances and their effects on human cells. In her book, she brings together both recently collected data about toxins and newly released data obtained from cancer registries. Travelling from hospitals to hazardous-waste sites and from farms to incinerators to conduct her research, she relates stories in a beautifully poetic style that's gripping in its scientific precision and through which she brings us face to face with decades of industrial and agricultural recklessness.

I found her human-rights approach to be most compelling and that in many ways it echoes mine; I quote her throughout the book. I believe that her argument about quality of life, as illustrated in the following two quotes (1997: 268, 269), will strike a chord for many people and not only for progressives and ecology activists.

When carcinogens are deliberately or accidentally introduced into the environment, some number of vulnerable persons are consigned to death. The impossibility of tabulating an exact body count does not alter this fact. A human rights approach to cancer strives, nonetheless, to make these deaths visible.

I think we can say with assurance that the transformation of a popular swimming hole into a cancer hazard and child's play into a cancer risk factor is a terrible diminishment of our humanity. And we can say that the agency's gesture of educational responsibility *[in 1993, a United States Agency for Toxic Substances and Disease Registry had dispatched a group of representatives to Chattanooga, Tennessee expressly to teach schoolchildren to stay away from the local creek, which happened to be surrounded by no fewer than 42 hazardous-waste sites]* is indicative of a vast national irresponsibility. A human rights approach to cancer would also speak out against other deprivations besides gross loss of life.

Steingraber pays tribute to Rachel Carson, who, in 1962, more than 30 years before her, had already warned people about the dangers of chemicals; the book was entitled *Silent Spring* (Carson: 1962) and was published by Mifflin. As a government scientist, Carson had access to reports in which it was revealed that eradicating pests by spraying them with pesticides had devastating consequences for both people and wildlife.

At the time, however, the key government officials were not willing to listen. Carson couldn't find one magazine or other periodical publisher who was willing to publish her research – in which she documented the problems connected with pesticides, from blindness in fish to blood disorders in humans – she decided to write her own book.

By using the word 'silent' in the title, Carson was alluding to the facts that her warnings were being silenced and that extinction of the sounds of birds, bees, frogs and crickets, and ultimately of the human race, was being threatened as a result of pesticidal warfare. The book is also about the complicity of the scientists who were aware of the dangers of chemicals yet kept silent about them. Carson questioned the cozy relations that existed between the scientific community and the corporate world, especially the chemical companies.

In 1960, at age 52 and in the middle of writing *Silent Spring*, Carson was diagnosed as having breast cancer. Her tumour spread to her bones, and even though she was left exhausted and weak as a result of her trauma, she continued writing (1962: 21):

The tumors in her cervical vertebrae caused her writing hand to go numb. Carson lived for eighteen months after finishing *Silent Spring*, long enough to smoke out a hornet's nest of ridicule and invective from the chemical industry, as well as to receive every imaginable award from the world of arts, letters, and science.

Steingraber poignantly underlines how, despite the fact that Carson's doctors were stating she had very limited time left according to her medical evidence, she kept hoping for a remission (1962: 21):

> She did not go gently or gratefully into any good night ... Carson appears before us again as a typical woman with breast cancer ... *[In a letter to her dearest friend, in November 1963, she writes,]* 'There is still so much I want to do, and it is hard to accept that in all probability, I must leave most of it undone. And just when I have attained the power to achieve so much I feel is important! Strange, isn't it?'

Carson had just started to indicate the connection between economic structures and the link between science, medicine and industrial interests when she was silenced herself. She left behind an adopted son, plans for books and her field-work. She died of breast cancer on 14 April 1964. Thirty years later, Steingraber is continuing the Carson tradition; however, the problems have become more acute. She asks (1997: 13),

> ... more than three decades after *Silent Spring* alerted us to a possible problem – why so much silence still surrounds questions about cancer's connection to the environment and why so much scientific inquiry into this issue is still considered 'preliminary'.

By 1962, Carson had already produced evidence through which the link between cancer and environmental causes was revealed. She drew a startling picture: creation, as a result of twentieth-century industrial activities, of sub-stances we have no protection against; atomic and chemical exposure in the aftermath of the Second World War; the increasing frequency with which cancer was striking the general population, most ominously children; development of tumours in animals; and the unseen inner workings of cells (1997: 28):

Carson predicted that future studies on the mysterious transformation of healthy cells into malignant ones would reveal that the roads leading to the formation of cancer are the same pathways that pesticides and other related chemical contaminants operate in once they enter the interior spaces of the human body.

Steingraber reveals that in the United States, in 1995, 1.2 million people were told they had cancer; that between 1973 and 1991, incidence of breast cancer rose by almost 25 per cent – 40 per cent among females older than 65, and 30 per cent among black females of all ages; that since 1950, cancers among children have risen by one-third; that at the time of writing, each year, about 8000 children were being diagnosed as having cancer; and that one in every 400 Americans could expect to develop cancer before they turned 15.

Like Carson, Steingraber is especially attentive to incidence of cancer among children (1997: 39):

Cancer among children provides a particularly intimate glimpse into the possible routes of exposure to contaminants in the general environment and their possible significance for rising cancer rates among adults. The lifestyle of toddlers has not changed much over the past half century. Young children do not smoke, drink alcohol, or hold stressful jobs. Children do, however, receive a greater dose of whatever chemicals are present in air, food, and water because, pound for pound, they breathe, eat, and drink more than adults do. In proportion to their body weight, children drink 2.5 times more water, eat 3 to 4 times more food, and breathe 2 times more air. They are also affected by parental exposures before conception, as well as by exposures in the womb and in breast milk.

In 1997, the same year in which Steingraber's book was published, another book was published in France, by Gilles-Eric Séralini, entitled *Le sursis de l'espèce humaine* (*The Human Race: On the Brink of Disaster*). Séralini also sounds the alarm. I was surprised at how similar the two books were, given that the authors, two researchers living in different countries, seemed to be unaware of the work their fellow author was doing. Their analyses are astonishingly consistent with reference to how environmental degradation has serious consequences for both the planet's survival and proliferation of cancers (Séralini: 1997: 11, 12, 13):

The entire human race might be said to be on probation today, and for the first time in its history is facing a situation unprecedented in its seriousness. Rampant pollution has reached into every corner of the world, into the bodies of children, via the air, water and food supply. They are absorbing these contaminants into their flesh, where they will accumulate in body tissues and trigger diseases of all kinds, including cancer. The youngest children are the most sensitive, but adults are also well within the danger zone.

What I say is not intended to preach or to alarm, but it is simply a realistic, scientific fact. To bury one's head in the sand amounts to a crime against humanity, and we need to truly understand what has gone wrong before a solution can be found. Likewise, for the first time in the course of human affairs, some of us are now able to genetically transform embryos, without fully imagining the consequences. Laws governing these matters are still quite muddled in nearly all countries, and we are about to hand down to the next generation a dangerous world. In order to better apprehend how the situation is evolving, I have proposed an up-to-date, across-the-board pollution report in terms of air, water and food production, as well as an explanation of the genetic risks involved and the effects of this overall situation on public health.

Since this problem is being raised for the first time in human history, and since world population is also at an all-time high, any delay in the ordering of our priorities will result in more shattered lives, ground down by hunger, thirst, cancer and wars that will result from the bitter struggle over the world's dwindling resources.

⌛

When I chose Elie Wiesel's quote to open the book ('To forget nothing, to efface nothing …'), the early readers of the manuscript had mixed reactions. I believe these mixed reactions will become stronger once the book is published, so I will justify my choosing the quote. I will start by briefly making some observations, as follows.

I'm not the first person to draw the parallel contained in the quote: in many of my readings, of, for example, Elizabeth Gille, Jeanne Hyvrard, Gilda Radner, Deena Metzger, Fritz Zorn and Ania Francos (Francos: 1983: 47), I found the same analogy reflected:

> I caressed my left breast, I rolled the lump under my fingers and I told myself it was at exactly the same place where my mother, thirty-seven years earlier, had sewed on the yellow star. Finally, it had hit us. The much hoped for punishment was here. Would the dead be resurrected?

I have come across the analogy more among French Jewish writers than among American Jewish people. First, I wonder whether the difference might have something to do with the fact that European Jewish people are more familiar with and physically closer to the reality of the Holocaust. Second, I wonder whether Americans' guilt about being both physically and morally remote from the Holocaust is a cause of their somehow feeling disqualified from using the Holocaust metaphorically when they're writing about cancer.

The person who most encouraged me to pursue this analogy is Monique Chajmowiez, a French Jewish woman whose family includes Holocaust victims and who is herself a cancer survivor. I am thankful to her for introducing me to Ania Francos, whose astounding work I analyse later in the book.

Alex Sorkin, who is a friend, an eye doctor, a cancer survivor and an American Jewish man whose family includes Holocaust victims, also spent a lot of time encouraging me to use the quote. However, he intimated to me that people who had not lived through the torture of undergoing heavy cancer treatment would find it difficult to understand what I was trying to convey.

Jane: But that's the point: there are fewer and fewer actual Holocaust survivors as the years pass, but the memory is kept alive through relentless efforts to inform new generations of this reality. People who have no direct experience of cancer must also be made to understand the reality of the disease.

More recently, in 1998, when I was putting the finishing touches on the book, Gloria Orenstein, an American Jewish friend who's lived in France for quite some time, brought to my attention a book published in 1987 and written by Jeanne Hyvrard, entitled *Le cercan*; I also quote from that book throughout this one. Uncannily, in her book, Hyvrard draws the same conclusions, makes the same analyses and calls for the same action as do I. Her comparisons with the Holocaust are strangely similar to mine (Hyvrard: 1987: 193):

A woman was talking about what she had felt during her treatment, and a man replied that what she said sounded very much like the kinds of things he had heard from concentration camp survivors ... As excessive as that statement might seem, it does give one pause. If hospitals might in some respects bear a resemblance to the hell on earth that was the camps, then there are some serious questions we should be asking ourselves. Not only with regard to the harshness of treatment and its many side effects, but something that has more to do with how the hospital functions. It is harder to frame the question in these terms, since everything becomes rather vague and subjective, and yet ... Without the effort of finding words to express things, the whole project of this book would be futile one.

Areas in which the cancer–genocide analogy obviously breaks down can be easily summarised as follows. First, Holocaust victims were specifically targeted, rounded up and executed as part of a systematic operation, whereas cancer deaths result from a disease that involves no *intent* by anyone to destroy. Cancer is 'simply' a disease that medical scientists have yet to control: if its victims didn't have medical intervention, there would be many more of them. Second, in the Holocaust, there was a will to exterminate the Jewish people, whereas cancer's victims are random.

The key word through which the difference between the two types of victim is marked is perhaps hope: right or wrong, we continue to believe that modern doctors will eventually find solutions to even the most intractable diseases, whereas the question of whether evil exists, which is at the heart of the Holocaust, is in area in which not much hope shines.

Nevertheless, there are many similarities between the two analogies, as follows. Every year, hundreds of thousands, even millions, of cancer victims are claimed. We're being confronted with something that is tantamount to wide-spread massacre and mutilation, on the scale of the Holocaust.

Even if the political-power mongers are not actively pursuing a policy of extermination, they are responsible by default for the ever increasing toll of deaths, mutilation and disease. Even though statisticians have proven beyond doubt that not only is the number of cancers on the rise in industrialised countries but an accelerated rate of increase now seems unavoidable, the political-power mongers have failed to meet this serious public-health challenge by not establishing a treatment and prevention policy of the same scale. It is well known that scientific progress is above all a question of means: seek and you shall find, provided you have the funding. We need only turn to the recent conquests of outer space to conclude that that area of science has been given priority over the health of the people in the world's nations and therefore over the life and physical integrity of millions of people. What is absent is the political will to kill, although at present, what is equally absent is the political will to do something about cancer, and we could view the situation as being a kind of passive, random genocide – and there's nothing apolitical about that!

As was the case in the Nazis' extermination of Jewish people and other European minority groups, after which many perpetrators either went into hiding or denied they were individually responsible for the mass murders, people now exist who lay the blame for our environmental degradation on an impersonal system: they won't have it that we are individually responsible for the decline in quality of life that's an inescapable factor in cancer development. On a larger scale, individual industrial polluters can therefore refute accusations that they are responsible for an industrial, technical and scientific system that has nevertheless been built by and for them. Also, in an even more diffuse way, the larger commercial, administrative and academic bureau-cracy that's been spawned by industrialists operates at so great a distance from the actual industry sources that it's impossible to claim any collaboration whatsoever in pro-ducing the industries' ill-effects. The whole mechanism is regulated through an impersonal, blind law whereby the law makers can no longer claim that industry is more ratio-nalised and efficient (Hyvrard: 1987: 173):

> No, the truly astounding topic is that of the 'side' side effects, in fact that term had to be invented so that we could talk about them. This is what we call the effects that last beyond the completion of treatment. Testimonial books do not address this issue. Yet this is what seemed to us the most painful aspect of the whole business. And the situation is made all the more unbearable by the patient's immediate cir-cle of friends and family, as well as the medical establishment who do not wish to hear about this aspect. Family and friends are afraid of bursting the bubble of the 'miracle cure' which shields them from their own anxieties, and the medical estab-lishment would rather not have to face yet another unknown. It took four years of obstinate collecting of testimonials for us to be heard by one doctor who came forward with this com-mon sense response: 'In the past, patients used to die. We did not worry too much about the consequences of treat-ment. Now people are cured more and more frequently, and the aftereffects have become a new problem.'

Again as in the case of the Nazis' campaign of extermination, a conspiracy of silence surrounds the massacre and mutila-tion of masses of people. Everyone knows and doesn't want to know; sees and doesn't want to see (Hyvrard: 1987: 31):

> It is all happening as if society as a whole knew very well what cancer is, but that in order to cast it back into nature's magma,

society forbids itself to talk about it, blaming the carriers who thus serve first as scapegoats and then as sacrificial victims. It was not that long ago that human sacrifice was still in practice. Perhaps there remains something of that need, beneath the guise of asepticized medicine.

First and foremost in the 'Denial' category is the medical establishment through which patients are surrounded with soothing words, such as 'No: the increase in the number of cancers isn't real; it's only due to the fact improvements have been made in diagnosis and statistics gathering, to the fact that more women are living longer, to the fact that you're living in an academic environment in which everyone knows everyone and word gets around quickly. No: estrogens are not the cause of breast cancer, and even if they were, their effects are so positive for so many other ailments and diseases that it's well worth the risks to use them.' In this reasoning, patients who are facing cancer are isolated by way of making their family history a central question whereas heredity has practically lost any meaning with reference to the disease (Steingraber: 1997: 260):

Cancer incidence rates are not rising because we are suddenly sprouting new cancer genes. Rare, heritable genes that predispose their hosts to cancer by creating special susceptibilities to the effects of carcinogens have undoubtedly been with us for a long time. The ill effects of some of these genes might well be diminished by lowering the burden of environmental carcinogens to which we are all exposed. In a world free of aromatic amines, for example, being born a slow acetylator would be a trivial issue, not a matter of grave consequence. The inheritance of a defective carcinogen-detoxifying gene would matter less in a culture that did not tolerate carcinogens in air, food, and water. By contrast, we cannot change our ancestors. Shining the spotlight on inheritance focuses us on the one piece of the puzzle we can do absolutely nothing about ... Risks of lifestyle are also not independent of environmental risks. And yet public education campaigns about cancer consistently accent the former and ignore the latter.

Ordinary citizens also either keep quiet or talk about the disease only in whispers, fearing they will conjure up the ghost of collective death: a fate that the earth is dragging all its inhabitants towards as a result of our continued poisoning of the earth. These ordinary citizens speak in whispers, if at all, because they live in a society in which their extermination has been programmed in advance, and yet they remain dumbfounded in the face of the future calamity. In reality, they're similar to the members of ancient societies who dared not say the name of diseases in order to avoid bringing forth mysterious, uncontrollable and evil forces. This fear remains in the Middle East, in which Arabic-speaking people refer to cancer as *Al-marad illi ma btitssamma*: 'the disease not to be named'. It's as if by saying the word, people would bring the disease upon themselves and/or their loved ones (Hyvrard: 1987: 29):

To keep silent *[in France as well]* is to keep living in some archaic past. When words are taboo, we are forbidden to talk about their referent. Society carries on according to the strictures of some bygone age. It fosters anxiety and panic, perpetuates the policy of burying one's head in the sand, which is what leads people to flee the kind of medical screening that remains their best chance for cure.

For me, contemporary cancer treatment amounts to medicalised massacre and mutilation of diseased people that is regulated in a medical establishment in which practitioners blindly apply standardised protocols. These practitioners betray their ignorance and arrogance towards their patients by treating cases statistically and hiding the consequences of their applied treatments of their patients, who they consider to be objects.

Cancer victims either enter or are pushed into a space I call a *zone of illness*, in which they lose control of their life and are no longer free to choose; this state also resembles the state of concentration-camp victims. Patients enter an organisation that's been designed to be a rational machine: an industrial machine that's been created to treat the disease whereby patients aren't able to consciously choose but are instead oriented towards a programmed direction. They aren't warned about many of the consequences of the treatment they're to be subjected to; instead, they discover the consequences while travelling down the treatment path: castration; mutilation; loss of use of limbs; pains; threat of contracting other, treatment-induced cancers; weakness; debilitation; fragility; and risk of death (Hyvrard: 1987: 186):

> Treatment against cancer also has the unwanted side effect of making impotent or frigid those who were not, prior to the treatment. It is symptomatic that our group debates began by addressing this theme, and that we were unanimous as to our diagnostic. We seemed to recall that in the Middle Ages, lepers were castrated, and we find many similarities between their state and ours. Over the years, the situation has taken hold again under many guises, depending upon the individual.

Accompanying these consequences are others that the patients are often warned about but that are minimised as being 'secondary effects' whereas they're actually very central: baldness; nausea; pain; muscle weakening; heart-muscle damage; loss of appetite; burns; and tiredness.

Alex: Sometimes devastating food allergies.

People such as my friend Alex can no longer eat as they choose, and constantly have to either deprive themselves of the foods they love or suffer painful consequences (Hyvrard: 1987: 34):

> Anyone who is known to have been ill, even once cured, will find it hard to shift into another mode of existence, and will gradually resign himself to inferiority. He will henceforward wear the yellow star of the sick, and will discover that it will be in his interest, and for the sake of his own peace of mind, to conceal even any mention of his illness in the past tense, despite all the pain he suffered to attain full recovery. He will in turn contribute to maintaining the secret, the archaic social norm, this site of obscurantism and terror of a disease for which he should have represented the living proof of a positive outcome. We are well advised to reflect upon this paradox which, for us, no longer is one. In addition to their loss of health, cancer victims are also enclosed in a social function that turns them inexorably into scapegoats.

Because I'm comparing cancer with concentration camps, I'll undoubtedly be subjected to yet another critique from the victims of Israeli violence in the Middle East. The victims will ask why I, an Arab Lebanese woman, would use the same image that Israel continues to evoke in order to justify its massacres, bombings, shellings, invasions and occupations?

First, I affirm that memories of the European concentration camps do not belong to Israelis only: the Holocaust is the paradigm of modernity gone horribly awry; it's the paradigm of what feelings of superiority can lead to, whether they're inspired by an ideology of race, religion or science; it's the paradigm of where existing trends are leading to in this world that's coming apart at the seams; it's a paradigm we have to keep in the foreground of our collective memory to warn us against giving in to the impulse to dominate by any and all means.

Second, as Yolaine Simha, a French Jewish woman herself and a cancer survivor, rightfully reminds me, genocides have involved not only Jews but groups such as Amer-Indians, Serbs, Armenians, Ruwandans and Bosnians, in a seemingly unending stream.

The concentration camp, therefore, serves as a double-sided mirror: it reflects both the Nazis' horrors and also the present-day injustices. Israelis have to be courageous and honest enough to gaze into both sides of the mirror and recognise that they, too, are perpetrators of terror. As my friend Alex rightfully points out, Israel is itself a creation that grew out of Europeans' cynicism and collective guilt about the fate of the Jewish people. In this tradition of cynicism, Israelis can't continue to justify their present-day abuses by conjuring up the spectre of the concentration camps.

We must recall the image of the concentration camps whenever we see perpetrators systematising liquidation of groups of people. We must unveil and talk about the hidden problems as the first step towards finding solutions to our present-day tragedies. Today's victims often become tomorrow's torturers. To talk about all forms of oppression, wherever they might be, and make the connection between them – in other words, to remain lucid in the face of the contemporary world's miseries – is to go beyond those miseries.

Having lived through both the war in Lebanon and cancer in my body, and having witnessed the death of loved ones, some killed by shells and others by cancer, I can attest to both horrors. Throughout the book, I make parallels between my war experience in Lebanon and my struggle to survive cancer.

If, in writing these lines, I can be of help to someone, I won't have suffered in vain. Sometimes what I say might seem excessive; however, this excessiveness is only relative in a society that's going numb, in which lethargy is promoted in the discourse of governments, corporations and the media whereby we're made to believe that everything will always be the same. Because I was hit with the disease of cancer, I was forced to open my eyes.

I share with you not only some of my thoughts and painful experiences but the joys I encountered as my cancer life was unravelling during my travels through the dark valley.

1

HORMONES AND BREAST CANCER
WHY ME?

'It was the same in the camp,' Aunt Rivke said to me. 'We were always sad at the death of one of ours, but at the same time, we would say: well, I'm still here. They haven't got me yet.'

She, the survivor, repeats to me regularly: 'To live is a sacred duty. Act as I did in Birkenau. Tell yourself: what I am seeing is a film, a book I am reading.'

Yes, I know: it would be better if I wrote instead of bullshitting. 'Do it for me, Lola,' you used to say. A lawyer is also someone who can bear witness. Will no one remember us?'

I could whisper to you these words written on the neighbor's tomb: 'See you soon'. But it's wrong. I don't feel at all like going there yet. Give me one more minute, Mister Executioner. (Francos: 1983: 14)

Urbana, 20 February 1994

VZ, my doctor, calls me on this Sunday morning, saying she has to talk to me and that it would be good if Alban were there also. Feeling something in her voice but also in her strange way of approaching me, I conclude that all isn't well.

She arrives on this grey and rainy Sunday, and right away asks, perhaps by way of introduction, although the request

34

is absurdly trite, or perhaps out of habit, for a box of Kleenex, in anticipation of the drama to come. She sits down and tells us that according to my mammogram, I probably have breast cancer. I ask her how she can know this with so much certainty. She isn't very clear. However, Alban and I understand that the evidence is clearly shown on the mammogram, which VZ hasn't seen: the edges of the mass that for a few weeks has been weighing inside my breast. VZ has made an appointment for me to see a surgeon tomorrow, and he will tell me how to proceed. She adds that it would also be good if I saw an oncologist. She seems so sure I have cancer that I burst into tears. She tells me that crying is a normal reaction: she must have expected it, because she asked for the box of Kleenex. She must have had a deep knowledge of patients' psychology, and knows how to proceed in difficult circumstances such as mine.

Alban, my wonderful love, is with me. He can't accept the diagnosis: he says it can't be true, and doesn't believe the cancer is possible. He thinks a cancer can't be developing so quickly it will become as big as a fist in fewer than two months.

When I insist on asking VZ more about how she can be so sure about what she's telling us, she finally says, 'It is my opinion.' In my naivety, I think her answer is strange and unscientific, and unworthy of a doctor.

Later, once I have time to think more about the diagnosis, having consulted with many doctors both in Urbana and overseas, I also think VZ has been too ready and not cautious enough in prescribing me hormones – estrogen and progesterone – at a time when it remains unclear how useful they are, especially because I didn't yet have any symptoms of menopause, although according to my blood test, my hormone level was unusually low. VZ believed it was necessary for me to have Estrogen Replacement Therapy – ERT – in order to prevent me from suffering the osteoporosis my mother suffers from. However, I ask, *Why hadn't she ordered more tests – blood and other tests – before she prescribed the hormones?* In every article I read about ERT, the writer seems to indicate that cancerous cells can be activated as a result of the therapy. All the doctors I later consulted were astonished that hormones had been prescribed to me in so cavalier a way. However, all of them consider the risks run by patients who use the therapy from a statistical angle. Astonishing! Why has thalidomide been forbidden? Why so much fuss and screaming about 'mad-cow disease' when the number fatal consequences is relatively small? Medicos and scientists are so inconsistent! Doctors aren't responsible enough, and medicine and the pharmaceutical–medical complex is a huge profit-making enterprise!

Hormones are prescribed to almost any woman, both before menopause, in order to prevent conception, and during and after menopause, in order to slow down the ageing process.

Bettina: These hormones are called birth-control pills. Women who take them and smoke run huge cardiovascular risks, a fact that isn't emphasised enough.

Women pay a lot of money for this treatment, which is partly paid for by way of their insurance, an industry sector in which sizeable profits are made at the expense of women's health. It doesn't cost much to produce the hormones, but they're sold at high prices in the industrial capitalist countries. In the so-called Developing World, they're dumped at lower prices and are often of a harmful quality, in the name of 'providing aid to developing countries'. On top of this, women enter – or rather are pushed – into a medical system in which they lose control of their body. Hormones have many side effects, and the women who are prescribed them have to have various types of follow-up treatment so the medical machine continues to function economically. All this is sickening and upsetting! Women are losing control of their body, their money, their health, their life!

27 February 1994

Since last Sunday, I've been feeling as if I'm being precipitated into a chain of events I have no control over. It's like being thrown over a cliff. I'm terribly anxious. One of the sources of my anxiety, which I'll come back to later, is the slowness of the medical machine and the feeling I'm being forgotten.

Bettina: This is what so many patients feel!

Jane: Paradox: the patient is 'precipitated', rushed into a decision, while at the same time experiencing 'the slowness of the medical machine'.

I must recall some of the events that preceded the catastrophe. In the middle of November, I'd gone for my annual medical check-up. At the beginning of December, my doctor, VZ, was prescribing estrogen – 6 milligrams for a period of 25 days – and progesterone – 10 milligrams for a period of 10 days – and was telling me that according to my hormone level as determined in my blood test, I'd entered menopause. As yet, I didn't have any of the symptoms that apparently can characterise menopause: no hot flashes or cessation of menstruation, and so on. However, VZ said I had to take hormones in order to prevent me from suffering the osteoporosis that was afflicting my mother. When I asked her to give me the lowest possible dose, she assured me that the lowest dose wouldn't be effective against osteoporosis, and that I had to take megadoses.

Bettina: It's very important to warn people of the importance of dosage. How much each person takes has to be studied carefully, after many tests, and not given systematically; in fact, hormones are given when peri-menopausal or real-menopausal symptoms are present, never to prevent them!

I followed VZ's recommendation. She hadn't told me to follow my hormonal menstrual cycle; instead, she'd told me to start the treatment on the first day of the month: 1 December 1993. On the fourteenth day of the treatment, which happened to be the day I should have gotten my period, I was to start the progesterone, but I started bleeding like never before.

I was in Paris, receiving the France–Lebanon literary award, for one of my books. Conferences, meetings, debates, concerts and radio talk shows had been programmed. I continued taking the progesterone and estrogen. The bleeding became a hemorrhage accompanied with terrible pains. I immediately called Dr EL, a psychologist and gynecologist and one of the pioneers of France's feminist movement, and explained to her what was happening to me.

She said I must have been prescribed too strong a dose of the hormones, and advised me to reduce the dosage and take an anti-hemorrhage medicine, which she prescribed for me over the phone, because that evening I was to have a panel discussion about my book. She told me she no longer practised gynecology, but that her daughter practised it and that I could go and see her. That evening, she came to the debate and actively participated in it. I was very touched to see a woman I admired so much. She's written a book about women turning 50, which I must get.

I then left for Lebanon, to spend Christmas and New Year with my family. The hemorrhage had stopped, and I'd reduced the doses of hormones. In Lebanon, I contracted a terrible flu that wouldn't go away. I was with my dear parents, both of whom were ill: my father was dying of prostate cancer, which had metastasised to his bones, and my mother had the osteoporosis I'm supposedly heir to, as well as Parkinson's disease and all kinds of other health problem.

Already I wrote in my diary that 'I was absorbing all of their illnesses inside of me: the suffering of my dear father, his courage; all of Adelaide's abnegation, courage and care.' And it was my sister Adelaide who was taking care of my parents at that time. I felt so weak in the face of their ill-nesses; of my own flu – I wrote 'illness' – which would not go away; of life that was so full of suffering. Already I wrote, 'How much strength and courage one needs to live, and especially to live differently.'

Little did I know what was awaiting me, nor how prophetic my reflections were. Did my subconscious know? Can we really avoid these problems by listening more to our inner self, receiving our body's signals and learning to be more cautious? Have I learnt the lesson?

Bettina: There is always an anxiogenic terrain for cancer: encourage your readers to try not to internalise their problems – women in particular, especially women from the Middle East [Bettina has Middle Eastern roots], who tend to keep it all to themselves.

When I returned to Urbana, on 15 January, I wrote that I wasn't feeling well. The weather was freezing, and I came down with another cold and flu symptoms. These relapses were quite unusual for me: I'm not used to getting sick like that so many times in a row.

I surrendered to my sickness, to my sorrow, to the suffering that life seems to require of all humanity, to the fact that life ends in death! Why did I have such dark thoughts? I wrote that it was as if I'd absorbed all my parents' illness and suffering as well as Adelaide's courage, complaints and suffering; it was as if I were still bearing the weight of all this, irrevocably – and I'd underlined that adverb. It's the same word Gilles had used, in one of his letters, to describe the death of his only daughter, Florence, in her sleep, at age 30, from an aneurism: a blood vessel that had burst in her brain. I'd felt this death as a terrible injustice. I used to like seeing these friends when I visited my parents, in Switzerland. I haven't felt like going back to Switzerland since my parents have left there.

Bettina: For sure you absorbed your parents' illness! A disease like cancer is never by chance: the emotions send signals. If they're negative, and if the body is tired, it can get translated into a disease. It's also a way to put a stop to negative waves.

'I hurt all over these days,' I wrote. 'After the warmth, the beauty of Lebanon, the kindness of its people, it is difficult to be back in the Western world, so dehumanised, so cold, so stressful and cruel.'

I went to consult the advisory nurse, because my doctor, VZ, hadn't yet returned. The nurse told me to reduce my intake of the estrogen, but not of the progesterone, and to have a mammogram because of the unusual hardening in my breast. I'd also noticed the hardening, but wasn't alarmed, because my idea of something to worry about was a round lump rather than a hardening.

Bettina: Insist on this aspect, which many women are unaware of: we're taught to look for a round lump, not a hardening.

I thought the hardening was due to the hormones and that it'd disappear when I got adjusted to them. The nurse also advised me to reduce my coffee intake – which is already quite minimal – because it's associated with incidence of cysts and fibrosis in the breasts.

Bettina: It doesn't make any sense to be blaming my condition on coffee instead of on the hormones.

I've since found out that in French medicine, caffeine and alcohol aren't connected to breast cysts, in contrast to the fact that in the United States the connection is made routinely.

I'd seen the advisory nurse on 21 January. At the beginning of February I started bleeding again, when it wasn't yet my period time but rather my ovulation time. I called the nurse again. I had a hard time getting hold of her. I must recall how hard a time I usually had getting to see a doctor. I asked several times for a doctor – a specialist, I'd specify, only to be told there were no specialists! – and couldn't have appointments with a doctor until May: more than three months later! It's appalling how difficult it is to see a doctor in a city the size of Champaign–Urbana, which has two polyclinics!

However, I insisted. I told the nurse who'd suggested I reduce my coffee intake, and who finally got back to me by phone, that I'd started bleeding again and wasn't feeling well. She advised me to have an endometrio-biopsy because my bleeding could signify cancer of the uterus. She could get me an appointment with a doctor in Champaign. In the meantime, Dr VZ had returned, and I preferred to see her first.

When Dr VZ found out what was happening, she told me to stop taking estrogen altogether but to continue taking the progesterone, and gave me a 16 February appointment to have the endemetrio-biopsy. That little operation turned out to be painful, and I didn't like the intern, who performed it in front of VZ. However, when VZ saw the hardening in my breast, she told me to stop taking the progesterone altogether and to immediately have a mammogram. She warned me that if I stopped taking the hormones, I'd provoke bleeding. And it was provoked.

On 18 February, I went for the mammogram, which was

painful because of the hardening in my left breast, and on the Sunday, Dr VZ stopped by the house to tell me I had breast cancer. The next day, I went to see the surgeon, who did a needle biopsy. On the Tuesday, he called me to say that the lab technicians were unable to detect whether it was cancer, because I had too much fatty tissue. In the report, I read 'lipomas', a word that at the time caused me to be both intrigued and worried. The surgeon had to do another biopsy, by opening up my breast while I was under general anesthetic, but he wouldn't be able to do it before 2 March, which would be in about two weeks' time.

Since then, I've been feeling as if I'm caught up in a frightening whirlwind I have no control over. Last Sunday night, after Dr VZ came with her announcement, I couldn't sleep: how and why can she be so sure? I'm completely disoriented, and so thankful that Alban, my love, is here with me. I'm very scared: it's terribly cruel to have to wait two weeks when you've been told you probably have cancer!

Yesterday, I saw an oncologist I didn't like at all. He made us wait 45 minutes and didn't apologise for the wait; Alban thought he'd probably gone to lunch. The man seemed arrogant and self-satisfied. He hadn't read my dossier, and barely examined me. He was more interested in ordering all kinds of pre-operation tests. Later, I found out that when doctors order tests, they're enabled to raise their fees considerably; in fact, the oncologist charged me a huge fee: $225 for a 15-minute consultation.

Bettina: It's good you're raising this disgusting aspect of some 'cash box' doctors!

I was appalled. Even though my insurance company would pay the bill, I wrote to the office of complaints to have the amount reduced. The official obliged, and sent me a letter of thanks.

The rapid birthrate of new synthetic products that began in 1945 far surpassed the ability of government to regulate their use and disposal. Between 45,000 and 100,000 chemicals are now in common commercial use; 75,000 is the most frequently cited estimate. Of these, only about 1.5 to 3 percent (1,200 to 1,500) have been tested for carcinogenicity ... Thus, many carcinogenic environmental contaminants likely remain unidentified, unmonitored, and unregulated. Too often this lack of basic information is paraphrased as 'there is lack of evidence of harm,' which in turn is translated as 'the chemical is harmless.'

According to the National Research Council, only 10 percent of pesticides in common use have been adequately assessed for hazards; for 38 percent, nothing useful is known; the remaining 52 percent fall somewhere in between.

According to the most recent TRI (Toxics Release Inventory), which is about the size of an average telephone book, 2.26 billion pounds of toxic chemicals were released into the environment in 1994. Of these, 177 million pounds were known or suspected carcinogens. (Steingraber: 1997: 103)

Jewel in the crown of industrial pollution, chlorine and phosphorus-rich pesticides, once ingested over long periods, are carcinogenic poisons that deaden or destabilize the central nervous system and irritate the digestive system ... When all the various causes of problems start to mingle and get overlaid one upon the other, it is hard to clearly identify any one in particular, and these pesticide-driven causes can practically go unnoticed when things get beyond a certain point, and our society is rapidly reaching just such a point. (Séralini: 1997: 86)

2

DEATH OF FATHER
HAIR, OIL AND MOURNING

Like a jury's verdict or an adoption decree, a cancer diagno-sis is an authoritative pronouncement, one with the power to change your identity. It sends you into an unfamiliar country where all the rules of human conduct are alien. In this new territory, you disrobe in front of strangers who are allowed to touch you. You submit to bodily invasions. You agree to the removal of body parts. You agree to be poisoned. You have become a cancer patient.

Most of the traits and skills you bring with you from your native life are irrelevant, while strange new attributes sudden-ly matter. Beautiful hair is irrelevant. Prominent veins along the soft skin at the fold of your arm are highly prized. The abil-ity to cook a delicious meal in thirty minutes is irrelevant. The ability to lie completely motionless on a hard platform for half an hour while your bones are scanned for signs of tumor is, conversely, quite useful. (Steingraber: 1997: 31)

Urbana, 3 March 1994

I have the operation, during which several biopsies are done: I do indeed have cancer. I'm frightened, but at the same time feel at peace. Do I feel at peace because I no longer have the choice, and because I know that in these circumstances it's better to be calm? Until now, I was uncertain, and uncertainty is a very strong cause of anxiety: not knowing what to expect was painful and extremely torturous. Uncertainty is unbearable – now I know what I have, I can start defending myself.

I'm told that in the United States, one our of every eight women gets breast cancer, and I later learn that the proportion is now much higher and increasing; in some regions of the States, for example Long Island, the proportion is one out of every four women!

By phone from Beirut, my sister Adelaide tells me that cancer is a Satanic disease – just what I want to hear! She asks me whether I've had myself anointed with oil and been prayed for. She says she'll send people from her church to pray with me. I know she means well, but why does she always introduce religious connotations and dramatise situations by using metaphors though which life is painted in black and white, as if to reassure herself that her beliefs are justified and actualised and that her system of thought is thereby reinforced? She locates illness in a magical world of struggle between good and evil: between the Devil and God. On the one hand, illness becomes located in the spiritual world, so its biological reality is cancelled out, and on the other, the spiritual world is a dichotomised, 'either/or', system.

Adelaide's words must be upsetting me more than I think, because when I phone Milwaukee to speak about my illness with Pastor Eriks, who's also a medical doctor as well as a friend of Adelaide and my brothers Théophile and Pierrot, I mention what Adelaide has said and ask him for his opinion. He says that cancer isn't a Satanic illness but is a very bad disease, and that in the United States it's a real epidemic these days. Adelaide's words must strike a chord with me, whereby some of my ancient beliefs are revived, even though I'm only semi-serious when I ask the pastor about whether cancer is a Satanic affliction. Proselytisers often use individual or collective hardship to shamelessly exploit people who are in a position of weakness.

Bettina *[who doesn't mince her words!]*: To make a person feel guilty because he or she is sick amounts to utter stupidity. Adelaide must have things to reproach herself about, and probably needs more reassurance than you do, Evelyne!

Some day, I'll have to write about father and his illness: how he's made to feel it's evil, that it's through his sins that he's brought it on himself. I must write of the bouts of soul searching he experiences because he can't sleep between midnight and 4 a.m. Pierrot is certain the situation is linked to the fact that father used to look at pornographic magazines when my mother was asleep.

Cancer: a disease that kills. According to Adelaide, it's Satanic because it eats up a person's insides. This analogy of the internal being, whereby the illness is located in the body and originates in the soul, is the expression of a very archaic way of thinking. We all carry evil within ourselves, evil that some of us don't accept, don't want to see and refuse to recognise. Evil is its own entity: it conceals itself within some beings, and occasionally manifests itself in the senses, through, for example, illness. Proselytisers thereby explain that illness stems from some evil force that dwells within us, whereas the evil force is in fact exterior to us. When an illness is dressed in the guise of evil, it becomes more acceptable and easier to bear, and we are more comforted. Once it's become identified with an alien entity, we can better fight against the evil by participating in rituals, expiation and prayer.

In the third and fifth centuries, Manicheism was a religious system in which Satan was represented as being co-eternal with God. My sister Adelaide requires a Manichean explanation for my illness, so she invokes the occult dual powers of

Good and Evil. She sets herself up as a self-righteous, self-proclaimed judge: a kind of exorcist, and views everything as being either good or bad, black or white, with no shades in between.

Between Chicago and Nashville, 4 March 1994

I'm on a plane travelling between Chicago and Nashville. Now I have cancer, will I be better able to ask essential questions about life and to seek new answers?

Bettina: Any painful experience in one's existence makes one want to live more intensively: this is the positive of the negative.

I'm traveling with my love, Alban. This trip to Alabama and New Orleans is like a honeymoon for us. All our trips – before, during and after my illness – we call a honeymoon. We've had so many of them. Our relationship is always like new: it evolves and matures with time, yet retains the excitement of the first moments we had together.

I wonder how my body will react to the treatment. I know that my mind and spirit will also have to move along with the treatment.

As I sit in the plane, my mind again wanders to my father's bedside. He's dying, and his children are harassing him by making him confess his sins – my poor father, who was supposedly looking at pornographic magazines between midnight and 4 a.m.! They've made him confess. Mother was astonished and is now wondering now whether she was the woman he needed, the right woman for him, although their whole life, too, has been a succession of honeymoons! My father is being eaten up by both suffering his cancer and having his conscience forced on him! My poor father: suffering in both his body and his soul.

Children who haven't come to terms with how best to relate to their parents, who are burdened with confused and murky feelings, project their own frustrations and guilt feelings on to their parents.

Mobile, 5 March 1994

When life is threatened by death, everything becomes very intense.

We're in New Orleans. What a good idea it was to come here despite my disease. We meet my friend Caryl, who's invited us to deliver lectures and do a reading of my novels at her university in Mobile, Alabama. I decided not to cancel this trip: my life has to go on. I don't want to stop being involved in my activities just because I've been diagnosed as having breast cancer; actually, I feel split between the temptation to yield to the illness and the will to resist abandoning myself to it.

Caryl is wonderful. She tells me she went through having thyroid cancer several years ago: I probably wouldn't have known so if I hadn't been hit with cancer myself. Because of my illness, many people who otherwise would have kept quiet reveal their experiences to me. I'm discovering that cancer is much more prevalent than I'd ever imagined, and that many more people than you'd ever think possible either are suffering or have suffered from the disease. Caryl helps me a lot by telling me stories about how she overcame the disease and its treatment, and how she struggled against the odds. Her stories are so lively.

She tells me you have to be aggressive, and not let yourself fall into either despair or the medical establishment, in which the practitioners try to dominate the situation, neglect to do some things if you aren't cautious and prevent you from taking charge of your body. She tells me all kinds of stories through which I'm able to glimpse how widespread the disease is: she 'de-dramatises' it so it seems less sinister and I'm less fearful.

Jane: The word 'de-dramatise' doesn't occur in the Random House dictionary. It translates from the French into 'to make something less dramatic'. I'd prefer a word like defuse, which means '1. To remove the fuse from a bomb, mine, etc.; 2. To make it less dangerous, tense or embarrassing: to defuse a potentially ugly situation.' This verb fits nicely into your pattern of words that are borrowed from the language of war. I see a connection with the movie version of *The English Patient*, in which one of the characters, the Sri Lankan, spends his time defusing bombs and land mines, but also 'defused' Helen, the Canadian nurse, played by Juliette Binoche, by loving her in the right way. Before that, she'd believed she was a destructive person: that anyone who got close to her would be destroyed.

Caryl has a friend who'd recently had a double mastectomy. The woman immediately underwent breast reconstruction and asked that each nipple be sculpted into a heart shape. She celebrated by inviting all her friends to come and look at her new, heart-shaped breasts. The story makes me laugh.

I need to hear these stories rather than have people start crying when they see me; or feel sorry for me; or act as if I were stricken by plague, a victim of some curse. I absolutely must see and hear women such as Caryl and her friends, who struggle for theirs and other people's life, for different values, for more justice in this world. As for Caryl, she works to revive the memory of forgotten women: the memory of oppressed women and women who have in some way suffered. She describes and analyses all this by way of choosing the literature she teaches and the authors she brings out of oblivion, as well as in her own writings, in which she interweaves poetry and commitment. She believes that getting angry is sometimes necessary, because we thereby take charge of our life.

Last night, Alban and I make love passionately, in the magnificent room of our beautiful little hotel, located on the outskirts of the old quarter of Mobile's harbour. We're staying in an old Spanish villa that has a fountain; an interior courtyard surrounded by arcaded galleries; an avenue covered with tufted, hundred-year-old oaks; rosewood-coloured marble; and big, gold-leaf mirrors. Alban and I feel so good together: we're so well when we're with each other. Everything's so intense when we're together.

Later, he tells me that while we were making love, he was thinking about my breast, which was getting bigger by the day, and that he was wondering when and how the growing would stop. He's panicking.

6 March 1994

It's my father's birthday. Alban and I have returned from New Orleans, in which we spent a marvellous 24 hours with Caryl and her husband Craig. I almost forgot all my worries: father dying; my breast cancer; which treatment I'll have to undergo – I don't yet know what it'll be. I'm afraid, and worried that in Chicago tomorrow, when Alban and I will have to say goodbye, I'm about to find myself alone with the illness.

I'll have to write about all that's happening; what I'm learning, reading and discovering; how I'm dealing with this illness, the plague of the so-called modern twentieth century; and how other people are dealing with it. I must write for both myself and other people: the ones going through the same ordeal and the ones who will go through it.

Later, when I ask Dr VZ how, once we knew it was cancer, she could be so sure, she replies, 'It was just my opinion!' Is this something a serious doctor should say? And later again, when she finally answers the message I'd left on her answering machine, and I say, 'I hope I'm not disturbing you with all my questions and anxieties,' she replies, 'I wouldn't answer if I didn't want to.' What huge differences exist between our two cultures! I have to be reassured, listened to and taken care of by my doctor; she, on the other hand, has to affirm her individuality: her American, Western attitude of 'Me before anyone else!'

Jane: This is usually said as 'me first'. The Reagan generation of youth were called the Me First generation – but you don't need to explain this to your readers: it's common knowledge.

I agree with Jane; however, I'm not writing solely for people who've been exposed to mainstream American culture: my readers will hopefully also be from European, Arab and other cultures.

When I hear the doctor's words, I'm deeply hurt and shocked.

Bettina: Urge your readers not to hesitate to consult another doctor when they're unhappy with the one they have, because a good doctor–patient relationship is the best medicine.

In the year after I'm treated, I do consult another doctor. In the meantime, I change my medical-insurance company to one that allows me to choose doctors and places for therapy located anywhere in the world, whereas at the time I'm diagnosed, I'm limited to the group at Share, one of Champaign–Urbana's polyclinics. I'm one of the lucky ones: because I'm employed at the University of Illinois, I can choose my insurance company. I'm not limited to a HMO, which stands for Health Management Organization. I find out that some people aren't limited to having restrictive insurance, but that people who have a pre-existing condition such as cancer won't find an insurance company that's willing to insure them!

⧗

What a wonderful stay Alban and I are having here in Mobile, Alabama. He's so tender, so affectionate. We're so much in love. The Malagua Inn, which we're staying in, is a dream hotel. The sun is shining. We're on the 'Pacific Bay' – it's actually the Gulf of Mexico, but Alban, who has a great capacity for fantasising about places, has named it the Pacific Bay. We've forgotten our worries for the time being. It'll be difficult to part tomorrow: we're trying to forget.

Caryl thinks we're very much in love, Alban and I, and it's so true. What a courageous woman she is. They removed her whole thyroid gland. She underwent a cobalt treatment and an operation. She explains to me how she had to affirm herself by asking for a copy of all her medical reports, taking charge of her life and affirming her sovereignty over her body. Her family members also tried to use her disease to dominate her by telling her things they'd never have dared mention if she hadn't been ill. Craig and she reacted vehemently by threatening to never see them again if they persisted in adopting their attitude. Caryl's account reminded me of the comments my sister Adelaide made about my illness. I wonder whether everyone who gets sick has to face similar situations created by their loved ones who allow themselves to preach to the ill person because he or she is weak, dependent and helpless and in a situation that's probably painful and unacceptable.

Yesterday, at night, Alban and I walked in the city of Mobile, first near the port and then in the centre of town. The place was completely deserted, a frightening void: not a single passer-by, only cars and cars and cars. We found a magnificent building: the Convention Center, near the bay. We went in through forbidden doors and were able to reach the balconies overlooking the bay. It all seemed to be too empty. Then, inside the building, we came across a room of animated people, at a bowling convention. We ordered some pizza and beer, and had a sumptuous picnic overlooking the bay ... beautiful moments I felt I needed to capture as never before.

I watch my sweet love, crossing the Malagua Inn's garden, with its little water fountain in the centre: my sweetheart, so elegant, his beautiful hair flowing around his intelligent head, filled with softness and kindness. I marvel at this love that carries me across time and space. It'll be hard to part tomorrow, but he will return in April ...

Each of us has a cross to bear. My old beliefs are now resurfacing and haunting me, and I'm trying to be soothed by them. I notice this phenomenon, and will try to analyse it later. Often when difficulties arrive they all arrive at once. My previous crisis occurred in 1974–75, when the war broke out in Lebanon and my ex-husband Jay left me. Do crises occur every 20 years? What will happen in 2004–05: 10 years from now, or in 2014–15: 20 years from now? I'll be 70 and Alban will be 90. Time passes so quickly. I already knew it before my illness; now, with my parents' imminent death and my own disease, I feel it even more.

On the plane for Champaign, 8 March 1994

We've just parted, Alban and I: a painful separation. Yesterday, we have three sessions at the university, two of which involve reading, singing and answering questions about my work, and one of which is a public lecture in which Alban and I speak about our research into the city of Cairo.

Lots of attendees react to the session about Cairo, especially 'fascist' men who would like us to deliver the usual cliched lecture about Arab women, seeing as our conference's title is Women in Islamic Societies. Instead, we take the discourse of

women who live in Cairo's popular districts. We're especially attentive to the discourse of Umm Ashraf, who has some
particularly pertinent things to say about contemporary daily
life as lived in Cairo's poor and working-class districts. She
talks about her miseries; how hard it is just to scrape by from
day to day; and how, as a woman, she has to share her husband with another woman. She also tells of matters such as
her financial problems and how she copes with them, and of
her experiences in the judicial system, with doctors and in the
black market. Umm Ashraf is an incredible woman whose
self-assurance comes across clearly in her voice. Hers isn't a
pitiful discourse: her life is one of struggling until she's
exhausted, never letting go and trying to get ahead.

The room is full: the crowd must have been attracted by
the title. I'm upset by a young Lebanese man who says the
title is misleading and wonders how we can claim to be talking about 'Women in Islamic societies' when we're talking
about only a few women from some poor Cairo neighborhood. I feel I need to support Caryl, who's given us the title,
and tell the angry young man that it's precisely the title
that's brought us the crowd we have. Why, I ask him,
shouldn't Umm Ashraf's discourse – her voice – be as important, if not more so, than the usual discourse we could have
given about the subject? We wanted to see things from a
fresh vantage point, to promote a different viewpoint that
was outside all the cliches perpetuated by the media. Umm
Ashraf is an authentic voice through which we're being
given an authentic image of contemporary Cairo: she's the
real speaker at our academic conference. I add that I would
like to have heard the voices of women in the audience, voices that didn't dare rise above the palpable aggressiveness
and domination of some of the men present.

Alban also gets upset. Later, he tells me later he had a lot of
fun responding, and that it was very amusing to hear these
males who'd just been dispossessed of a counter-discourse

that would also have consisted of cliches: we'd literally cut the ground from under their feet. I love it when Alban gesticulates when he's speaking: when he gets excited and talks passionately.

Jane: Americans consider punctuating one's speech with gesticulation a quaint cultural trait among the French! But for French people it's considered an Italian characteristic!

Alban also wants to support Caryl, who'd felt obliged to excuse herself for suggesting the title: 'Why,' he asked of the males present at the session, 'do you always want quantitative analysis – numbers etc.? The discourse of Umm Ashraf gives us a quality, another vision, worth thousands of so-called scientific data.' It was a very lively session.

Between my morning presentation and our afternoon talk, I return to the magnificent, Spanish-style hotel, at which Alban is waiting for me. We make love passionately, as if for the first time. Yes, on that trip, we make love so many times, and it's so wonderful each time. We're far from imagining that these are probably the last 'normal' sexual acts life will allow us to enjoy, the 'un-nameable disease' having hit both of us in a part of my body whereby, unfortunately, there are huge sexual repercussions. It's so good: this love in my life is so uplifting, and is a love that I always feel is present, even during Alban's absences.

I'm also helped a lot by meeting Caryl and witnessing her courage, her lively stories and her struggle for life. She tells me that when she was undergoing the cobalt treatment, she found she was pregnant. The doctors hadn't warned her that she could become pregnant. She was on her way back from a treatment when she and Craig decided to go off somewhere together, to simply forget about it all. They made love in the bushes by the roadside, like a crazy young couple. When life is threatened by death, everything becomes so intense and is marked with a craziness, a joy, a passion for living. I also saw this phenomenon in Lebanon during the war, and many writers have described scenes such as this in their novels.

Caryl also tells us about an operation after which she was left with a huge scar on her abdomen. To assert herself over her fear, she asked Craig to go with her to a Florida nudist camp. At the camp were lots of elderly people who'd also had a deforming operation. They rubbed suntan lotion on Caryl's scar, and their kindness made her feel good, as if she'd overcome her wounded body. She tells us that Craig, who seems so reserved, played the game with her. She even has pictures of him reading a history book, wearing only his glasses.

I love how this woman overcomes her anxieties, her fears and her body, which must have hurt so much. I love her audacity. I needed to meet this woman in order to exorcise the demons of my own anxieties and to see how I'd face what was awaiting me.

Jane: What an angel was sent for your 'Satanic' disease, to use Adelaide's term.

Urbana, 12 March 1994

I'm back in Urbana. Zohreh, my dear friend, who's so wonderful, is waiting for me at the airport. She takes me to her place to have some of her good soup and then insists on accompanying me to the oncologist. Diane also comes with us. Both women take notes. I like the oncologist, Doctor JE: she reminds me of Huguette, my sister-in-law – direct, full of humour, human. She asks me lots of questions about both my health and my life in general. She takes notes. Then come the diagnosis and treatment options:

Diagnosis: *Infiltrating lobular carcinoma; biopsy removed 3 cm; margins were positive. It is a large tumor: T3No (Stage III) breast cancer.*

Treatment options:
(1) Modified radical mastectomy. Surgery removes breast, and nodes under the arm. Usually, no radiation, but for very large tumors, this should be considered. Chemotherapy would be given [in my case before surgery]. *Breast reconstruction could be done immediately or later.*
(2) Breast-conserving therapy surgery removes tumor and small area of normal breast and nodes under arm. Radiation to the breast; about six weeks of daily treatment. Chemotherapy would be given [in my case, first – before surgery].

Because of the size of tumor, chemotherapy should be given before more surgery. It is possible that the tumor can be made small enough to do breast-conserving therapy.

Chemotherapy: *Adriamycin and Cytoxin, intravenously every three weeks, four times. Side effects: Hair loss (temporary); nausea; mouth soreness; bladder irritation; blood counts lower: white cells (danger of infection), platelets (danger of bleeding); cumulative limit to lifetime Adriamycin dose.*

Tamoxifen: *anti-estrogen pills, to be given later, for probably five years; side effects: menopause symptoms.*

Cindy: How ironic: the opposite of VZ's treatment!

Several studies show equivalent survival for mastectomy versus breast-conserving therapy.

To these details recorded by the doctor, my dear friend Zohreh adds her own notes, as follows.

Chemotherapy has to be given for something of this size, before surgery so the lump can be contained and reduced.

The doctor says she's worried about the fast growth of the tumor.

The 'yucky' part of chemotherapy, the side effects, are no fun – repeat: no fun. Added to the ones enumerated above, the lower blood count in white cells and platelets could weaken the heart muscle! The advantage of chemotherapy is that it prevents the spread of the cancer.

The doctor predicts that chemotherapy can end in May. Surgery can then follow in 3–4 weeks. And radiation follows after I can lift my arms.

Prognosis for lobular cancer is good.

Dr JE thinks she's giving me some options. She tells me to take time to think them through, and to let her know which one I decide to take.

I don't realise it when I'm with the doctor – it's all too much of a shock – but I'm actually not given some options, because there aren't any: it's the usual 'Poison, cut and burn' treatment that breast-cancer patients know only too well. I burst into tears, suddenly realising I won't be able to do the things I usually do: travel between Paris, Tunis and Beirut; visit my ageing and dying parents in Beirut; see my friends everywhere, but especially the ones in Tunisia; do my writing; be with my loved ones in Paris. I suddenly feel that my life is coming to a stop. I'm entering a zone of illness, doctors and hospitals.

Dr JE, unlike Dr VZ, does not provide Kleenex. She mumbles something to the effect that she's used to seeing her patients react in this way but she's come unprepared. Zohreh hands me a Kleenex.

I'm writing this account a year later, by reworking the notes I took during the consultation. At this moment, my dear friend Zohreh is undergoing chemotherapy for ovarian cancer, and I'm not at her side to offer her the help and support she gave me during my trials. It's breaking my heart to know she's having to travel the same 'road to Calvary'. We didn't know about her illness a year ago, and what else didn't we – don't we – know?

I wonder how my body will react, how my mind and spirit will react. I hope I learn new things about myself and other people, so I'm better able to grow and to forget about myself in favour of concentrating on other things. I stop crying, and peace settles deep within me. I have to cross this dark valley. There's hope at the end of it: I know it.

I don't really have options: I have to undergo chemotherapy right away, to prevent the cancer from spreading.

Later, I reflect on this moment and on what this doctor was offering me: she was either ignorant or fooling me. Given the size and nature of my tumour, she should have known, first, that it was impossible to reduce the tumour to the point that I'd be able to choose between two options for surgery, and second, that chemotherapy couldn't have much effect and was therefore unnecessary. In reality, because she was either ignorant or afraid to tell me things and was therefore dishonest, first, I had to undergo a useless bout of chemo, and two, I had to wait three months for a surgical intervention that she should have known was unavoidable. Beyond her, the whole medical establishment was what was on trial. I return to this facet later in the book.

Yesterday, I start it: 'the poison', as cancer patients call it. I attend my first session with my niece, Anaïs, who's come to take care of me. She's as light as air – a free spirit. What a treasure she is, this sweet young woman! She meets Dr JE, who all my friends like. Dr JE measures my body, because

the drugs – Adriamycin and Cytoxin – that have to be injected into it intravenously are measured according to the
body's surface area. She measures my tumour: 12 centimetres! It feels enormous to me, and I can hardly believe its
size: how could it have grown so fast?

16 March 1994

I have a friend named Zahra, and I call her *Petite-Fleur*, both
to distinguish her from Zohreh, my other friend, and
because in Arabic the word *zahra* means 'flower', which
seems so right for my friend, who's pretty and delicate.
Yesterday evening, Petite-Fleur, Anaïs, Youenn and I go to a
bar called the Embassy to hear some blues. Keith Harding is
playing the guitar and harmonica as well as singing. He
says, 'I want to sing this song for Evelyne.' It's Leonard
Cohen's 'Suzanne'. How can he remember that I like the
song? It pleases me so much! Everything takes on such
intensity when you're hit with a life-threatening disease.

Bettina: Cancer is a disease that can be fatal, but breast cancer
can also be cured nowadays.

I want to 'go down to Suzanne's place on the river', as the
song goes, with my love, Alban … Oh, how I want to go
with him and be healed.

Today, I'm rereading some books about cancer. I get
frightened when I read some accounts and statistics. It's
good that Séverine has come by and brought me some beautiful yellow flowers. There's something very special about
Séverine, and I'm glad we're getting closer.

I used to like my body; now I'm afraid of it. It feels foreign to me and capable of hurting me, of abandoning me,
of betraying me! Tonight, Charlotte and David Bruner
phone me, and I'm very touched to hear from them. I find

out that Charlotte has undergone two mastectomies, and that her daughter had breast cancer last year. It's been 10 years since Charlotte had the operation, she remains enthusiastic, full of energy and involved in many projects. What a woman! I've known the Bruners for more than 20 years now, but it's the first time Charlotte has told me about her cancer. I need to hear their voices tonight; they're such wonderful people. David is more than 80 and Charlotte is 77, but they're active participants in life, even though David has had to slow down and is weak from recently having had an operation; they don't tell me what for. I need to see them, to talk to them and to share with them our physical struggle and hopes for a better world. I hope they pass by this summer. They're such good friends, and I'm comforted to hear from them.

I've been receiving many phone calls, cards, flowers and special attention. However, I don't get the same pleasure from all of them. It's strange how some people project themselves on to me: how they often react as an expression of their own fears and anxieties, of their own sense of tragedy, and of their feelings about life and death.

Bettina: Unfortunately, these reactions are very common, but they often come from people who are ill at ease with themselves.

Yesterday, after taking a few phone calls during which I have to repeat in detail what treatment I'm receiving and how I'm feeling, and in return have to listen to the expressions of emotion and anxiety that my condition is bringing about, I don't want to pick up the phone any more; instead, I let people leave a message on my answering machine. I need to be surrounded by joy and happiness. I decide to keep the 'out of the ordinary' words and cards through which something deep is truly expressed.

As I'm writing this journal, I'm jotting down some of the relevant thoughts, feelings, encouragements and emotions that my friends have expressed. Following are some extracts from the letters and postcards I've kept.

Kristin Stiles: *I still have your song in my heart, your sharp mind in my thoughts, your dancing eyes in my soul and your human glow in my memory.*

Cheris Kramarae: *You have been well trained to be kind to others. Now we need to give you encouragement to be very good to yourself. It's a kind of training most women have't had a lot of.*

Caryl Lloyd: *Among the many things I wanted to thank you for during your recent visit was for bringing poetry back to my life … Your songs and texts have had such a salutary effect, allowing me to feel the strength of the bonds that connect us all.*

Consuelo: *From my experience, I see very few senior academicians who take time out to be caring. And you remind me that to have a full life, this is essential.*

Mary Lee Sargent: *Since I imagine that you can use lots of encouragement and positive energy to enhance your recovery process, I send this to remind you that women around the world honor you and are at this moment sending prayers, incantations, exhortations and explicit orders to our special goddess asking that your anxieties be lifted and your breast healed now, if not sooner.*

Lezlie Hart: *A friend of mine here is also undergoing chemotherapy for breast cancer. My heart goes out to you both, and I feel a sense of rage and helplessness at the same time … Even though we see each other rarely and fleetingly, you are an important part of my life, and I love you for the woman you are and for all you have given me.*

Cindy Hahn: *You know, your cancer has made me think a lot about my situation, my health, etc., and I am going to try to eat better and to make a bigger effort to lead a less stressful life, etc. You have always had a good influence on me, Evelyne, even when from afar! You are so courageous, and I admire you so much ... I hope that the package I sent you contains something that can help you; at any rate, I am with you mentally. I am trying a meditation that helps me sometimes and that could help you also: You imagine your body with a white light in movement inside yourself, where you see dark spots. You push them away with the white light. It is as if you are 'washing' yourself mentally of all the obstructions, and you imagine this light like a strong energy that uplifts you, heals you and gives you peace. Don't worry if you are too tired to write me.*

Amel Ben Aba: *I heard you had tried to call me yesterday evening. I was sad not to have been there. I was at a lute concert with Rachida, and we thought of you. It is Ramadan right now, and there are all kinds of shows at night. I hope you do not have any bad news about your parents and Lebanon.* [She didn't yet know I was sick, and I'd called her to let her know so she wouldn't learn about the illness through someone else.] *Evelyne, your letter is steeped in the smells of the sea, of the mountains.* [I'd written to her from Lebanon.] *It is scented and filled with your future book, which I know will be good. Thank you for the voice of your brother Lucien in that little church near the sea. Thank you, Evelyne, for sharing with me this love, these loves. You know how I love Lebanon already. If it can be in mid-June, I will be so happy to join you there. I read in* Peuples Méditerranéens *the article on the violence in Lebanon, by Fawaz Traboulsi. I had to stop several times it was so unbearable. It is true that we have not thought enough, analyzed enough, this theme of violence. It would be wonderful to reflect on it in a writing workshop. What is going on close by, in Algeria, is horrible ... Evelyne, sometimes I close my ears. It hurts so much, this continuous violence, this arrogance of the strongest, this anesthesia of consciousness. During the five days spent in Rabat, I saw Algerian women exhausted and closed. I would like to have given a massage to one of them, but she was not ready to let anyone touch her ... I miss you ...*

Julie Miesle: *I will come with pleasure to keep you company if you feel depressed or need someone to tell you silly jokes; I can run to you with good records and tons of chocolate ... I would like to help you overcome this disease, which I want to believe is only temporary, because it is essential for me to have my daughter know you. She will be able to learn so much from you, and I would like her to feel all the things I prize in you.*

Gilles Steudler: *When I was in Urbana, I had thought of creating a small collection of poems, one of which would have consisted of a picture of a train station in a corn field; I would have entitled it 'Melancholic Illinois' ... Those years when I thought I was unhappy ... I did not know what unhappiness was, which I have just found out, irreparably.*

Andrée Chedid: *So many thoughts flow to you, Evelyne. Thoughts that resemble you full of vitality, of the sunshine within, of invention, of renewed images. Everything will be alright – I feel it, and soon you will be here in Paris for a beautiful sabbatical year. What a joy for your many friends. I kiss you in all tenderness.*

⧗

Diane is here tonight. She's talking to Anaïs about her miseries, her anxieties about life, and Anaïs is listening to her tenderly. I find them both so moving. Diane has so much talent, intelligence, strength and sweetness, but lacks self-confidence. She's so vulnerable. I don't know whether I should tell her to trust her intelligence or whether I should just shake her.

Fortunately, Anaïs is here to listen to Diane, to feel with her and to encourage her. She's wonderful, my little Anaïs: a real jewel. She reminds me a bit of how I was at her age. I was also very closed in. Already married, I wanted a life out of the ordinary. Little did I know, or ever think, that I'd go through the pain I have to go through now. None of my female relatives have had breast cancer, so why would I have thought about it as being something that could happen to me? Will my nieces be more prepared now they've seen what I've had to go through? I hope that milder and more-effective cures for cancer will have been found by then.

I go back to my past, remembering how I was at Anaïs's age. I wanted a life that was different from other people's. That's why I married Jay: he was different from other men. Unlike most men I'd known, including my overly authoritarian father, he attracted me because he had an artist's sensibility. I didn't know he was gay; nor did he, at the time. It's likely that I unconsciously liked him because he was gay: his softness and sweetness were promises of a different kind of life. And in any case, homosexuality isn't an essence; it isn't inscribed in our genes, and the choices that people think are implied in it are very much dependent on circumstances. Personally, I've never either associated it with failure or nurtured that feeling in other people.

Jay calls me tonight, and is worried and tender. He reminds me that before our wedding, I permed and completely ruined my hair, and that I had to buy fake 'bangs' and pony tails to cover up the disaster. Now I have two wigs: one red, the other black. I'm prepared. Jay says my features are good enough: my head well shaped enough, even to go bald! I trust his judgement, because he's an artist I admire. He's concerned, and I'm touched by his phone call.

17 March 1994

I'm reading a lot of articles and books about cancer, and some of them are depressing, such as the ones I'm reading tonight. All the statistics are frightening, and sometimes I'm scared. Emma, a friend of Anaïs, comes for dinner tonight. She talks about how she sees me in relation to the rest of my family members, who she describes as having 'a religious spirit' rather than a faith. To describe me, she uses the image of a vessel that doesn't contain much oil, and she tells me she's praying so the vessel will grow larger and contain a lot of oil. I like her image of the vessel that contains oil, even if the metaphor isn't very poetic, and hope that her wishes that I open up to more blessing – the oil prescribed by Adelaide – and have more spirituality in my life become a reality. However, I think that Emma, like Adelaide, remains too closed within her dogma, which includes the ideas of good and evil.

I have just talked to my brother Pierrot. I'm revolted by his stories about the so-called pornography my father used to look at and by the fact that he made my father confess to looking at it before he died. He'd urged my father to ask my mother for forgiveness – as he'd done in the case of his wife, Marilyn, because he himself used to look at pornographic magazines and watch pornographic movies.

Pierrot is full of 'good' feelings, and attempts to express a lot of love – but are these enough? Some of his remarks, such as 'We carry our parents' chains,' could be pertinent. However, it's hard to accept his perspective about things even when his analysis is accurate. Listening to him, I'm taken back to the dogmas of my childhood: to everything that made me angry and anxious to leave, to what I revolted against and found unacceptable.

Pierrot is both right and wrong: right that we all bear a legacy, but wrong about the legacy's content, because I believe that the legacy isn't necessarily expressed from one generation to the next. No one is an exact replica of his or her parents, and we can either accept or refuse the legacy. Why should we carry our parents' chains? It's a childish idea. My father's 'trial' is sordid: where is love in all of that? It's hatred of the father that's being expressed, and we're right in the middle of the Oedipus complex of a boy who hasn't yet grown up. To top it off, the 'we' he uses includes me, because for him, my relationship with Alban can be only sinful.

18 March 1994

Is the problem Dr VZ's negligence or my misfortune? Why won't she call me back even though I've left a message on her answering machine, telling her I need to ask her some questions? She hasn't called Diane back either, and Diane thinks she must feel guilty because Sue, VZ's lover, is very 'anti-hormones'.

According to everything I'm reading, cancer can be provoked if a person takes estrogen, and 'people at risk' must never take the hormone. However, how can you know who's at risk, especially if hormones have never before been used in your family? In fact, this whole business of taking hormones is such a fad, a postmodern way of treating the body; I remain unconvinced it's a good one.

Bettina: It might even be dangerous, especially in megadoses. If they must be used, it's after many tests, at the right dosage and using precautions.

My thoughts are going in all directions. In order to speak about cancer, we have recourse to military metaphors: 'the war on cancer', 'the fight against the disease', 'losing the battle with cancer', and so on. I don't like these images of violence, yet feel as if my body is being invaded by foreign elements: cells dividing rapidly; capable of eating all my other cells; killing me. It's a frightening thought. Pierrot asks me whether my tumour could resolve itself; I haven't read anything to indicate it could. However, I ask myself, *Why not? Why couldn't it go away as fast as it's come? Is this only wishful thinking?*

Dr Wend, who's one of the doctors at Pastor Erik's church in Milwaukee, tells me that when the prognosis is of a cancer such as mine, the best thing is to proceed immediately by having a mastectomy, and that my type of cancer often spreads to the other breast. I read that between about 7 and 10 per cent of all breast cancers are a 'lobular invasive carcinoma' but that it's an aggressive type of cancer.

Later, I read that it's less aggressive than other types of cancer: one of the many contradictory statements I come across.

Why am I being hit with this type of cancer rather than another? I've been very diligent in examining my breasts carefully every week – even more than once a week when I've gone swimming and showered at IMPE, the university's Intra-Mural Physical Education building. I think I would have felt even a small node. Why did the mass form so suddenly? Why is it linked to my visit to Lebanon, in which I couldn't examine my breasts as easily as I do in the States, and in which my father was dying of this horrible disease: prostate cancer, which had metastasised to his bones? His whole body was suffering, and he was even feeling pain in his bones: my poor father, who called himself a 'felled oak'. Only a year ago, he was full of life and energy, and was engaged in projects. It was my mother who was very ill, and who we thought would die within the year. Is it because of her that my father let himself decline and didn't fight harder to overcome his illness? I believe there's a connection between his illness and my mother's, as there is between mine and theirs, along with other factors that I analyse later in the book.

Later, these intuitions are reinforced in my readings.

Bettina: Underline this factor: one cannot remain insensitive to the pain of loved ones; on the other hand, one can get help to overcome the suffering.

Last Friday, I have my first chemotherapy session. I'm full of anxiety. Fortunately, my wonderful niece Anaïs is with me, and holds my hand. She reads me stories I can't follow: something to do with a myth, as told by the writer C. S. Lewis. The chemotherapy session takes the whole morning: first, the visit to my oncologist, and the explanation by her nurse, Amy; then, the whole ordeal of having the needle put into the vein of my right hand, including, for starters, an anti-vomiting liquid; then, the reddish Andryamicin; then, the Cytoxin; then, more liquid. I feel bloated and uneasy.

In one way, I'm happy to take these drugs, knowing they'll destroy the cancerous cells; on the other hand, though, I'm frightened by all the vicious liquid, which contains so many poisonous elements I have to absorb: poison that causes you to be nauseous; makes your hair fall out; and travels into your body, killing both the good and the bad cells.

Even writing about it now, a year later, I still have nauseous reminiscences.

19 March 1994

It's four o'clock in the morning, and I can't sleep. Yesterday, Anaïs, Petite-Fleur and I are invited to Samira's. Petite-Fleur seems very sad. We ask her what's wrong, and she tells us she feels she's done poorly in her exams. She's doing too many things: babysitting, which barely covers her expenses, and all the courses she's taking. She's exhausted; she cries; she isn't used to doing exams, especially in English. I listen to her while I'm touching the tumour in my breast, wondering whether the bad cells are eating the good ones. It's frightening!

The evening before, it's Diane who expresses her anxieties about her exams, her incompletes – 'Excused' grades whereby students are given more time to complete their course – and her fear of failing. I go into the kitchen to talk to Samira while Anaïs consoles Petite-Fleur. I remark how hard life is. At Petite-Fleur's and Diane's age, I also lived with these problems of whether I'd succeed or fail, and did so until I became a full professor, only a few years ago. Since I've overcome that nagging inner dialogue, I've had to deal with health. What's worse? Is health the most precious gift of all? Poor Petite-Fleur: she must face both problems – health concerns and academic challenges.

Bettina: May people reading you who are in good health realise how lucky they are!

My Anaïs is present to console both Diane and Petite-Fleur. She's so sweet, and sympathises with other people when they're having problems. I say to her, 'You're wonderful, the way you're helping my friends.' She replies, 'But they're also my friends.'

In the morning, Dr JE phones to tell me that according to the results of examinations of my biopsy that were more in-depth, the hormone receptors are negative; however, she believes the results aren't conclusive, because my cells might have been too estrogen saturated for her to determine how accurate the results are. I don't quite understand what all this means: I'll have to investigate the situation and read more. I ask her whether it's possible for a tumour such as mine to disappear as fast as it's come. She says, 'Yes: I've seen it happen before.' I wish so much that this happens to me, especially because I'm feeling as if my body's going back to how it used to be before I took the hormones.

Much later, thinking about Doctor JE's call, and having read both the biopsy results and about how important this analysis is, I wonder why the doctor didn't mention the other results, which included the 'S-Phase fraction': the indicator of how the cells are dividing. If a lot of cells are dividing, the S-Phase fraction is high and the tumour is behaving more aggressively than if only a few cells are dividing, in which case the S-Phase fraction is considered to be low. Nor did the doctor mention the 'ploidy status', whereby if the tumour cells have the correct amount of DNA they're called *diploid*, and if the amount of DNA is abnormal, they're called *aneuploid*. Tumors the cells of which are aneuploid tend to behave more aggressively. These tests are much more crucial for predicting how the disease will evolve.

I'm reading that if doctors were to analyse biopsy results more attentively, they'd be able to avoid prescribing unnecessary drugs and treatments. This would be the case in my situation, because according to the other results, the tumour is very bland and slow growing. Why has Dr JE chosen to mention only the hormone receptors, whereby a test is involved to determine whether the tumour is sensitive to hormones, for the purpose of eventually prescribing therapy? Evidently it must be because, in her view, the hormones have something to do with what's happening to me, and have been irresponsibly prescribed to me! Also, perhaps she's trying to hide the fact that the chemotherapy she's ordered is useless, while she's simultaneously denouncing Dr VZ as being the person responsible.

I'm reading Bernie Siegel's book *Peace, Love and Healing*. He's a surgeon who shows how patients can influence their own healing by paying attention to their own peace and inner struggle.

Bettina: It does play a big part!

It's a very beautiful book. I want to develop this inner peace and overcome the disease. At the same time, though, I find it revolting to always project responsibility on to the patient without talking about the political and environmental factors that are so obviously involved.

I come back to Siegel's book and to my mixed feelings about his message.

Dr VZ calls me: Dr JE must have told her about my biopsy results. We're able to speak frankly. She tells me it's been hard for her to witness what I'm going through, because she knows me personally and prescribed the hormones that seem to have turned my whole endocrinal system upside down. She says, 'It's easier when doctors don't know their patients personally.' I tell her not to worry – but why do I tell her that, when in fact, deep inside, I'm very angry with her? Why haven't I yet learnt to deal with my anger as soon as it happens? I know it stems from the way I was raised: in the spirit of charity and Christian love, to 'turn the other cheek' rather than demand 'an eye for an eye'. I'm reading that one of cancer victims' characteristics is that they keep things inside rather than express them. Even if, *a priori*, it seems hardly convincing that patients' decrease in immune resistance could be attributed to their suppressing their problems, once again – and I have occasion to point this out at many other times – it *is* a way of blaming the victim.

Jane: It's like Edward Said's *Blaming the Victims*.

This is a book edited by Said, which consists of essays by several writers who show that history has been written to make the Palestinians the culprits for the very crimes committed against them!

Rather than express my anger, I tell the doctor not to worry, that she's done what she knew to be best, thereby revealing that I'm always able to identify with the other person's problems and feelings! I sympathise with her, and tell her that I noticed how disturbed she was on that cold and grey Sunday on which she came to tell me I might have cancer. At the time, neither Alban nor I had believed the diagnosis could be true: it seemed so unreal. Now I've read the mammography report, I better understand that she could be that certain. She tells me it's been difficult for her also, because her own mother went through the whole ordeal some years ago, and that that's why, despite being my doctor, she was plunged into utter disarray.

Alban and Nazik: Was VZ not exaggerating a bit? Was it not a naive strategy to soothe me?

Jane: Here is a case of the perpetrator victimising herself, perhaps as a way of lightening her burden of guilt, by shifting it on to you and to circumstances beyond her control!

Antje: What happened to the objectivity of the trained doctor?

Oh, how I wish all this could belong to the past! When I asked VZ whether she'd felt anything in my breasts when she was doing my yearly check-up back in November, she said, 'No: nothing, and I did a very careful and thorough examination.' How could this tumour have started and developed so quickly? Why didn't the doctor order extra medical check-ups before she prescribed me those disgusting hormones?

Oh, you, whoever you are, in charge of the universe, please stop it! I know you still want me to live. There are so many things I need, and want, to write and accomplish.

Jane: Your prayer reminds me of Bess's dialogue with God in the Danish film *Breaking the Waves*. The film is both pre- and post-feminist – full of myth and reality at the same time.

20 March 1994

Anaïs and I speak to Pierrot, who remains obsessed with father's so-called pornography. My poor father! It seems my mother was very disturbed by his 'confession', and that Pierrot thought my father should ask her to forgive him: he told my father so in front of her. And my father, my poor father, exclaimed, 'Forgiveness – what for?' He'd forgotten about his so-called confession. And when Pierrot tried to remind him about it, he said, 'But it was nothing: they were medical books!' and went on and on about his grandfather, who was an unbeliever but had married his grandmother, who was a believer, and that his grandfather had been frivolous and looked at pornographic magazines, and that his own father looked at medical magazines.

Alban: Pornographic magazines didn't exist at the time!

According to Pierrot, mother was convinced that the books were medical works, and father didn't want to insist they weren't so she wouldn't suffer any more than she had to. Pierrot retorted that father was a liar, that he'd lied all his life, and that that was why we now had problems in the family and weren't free. Pierrot talks about the family when it's really himself he's talking about, and this trait is called projection identification with the family. He doesn't quite know who he is. He adds that lies and sins weigh heavily on the whole family and thereby prevent us from being free!

Jane: Such heavy family relationships remind me of the film *Secrets and Lies*, and of the American playwright Eugene O'Neill, who wrote scenes about these painful dilemmas!

Personally, I believe it's the whole system of dogmatic thinking, and of magical thinking, too, because in Pierrot's case, it's the magical thinking of childhood at work in him whereby the rest of the family is prevented from being free. Those of us who've managed to break out of this framework are now much freer. I think especially of Théophile, who's completely left behind these magical ways of thinking. When I let myself go into them again, I feel suffocated: imprisoned, whereas I usually feel so free.

As for my brother Augustus, when I tell him the whole story, he says, 'If father hadn't wanted to confess, he wouldn't have confessed. It probably made him feel good to do so!' How typically cynical of Augustus, who refuses to see the concrete situation of a dying man, whom they're trying to extract a confession from, and who won't admit that it's the inquisitor, not the so-called penitent sinner, who's in the wrong.

It could also be that Augustus was unconsciously wreaking revenge and projecting on to father, even, perhaps, identifying with the father, because now that father was dying, he was being extremely harsh with Augustus and making him promise he'd get married as soon as possible. At the time, Augustus was divorced and living with a woman, and father considered it sinful to be living with someone out of wedlock. He had major confrontations with Augustus, who came with his woman friend at Christmas time – scenes I'd found utterly unacceptable and ridiculous. I could only excuse father because of his disease. Perhaps Augustus later got married because, to use his own words, he'd wanted to do so anyway, and it probably made him feel good.

21 March 1994

I dream that Anaïs is leaving – she is, in fact, leaving today – and that I've forgotten to write dedications in the books I'm sending with her, for her friends. The dream reflects my anxieties about forgetting to write and about Anaïs's leaving. She's been so sweet and of so much help! I don't need to tell her what to do in the house: she knows exactly what to do, and in that way takes after her mother. She's also been so supportive, by going with me to the doctors and asking questions. She knows which questions to ask, because she conducts laboratory research into retro-viruses, which are believed to be responsible for some cancers as well as for AIDS, at one of the United States' most important cancer-research centres: the Hutchinson Institute, in Seattle.

Yesterday, we go to a concert given by a lesbian woman, Gayle Naylor, and then to a martial-arts demonstration by a group that Diane is involved in. I go mostly to encourage Diane, who also bakes cookies to collect money for the martial arts. Only women attend the Channing Murray Foundation, at which the activity is conducted. The singer has a few good songs, but also some boring ones. She seems very nervous, and I wonder why, because the audience's response to her message and songs is mostly favourable. During intermission, Doctor VZ comes over to say hello and hug us. She tells me she's worried about me, and that she's leaving on the first of April in order to go to Belgium to meet Sue. She'd like to have dinner with me, Diane and Petite-Fleur before she departs. Her words touch me. I believe I'm not upset with her especially but that I'm mad at the whole medical establishment.

Alban: Her attitude shows how immature and unprofessional she is: irresponsible, like many others.

I'm still reading Bernie Siegel's *Peace, Love and Healing* (Siegel: 1989). It contains some excellent passages, even though I'm similar to Séverine, in that we find his approach exasperating at times. Siegel really gets on Severine's nerves. He says that when you read about anti-cancer drugs, only the toxicity and the horrible 'side effects' are mentioned whereas the fight the drugs wage against the cancerous cells has a whole positive dimension. Patients should be more aware of these positive elements in order to participate in their own healing. What he says is probably true, but in his way of thinking, you're sent back to being individually rather than collectively responsible. And the victim is victimised – I agree with Séverine about that.

Yesterday, as we're going out, Nina brings me some beautiful yellow crocuses. She has tears in her eyes as we speak, and soon has me crying too. She's a Dutch-born journalist who wrote an article about me several years ago. Her articles published in *The Courier* are widely read, and are very sensitive and touching, as are the articles written by Claire Gebeyli, my friend who lives in Beirut and writes pieces for *L'Orient – Le Jour*. Nina had breast cancer about four years ago. She found a lump while she was having her shower. She went to Dr JE, had a mastectomy and was given chemotherapy treatment. I'd like to go and see her, because I need to talk to her.

Séverine also calls, and I feel her friendship and concern. Anaïs tells me that Séverine has asked her church to pray for me. That morning, Anaïs went with Julie to a church that Séverine attends. I feel good when I think about these kinds of prayer: they have nothing to do with the prayers of guilt and submission that Adelaide and Emma advocate.

Sandra Broom, a travel agent from Mid-America Travel, has died of lung cancer. It's a shock to hear the news: I thought she'd live much longer. She'd been a chain smoker, and her doctors hadn't given her much time to live, but I didn't think it would happen that fast. If young people were aware they're committing suicide by chain smoking, would they stop? Perhaps they're suicidal.

Bettina: Underline once more that the association of birth-control pills taken with tobacco is suicidal.

I remember Sandra: when I first came to Urbana, I went to her to arrange my airline tickets. I liked her: so full of life and busily completing projects. Her business really prospered over the years. It's so sad to see someone die at only 58!

23 March 1994

Yesterday, I go to the pool with Petite-Fleur. I've been thinking my tumour is diminishing, but at the pool, I'm no longer sure.

Manicha: You say 'my' tumour: you appropriate it, to tame it and make it disappear!

With Petite-Fleur, I try to measure it, hoping she can tell me it's much smaller. However, she doesn't want to lie to me: it's still very big! According to Bernie Siegel, I must be more confident, trust that it'll decrease, and believe it'll shrink; I must use positive auto-suggestion and be more courageous. However, I feel tired these days. I miss Anaïs: she's so sweet and tender, – a light and free spirit. I'm glad she said she'll come back at the end of May.

I lack strength and courage. The liquids they've poured into my veins scare me. I call on them to have a good effect on me, to eat up the bad cells, but I'm afraid they're eating up the good cells as well. Do we ever return to what we were before? What if my heart muscle weakens – an Adriamycin side effect I'm told I might have? And why do they call them 'side' effects when the effects are so 'central'?

Today, I see my accountant about my tax. He tells me that when his sister was 48, she died of colon cancer that had metastasised to her liver. He cries while he's telling me about it. Alban notices how it's extraordinary that I gain people's confidence; perhaps it's simply because I dare to speak about myself. In this puritan world, people are afraid to talk about illness, either because they think that talking about is immodest or illness has nothing to do with what society is geared towards: making money. When I open up to people, these feelings are suddenly unleashed, and people cry about a tragedy they've never before discussed.

Bettina: When one talks about oneself, one attracts confidences: people who talk about themselves altruistically attract beautiful thoughts.

Jane: People unknowingly may be 'dumping' their cancer stories on you, not only making you feel good or comforted that you aren't alone in your misery, but also depressing you at times.

Deirdre: Yes! I worry about the cloud of suffering and illness that surrounds you sometimes. I wish people would give you a little break. Of course, I also understand why they come to you. I know that if I ever became ill, you'd be the first to hear about it: I can't think of someone more understanding.

Suddenly, even my accountant has become more human. He thinks that cancer is caused by stress. That's my view, too, but only up to a point. Until now, I've led too stressful a life. Mother's and father's health has affected me more than I think. I find it hard to function in my family: I'm stifled by its rigid dogmas, yet I love them dearly. The divided loyalties I feel – being torn between my hate for their narrow ways of looking at the world and my love for their commitment to help other people – have always been a source of my anxieties. Fortunately, I've been able to heal from them through my writing.

The night before, I dream that Alban is going to pick up Olivier's sister, Alban's grand-daughter, at the bus or train station, which is located in the mountains. When I ask him whether he always goes to pick up all the people who arrive, he tells me he has to because there are no other means of transportation to where he lives. In my dream, I'm with him in his mountain house. However, he doesn't drive. Why doesn't he send someone else to collect the girl? The dream reflects my sadness at being separated from Alban, and my wish that he could find someone else to do the things he believes he must do.

Tonight, at 10.30, Théophile, my eldest brother, phones from Beirut to tell me our father has just died. I burst into tears. He doesn't tell me immediately, but when he phones – at 5.30 a.m. Beirut time – and says that mother is close to him as he's talking with me, I immediately understand that father has passed away. Yet, I find it hard to accept – just as I find it hard to accept my illness and to be so far away from the family at so difficult a time. This year is much too hard!

Father died in his sleep. Mother got up in the night to go to the toilet, and noticed he wasn't moving. She called Théophile. Father's pulse was no longer beating. Mother talks to me very calmly as I cry. She says, 'He is in heaven; he is waiting for us up there.' But I just cry even harder. I feel so weak in my illness. I find it hard to accept the human condition.

24 March 1994

Father dies during the night. After Théophile phones, I spend almost the whole evening, and part of the night, on the phone, talking to David, Anaïs, Pierrot, Adelaide and Diane.

Adelaide regularly talks to me, from Beirut. She tells me that my mother is often asking about me, as if she knows I'm ill. She dreams about me. In her dream, I'm coming to see her and my other family members. They're meeting me at the train station in Neuchâtel. I'm carrying a big bottle of olive oil, which is spilling all over my clothes and skin. Mother is asking me why I haven't wrapped up the bottle before getting on the train. It's Adelaide telling me the story of the dream, which is marked by exorcism; extreme unction of the dead – a religious rite during which the dead person is anointed with oil; rites of passage; the fact that Adelaide had asked some of her friends to come and anoint me with oil; and Emma's reference to me as being a vessel that doesn't contain enough oil!

Jane: All this oil imagery is amazing!

Manicha: To dream, to absorb dream into reality, so as to change the situation …

She's marvellous, my sweet mother. She views me as being someone who's overflowing with oil – benediction, spirituality – from everywhere. She wants to protect me from wanting to help everybody at my own expense and thereby endangering myself. She tells me to wrap up my talents, to hide them and keep them to myself, and to open up at only the most propitious moment rather than expose myself to all life's contingencies, especially while I'm travelling on a train with strangers. This 'passage' is all very mysterious: reality, dreaming about myself; dreaming about my mother;

and the significance of talent, hiding, unveiling and favourable moments.

I make the connection with Emma's dream, in which she viewed me as carrying only a small amount of oil in a small container. I don't think about it at the time, but now believe that Emma is being somewhat judgemental, even though she tells me that she views me as being more gifted than the rest of the family when it comes to helping people and being of service to God: 'You're spoiling your religious vocation, my child. Come back to God – take advantage of this illness, which is a sign from God.' Her words remind me of Françoise's reminiscence: 'Did you hear God's calling, my child?'

Jane: A talented script writer could do a very interesting film based on your experience: it unwinds on three continents, and has a multiplicity of religious, medical, family and political dimensions.

I believe that Adelaide is also being somewhat judgemental. She tells me she was hurt that I'd rather have Alban with me if and when I undergo the operation. She says she understands that I need to have the man I love near me – even if it isn't what God wants for me! She claims that she understands, accepts and doesn't judge, yet she calls on God to judge me and tell me that Alban isn't the right man for me!

This morning, I peel an orange. I open it. There's a whole, black part in it – round, like a tumour! I'm disgusted. Even though the rest of the orange tastes good, I can't eat it. Is the image connected to what Adelaide has said to me? Is my whole religious upbringing coming back, whereby I'm being given these signals that one rotten part in my life is causing the rest of the whole to be disgusting? Is the rest of my body disgusting me because of the cancer? However, the rest of the orange tastes good: I'm the one who's rejecting it, because of the image evoked in me. Am I so afraid of the dogmas, the biblical images, the metaphors that my childhood was saturated with? Am I afraid that I'm continuing to be bogged down by them and be depressed by them during my weak moments, such as this period of illness, during which I should be courageous and hopeful because I have a true faith?

Adelaide tells me that father is to be buried in the village of Theopolis. He asked that two pastors he trusted conduct the burial ceremony. Mother is happy with the two decisions. She tells Adelaide that she and father loved Theopolis and that it's where she also wants to be buried. How strong mother is!

Adelaide recounts how father was still very strong, even towards the end, but that it was a physical strength: according to her, mother has the moral strength. Sometimes father held Adelaide's hands so tightly that she couldn't free herself. It was as if he were trying to cling to life, this oak felled by a violent death when he thought he still had a long time to live.

Father has died. They're burying him today, and I'm starting to lose all my hair. I feel it's no coincidence that I'm losing all my hair today: I'm mourning my father's death, and grieving over the loss of part of a past that I cherish.

I'm in the shower at the Physical Education Building, having had a swim with my Petite-Fleur, and chunks of my shoulder-length hair start falling out. It's frightening. I remember that when I started reading Dr Love's book about breast cancer, I couldn't read about the effects of chemotherapy. I was terrified by the treatment, not knowing I'd have to go through it! I gently pull on my hair, and it stays in my hands. My hair is falling out all over the place, by the fistful, and I can see Petite-Fleur looking at all the mess, not budging, so she doesn't alarm me. When I'm leaving the leisure centre, I try to hide my skull and my massacred hair, which, until now, I've always been very proud of.

Jane: What a nightmare!

Manicha: To lose one's hair or teeth in dreams is unbearable – a real nightmare!

Can you imagine it in reality?

25 March 1994

Théophile calls me from Aïn-Saadé, our house located in the mountains. Father has been buried in Theopolis. A service was held at the Achrafieh church, in which Father was converted and ordained a pastor, and in which Jay and I were married. The crowd at the church was so big that more than 100 people had to stand outside during the service. It seems that Adelaide and Théophile both spoke, and the young people sang. Adelaide had to insist she be allowed to speak, because the pastor thought she'd burst into tears and wouldn't be able to continue – women there are treated as if they're children. Adelaide delivered a very moving testimony. She's very charismatic when she speaks before a crowd such as that, and I've often wished she be given more chances to do so: I'm certain she'd have developed differently and stopped moaning that her life is unfulfilling. Mother was there, and said, 'I am not going to cry, so as to be a good witness.' She meant that death is only a passage to a better place – the narrow path and door that lead to a better world – and that if you really believe it, you shouldn't cry. She's so strong and courageous. I also want to be strong and courageous in facing and overcoming my trial.

It's the evening of the 25th, and Petite-Fleur comes over. She cuts my hair, and on my skull puts olive oil mixed with a powder and spices from Morocco. I think, *Here's that recurring olive-oil motif back again! It keeps coming back to signify important things in my life. Even in the midst of despair there are rays of hope!*

Tonight, I feel the complicity, solidarity and tenderness that exists among women. What a wonderful gift! Petite-Fleur also gives me a massage – gently, softly and tenderly. I'm completely relaxed and at peace, and so glad she's come to share my pain and anxieties.

When I phone Séverine to tell her that my father has died, she breaks down and cries. This Monday evening, I'm going with her to the cancer-support group. It's a group that was founded several years ago by my eye doctor, Alex Sorkin. I remember when, about 20 years ago, he told me he had thyroid cancer. I wept at the news: at that time, like many people, I thought that cancer meant death; little did I know I'd have to go through it myself. Fortunately, Alex is still alive and has founded this group, which he's been directing for the 20 years.

Alex: I don't like the word directing!

It's true that the way he leads and has organised the group is completely unconventional and non-hierarchical, which is what I like about it.

26 March 1994

I wake up. Petite-Fleur has slept here. She's sighing and stretching. I'm comforted by her presence. I dreamt a lot, although I don't remember all my dreams. In one dream, I had to take pills and climb into a boat waiting for me at the harbour. Perhaps the dream means I'm finally going to get the rest my body badly needs, thanks to the chemotherapy that's been forced on me but that I've agreed to have.

Bettina: It's the image of crossing the sea on the way to serenity.

I welcome the thought.

27 March 1994

Today, I go to Peoria with Marianne Ferber, to meet
Marianne Burkhart. Yesterday, I'm invited to Michael's for
dinner. I wear one of my wigs: the long, brown-hair one
that looks most like my hair used to look. Michael's apartment is freezing cold. I borrow one of his sweaters. I think
it's the effect of the chemotherapy, but Youenn, who is also
there, is also feeling cold. Michael has gone through a lot of
trouble to prepare a very elaborate meal. I'd have appreciated it before, but I now think it's futile to make elaborate
meals. As well as being cold, I'm very tired, and leave as
soon as the meal is over. Youenn also leaves, to finish writing a paper.

I'm tired because I've done too many things today. I went
to the station to collect Marianne Ferber, who told me about
her husband's death. He had colon cancer, and died not of
it but of complications due to the operation he had. I find it
hard to hear cancer stories that don't end well. I like
Marianne a lot: she's courageous and steadfast, and believes
in justice and equity. I like the way she's dealing with her
life, refusing to give in to self-pity at having lost her husband so soon.

Today, I also talked to Diane about her mother's cancer.
The tumour is very difficult to localise, and Diane's mother
is having very high doses of chemotherapy. The people
around her are very pessimistic, whereas rather than make
her feel as if she's condemned, they should be cheering her
and surrounding her with positive vibrations. Fortunately,
though, Diane is with her, and is full of hope and of life.

Getting together with Marianne Burkhart is also very sat-
isfying. She seems to have found peace now she's joined a
convent. Before, she was in academia, in my university's
German department. She was always nervous, stressed out
and unhappy. Now, her face glows with inner peace. She

tells me she'll be praying for me. In contrast to the prayers proposed by Adelaide's and Emma's friends, I welcome her offer as being a gift.

28 March 1994

In one of my dreams, I'm with Alban, in a big lecture hall. We're sitting in the second row, and in front of us, two women, perhaps Samira and Zohreh, are talking. Lots of people are sitting behind us. The scene is a bit like a court-room. A woman – perhaps Suzanne Kepes – is sitting behind a table, like a judge. To the right, and on the plat-form, two people are sitting, but I can't see who they are. Alban is in a teasing mood. He starts smoking. I tell him that this isn't a good place to smoke – or rather, I'm disturbed by the smoke, although I'm not sure I come right out and say so. Alban asks the female judge whether he can smoke. She replies that she shouldn't tell him what he can or can't do. He continues smoking. The two women in front of us leave: I know they're disturbed by the smoke, but don't know how to tell Alban so. The dream reflects my anxiety that Alban isn't living through the latest events with me. I'm afraid he'll want to do things I can't any more, such as smoke, and that smoking will annoy me even now.

The dream also reflects a conversation I have with Eva yesterday, when she calls me and tells me she's happy to know that Alban will be arriving soon. It's the first time she's said something positive about Alban. When I tell her how difficult the whole ordeal has been for him, that I even saw him cry when I woke up on the operating table and heard cancer announced, she tells me she never thought Alban would react like that, and that she thought he'd have dropped me when my illness was announced. She doesn't quite say it this way, but it amounts to the same thing. However, why do I always have to justify my relationship with Alban, especially to Eva, and in the past to Emile, because they view him as being cold, distant and incomprehensible? Why do I feel uncomfortable when I have to explain my relationship with him?

Jane: They're jealous, and they want to keep you to themselves, Evelyne!

Later in the book, I come back to these feelings of jealousy and possession.

Yesterday, Elizabeth brings me some white tulips. I'm very moved when she tells me that it's often harder for the people around the sick person than for the person himself or herself. I think she must be especially talking about her husband. The patient, having made the decision about which treatment to have, lives in hope of getting healthy again, and trustingly goes about having the treatment, whereas the people around him or her live with the anxiety of seeing the person they love suffering as well as with the fear they'll lose a loved one. I tell Elizabeth I've talked to her husband, and that we've shared the fact that our attitude to life has been completely changed as a result of our cancer experience.

I feel as if I've crossed a new 'time zone', a new era of my existence. It has nothing to do with normal life: I'm no longer as I was. My priorities have completely changed. Once I'm healed, I'll no longer live my life as I did previously.

When I think about what Elizabeth has told me – that people are more worried about their loved one than they would be were they to go through the illness themselves – I'm reminded of the war in Lebanon: knowing that your loved ones were going through hell, it was more difficult to be 'outside' than to be 'inside' with them. I often think of my experience during that war in relation to my cancer: both

war and cancer are a twentieth-century plague, intractable
in both their complexity and their scope.

Bettina: It's good to put them in parallel.

Deirdre: Can other symbolic parallels be drawn between the
Lebanese war and your experiences with cancer? I think these
symbolic links might be richer and more personal than the
Holocaust one.

They're links I make throughout the book. Everything holds together: the Lebanese war; cancer; the Holocaust; all the genocides that
the planet has witnessed and that its population continues to be
plagued by.

On Saturday, my friend Mona calls me from Beirut. She
went to see Théophile, mother and Adelaide after father's
funeral. She wasn't told about the ceremony; otherwise, she
would have attended. She tells me that the 26th of March,
the day she went to see my family, was the anniversary of
her husband Fouad's death, the day he was killed in their
house, by shrapnel. My father's name was also Fouad,
which in Arabic literally means 'heart'; both men, in fact,
had a big heart and great vision. Mona also faced her sorrow courageously and with fortitude. For me, she's always
been a model of sweetness, intelligence and strength in the
midst of adversity.

Many people are phoning me. Clarisse is very warm
when she phones, and has talked to Assia Djebar, whose
brother-in-law was assassinated in Algeria: he hadn't taken
the threats seriously. These days, assassinations are occurring all the time in Algeria.

Manicha: Here is another cancer multiplying, increasing 10-fold:
crazy madness; brothers devouring brothers, and even babies.

Clarisse is going to send me some recipes and the names of plants and natural remedies for fighting the disease.

Ibrahim and Nazik phone me from Beirut. Their voices cheer me up, whereas some others sound hypocritical and out of place: those people ask so many indiscreet questions that their condolences don't sound sincere.

Bettina: They'll recognise themselves in these lines!

31 March 1994

Tomorrow, I go for my second chemotherapy session. I'm a bit apprehensive. I don't feel as if my body is a friend, the way I used to before I had the treatment. I have conflicting feelings about my body.

Yesterday evening, I go for dinner at Denise and David's. They're packing all their belongings in order to leave for Las Cruces, New Mexico. I must be unconsciously disturbed by their departure: it's so sudden. At other times when I've spoken to him, David cried about his wife's death from lung cancer. A lot of memories are being brought out as a result of my having cancer.

This dinner invitation is their last before they depart. They've invited people from my street, for me to meet: Pearl Goodman, who I sometimes run into at the pool; her husband, who's an urban planner; and the Hendersons, who live across from me – Mr Henderson has polio, so has to use a cane to walk. It's sad to have Denise and David leave for good.

When I get home, lots of answering-machine messages await me, and one of them is from Anaïs.

Because my hair is continuing to fall out, I think I'll shave it all off, as Zohreh has advised me to do. I don't yet know that head shaving isn't a simple operation, especially when your hair is still thick, even though I've cut it again, since

Zohra first cut it. I try to shave my hair by myself, and cut my ear slightly. Blood starts gushing, and I panic, because blood thinning is a side effect of chemotherapy. Fortunately, I'm able to call my friend Zohreh, who tells me to read the instructions I've been given at the Share clinic. According to the instructions, I'm to press on the cut. I press, and after a while the bleeding stops. I leave my head half shaven, and feel very depressed.

I'm also depressed after I've talked by phone with Anaïs. She's phoned to tell me she's coming for my third chemotherapy session. I tell her I don't really need anyone, because Alban will be there. I feel as if she really wants to come in order to be with Diane, and say to her, 'If it's for Diane, come and stay with her. As far as I'm concerned, I want to be with Alban right now.' I'm worried I might have hurt her. I believe she's very vulnerable, fragile and agitated at the moment. Is it Diane who's upsetting her like that? Diane is going out with Melissa: is she rejecting Anaïs? I don't want her to be hurt again: how can I protect her? Zohreh tells me it's good that I've made it clear I want to be with Alban, because Anaïs needs to see and hear about how important intimacy is for a couple.

This depression is also linked to sheer fatigue: I haven't stopped teaching any of my classes, in spite of the treatment. I want to continue being engaged in my academic activities because I'm thereby better able to avoid dwelling on the disease, and because I need to have contact with my students and some of my colleagues who've been supportive of me and given me uplifting energy.

Bettina: Not stopping your activities, and carrying on with a normal life to whatever extent is possible: that's the best possible medicine.

I also find help through participating in the support group. Dr Alex Sorkin arranges a special session for me to meet women who've gone through similar therapy for breast or ovarian cancer and been healed. Séverine and I go together. I'm the only participant who's just starting the cancer treatment. I listen to everyone's story, and am able to talk about mine as well as about father's death. Dr Sorkin remembers my father: he saw him a few times when my parents were visiting me in Urbana.

Alex Sorkin also tells his story, during which I feel chills going down my spine. He was only 31 when he was diagnosed as having what his doctors thought was a goitre: a small, ball-like enlargement of the thyroid gland, in the neck, which is often associated with iodine deficiency and can become cancerous. He was treated by being given thyroid medication. He went to the Northwestern University clinic, at which his doctor, who was the head of the endocrinology department, was considered to be the United States' best endocrinologist. Although the surgeons wanted to take out the lump, the medics wanted to treat it as a goitre. Student interns often discussed Alex's case in front of him; they didn't know that he himself was a doctor and could understand their medical terminology.

Alex: They knew I was an OD [an ophthalmologist doctor – an eye doctor], but ODs are regarded as low on the scale of doctors. The arrogance doctors have is incredible!

Occasionally, one of the students asked a troubling question, which the famous doctor quickly suppressed. One day, after having this treatment for two years, Alex found himself unable to wear a shirt and tie to a meeting, due to the size of his so-called goitre. The doctors decided to operate to remove the goitre, and *fast!* When Alex woke up from the operation, he felt very tired – he'd never felt so weak in his whole life. He was in intensive care, and could hardly open his eyes. Someone said, sarcastically, 'Well, here's the malignancy!'

Bettina: Unfortunately, even though med. students are required to take courses in psychology, remarks like that one can still be heard in hospitals; it's really disheartening.

He wanted to kill the guy who said it, but for some hours couldn't open his mouth to react. When he did wake up and told the nurse what he'd heard, she gave him a shot to tranquillise him and put him to sleep.

The surgeon came in later and said, 'We just had to take out a little muscle: the one that connects the sternum to the collarbone.' Alex felt too weak to ask questions.

When the doctor came back later and said they'd gotten all the tumour out, Alex asked him whether that muscle also went to the mastoid. He answered, 'Yes.'

Alex asked the doctor, 'Shouldn't you call this a radical neck?'

He answered, 'It was a partial radical neck – it could be more radical.'

Alex was angry, and wondered what he'd do if he ever left the place. They kept telling him, 'Don't worry: it'll all get back to normal.'

Most of his neck now gone, Alex painfully pondered his having been misdiagnosed and for two years having been treated for a goitre. Six months later, he sat in his parents' living room wondering who could have been so cruel as to say 'malignancy' when he wasn't yet awake. He knew the voice, and realised it was one of the doctors he'd heard discussing his case in his presence, before the operation. Four years later, he saw the doctor again and confronted him about overhearing his cruel comments, about the operation and about his doing the 'radical neck'. The nurses later thanked him for doing so: word had gotten around about the doctor's callousness. It was because Alex had the courage to speak out that the doctor started changing his ways.

This is how Alex realised how important it is to talk, and

why he decided to form a group in Champaign–Urbana for people to go to and talk to other cancer patients about their problems, worries and concerns. In the meeting I go to, he also tells us about a radioactive substance they gave him five years later and that they kept him in solitary confinement to find out whether the cancer was completely gone. The substance, which is absorbed through the small intestine, almost destroyed that organ. Alex now has a lot of problems with some foods. When he talks about it with his doctors, they deny that it's an outcome of the treatment. They respond by saying that it isn't a gastrointestinal problem; it's a thyroid one. Amazingly, Alex is able to joke about all this, and to tell the story in an amusingly sarcastic tone.

It feels therapeutic to be talking about all our wounds with these people who've gone through a similar experience, who've been healed and who are willing to share their experiences. Alex makes us laugh.

A recent pilot study found that one-quarter of private wells tested in central Illinois contained agricultural chemicals … Some of the pesticides inscribed into the Illinois landscape promote cancer in laboratory animals. Some, including one of the most commonly used pesticides, atrazine, are suspected of causing breast and ovarian cancer in humans. Other probable carcinogens, such as DDT and chlordane, were banned for use years ago, but like the islands in preglacial river valleys, their presence endures. (Steingraber: 1997: 5)

A lot goes in the 11 percent of Illinois that is not farmland. Approximately fifteen hundred hazardous waste sites are in need of remediation – a list that does not include several thousand pits, ponds, and lagoons containing liquid industrial waste – which, until recently, included pesticides – through five deep wells that penetrate into bedrock caverns. These geological formations are overlain by aquifers and farmland. Illinois exports hazardous waste but also imports it – almost 400,000 tons in 1992 – from every state except Hawaii and Nevada. In this same year, Illinois industries legally released more than 100 million pounds of toxic chemicals into the environment.

Like pesticides, industrial chemicals have filtered into the groundwater and surface waters of streams and rivers. Metal degreasers and dry-cleaning fluids are among the most common contaminants of glacial aquifers. Both have been linked to cancer in humans. (Steingraber: 1997: 6)

Lindane, chlordane, dieldrin, aldrin, heptachlor ... all are now classified as known, probable, or possible carcinogens. Many are still manufactured and exported. A chemical company in my hometown, for example, released several pounds of lindane into the air in 1992 and dumped several more pounds into the sewer system. (Steingraber: 1997: 9)

It is crucial to remember that it is over the last five decades that humans have done the most to modify the planet, and in such proportions as to change how all life on the planet functions. In order to foresee how we might continue to exist, literally for better or for worse, it must be understood that the pollution toll worsens from one year to the next, and that serious effects upon our health are now in the preparatory stages, for we are living on a little ball, enclosed upon itself, not an inch of which we haven't penetrated, and that little ball is the Earth. (Séralini: 1997: 22)

The planet's natural reserves are now highly polluted and poisoned, and are seriously jeopardizing our quality of life as humans. The three single elements that enter our bodies and make up our tissue or make our metabolism function: non-toxic air; clean drinking water; and wholesome food, or food,

The Wounded Breast

plain and simple – an increasingly urgent problem, given the tripling of the world population that is currently underway – are neither everlasting nor interchangeable. We cannot do without air for more than a few minutes, without water for more than a few days, without food for anything over a few weeks or a month. (Séralini: 1997: 26)

3

DNA REPORT AND S-PHASE
TAKE ME TOWARDS HEALING

I'd been getting phone calls for a week from Aunt Rivke's old women friends who knew everything there was to know about cancer: 'Oï! Veï! Kaïn horeh!' (which in Yiddish means 'Reject the Devil's eye' or more simply, 'Watch out!') Chemo is awful: 'But it's not Auschwitz anyway! Things at least went fast back there *[that's debatable!]*: zyclon B took effect in a few minutes. But Kantsser … that's slow agony.' 'That's just fine,' I answered. 'I'm in no hurry.' (Francos: 1983: 109)

Urbana, 1 April 1994

I'm staying with my wonderful friend Zohreh. She takes me to the hospital for blood tests and the second chemotherapy treatment, and reads to me as I'm having the transfusion. We laugh together; then she cries while she's reading the opening chapter of Rick Powers' *Prisoner's Dilemma* (Powers: 1988: 14), which I include an extract from as follows.

Impressed with the truth he has just spoken, the one about the place's one prejudice, he gives us a final glimpse of that closet romantic he will keep so perfectly hidden in later years: 'For all must into Nothing fall,' he recites, the poetry lost on me until I see it in an anthology, decades later, 'If it will persist in Being' … I feel cold, colder than the night's temperature, a cold that carries easily across the following years. Only the sight of my mother in the close glow of the kitchen window, the imagined smell of cocoa, blankets, and hot lemon dish soap, keeps me from going stiff and giving in … I pull closer to my father, but something is wrong. He has thought himself into another place. He has already left us. He is no longer warm.

I'm unable to truly concentrate: Rick is describing his father's death; I cry because Zohreh is crying, and because the words remind me of my own father's death.

Dr JE measures my tumour and says, 'It's shrunk quite a bit.' Writing in French, I originally use the French masculine pronoun *il*, even though in that language the word *tumour* is feminine and takes the feminine pronoun *elle*, because my tumour feels so aggressive it's taken on the masculine trait of aggressiveness. It's shrunk by two centimetres. I tell myself that if it shrinks by two centimetres for every chemotherapy session I have, it might disappear. I'm given hope and the incentive to work with all my mind's strength for 'it' to go away.

According to the biopsy report, because of the DNA content, the cancer is low risk. I don't understand the finding: beforehand, I'm told I have an aggressive type of cancer whereas now I'm told I have a low-risk type. All these reports are very contradictory: if the cancer is low risk, how could it have grown so fast? Do 'fast' and 'slow' have nothing to do with risk? I keep asking the doctors questions but am not getting any answers.

I've started singing and composing again. I'm writing the lyrics in French, because it's the language that comes most naturally to me, and melody doesn't have to be translated. Following is how I translate one of my songs: the one I write while I'm staying at Zohreh's.

I wait for your return:
Our love place.
I wait for the good days:
A sun of life.

Chorus:
Take me to the river running to the sea;
Take me towards healing.

Your hand on my breast;
Your body near mine;
Our nest of love
In the middle of the night.

Your presence is my joy,
Our understanding a refuge.
We walk towards hope,
Our bodies interlaced.

I wait for springtime.
The love of my life:
Beyond time;
Eternal return.

I'd like to sing in a Paris café next year: it's my deepest wish.

I'm re-reading, reworking and rewriting this text while I'm in Paris this year, and I haven't yet fulfilled this wish. I've been too busy running around in search of doctors to do my check-ups. I don't want to be stressed the way I used to be, so limit my activities as much as possible.

Bettina: Don't worry: it'll all happen in 1999. You'll sing of your healing and your lust for life. From 1995 to 1999: that's the five-year period that determines the cure.

I need and love to sing: I feel much better when I do it, as when I meditate. My friend Samira, who's a psychotherapist, is so wonderful: she comes and teaches me various techniques for meditating and visualising. I'm learning a lot of new things I never knew existed. I have so much help from so many people, and feel surrounded with love.

Séverine is also marvellous: she brings me many books. When I call her to ask her some questions about cancer, because I know she went through the nightmare two years ago, she comes right away. She's in remission now, but struggling daily with the memory that when her own mother was her age, she died of ovarian cancer. She overcomes the pain of knowing this by both helping other people and being very assertive and involved in the treatment she's receiving. I'm so happy we've become close again as a result of our mutual tragedy. She says, 'How unfortunate that it had to be through that,' and I reply, 'Fortunately, some good things come out of misfortune.'

Yesterday, Petite-Fleur comes to shave my head. I'm slightly worried she'll cut me, but she's so gifted, sweet and gentle, and expert with her hands. She does the job flawlessly.

I wait for her for two hours, having cooked rice and vegetables the Lebanese way: in tomato sauce and olive oil, and constantly re-heat the meal on the stove. I become a bit annoyed, especially because while I'm waiting, I'm reading a book about breast cancer and looking at its horrible pictures of women who've had a mastectomy. Why don't they have photos that are more aesthetic in these books? Not that a mastectomy can ever be aesthetic; however, I've since seen photos that aren't as frightening and ugly as the ones usually presented in these so-called medical books. Looking at that type of photo has depressed me terribly. Also, my morale is considerably lowered because of the way the female author describes and discusses cancer: I'm a bundle of nerves.

So, I'm anxiously waiting for Petite-Fleur to arrive. Samira phones just in time: she senses I'm upset and offers to come over, an offer I gladly accept. Petite-Fleur phones just after Samira does, to tell me her meeting has lasted longer than expected, that she doesn't have the money to call me from where she is in order to warn me, and that there's no one to drive her to my place. She has to return home on foot. However, the poor soul has problems with her legs and walking, and asks me whether I still want her to come. I tell her I do, but that I'm exhausted and on edge from waiting for her. She calls Samira to come and get her, and they arrive together. It's reassuring to see them.

My anxiety leaves me as the last pieces of hair are shaved off my scalp. I feel light and free now I have nothing on my head. Petite-Fleur says I have the head of a baby, and it's true: my head feels strange to the touch, like an infant's head. It's soft, and in a way bizarre and hard to describe: a strange sensation, the way its contours undulate.

Bettina: The image of a baby's head is very beautiful: it suggests that life is being offered to you again; it's like a rebirth.

Samira tells me to change my clothes because my T-shirt's wet. I put something on my head, and it clings strangely on the freshly shaven surface on which Petite-Fleur has massaged a soothing lotion. These two women, in giving me their attention, love and amusing presence – Petite-Fleur is talking about her love affairs, and Samira is also opening up – are uplifting me and giving me strength and courage.

I eat with Petite-Fleur while Samira vacuums up the hair that's left on the floor. Petite-Fleur does the dishes. Before, I wouldn't have accepted it if people wanted to do all these things for me, but now, I let myself be 'carried' and cared for. Acceptance makes all the difference! These women are marvellous. I must write about them and remember them in these lines I'm writing.

Manicha: Why insist so much? It's as if, once a misfortune is behind us, we cease to be sensitive to the solidarity, the warmth of some of the people who were generous and present for us back then.

3 April 1994

It's Easter Sunday, and I'm still at Zohreh's: she's told me to stay with her until I feel better from the effects of the chemotherapy. She's preparing an incredible meal in order to celebrate the good news about my DNA and my reaction to the treatment, as well as for Easter: roast lamb on a bed of onions; roast beef with garlic potatoes and broccoli; and all kinds of other good things. I'm touched by her efforts. At the same time, though, my stomach is uneasy: I feel strange and a bit nauseous. I hope the feelings don't get worse so I'm able to enjoy all the good dishes my friend has prepared.

According to the DNA report, the cancer is diploid and a 4.9 S-Phase, so it's in a more favourable prognostic category. However, according to another report, which was written after the operation, the cancer is aneuploid, the phase isn't mentioned. I'm astonished that there can be two reports that differ so much, and wondering what it can all mean.

When I'm at Zohreh's, Théophile calls me from Lebanon. What an example he is: so tender, loving, compassionate and committed. He tells me that many visitors from all over Lebanon are continuing to come in order to mourn father's death: people who are coming to tell the family what father did in their life and how much he meant to them. I tell him that perhaps he and Adelaide should write down what they said at the funeral. The words could be placed at the beginning of the almost completed book that father left behind and that I intend to make publishable as soon as I'm over

this treatment. He agrees to follow through on my suggestion. He's just been elected the director who represents the
bible societies located in Europe and the Middle East. I'm
very proud of him. He asks me whether there's a chance the
tumour will go away without my having to have an operation. I say that if it diminishes by two centimetres during
every chemotherapy session, it definitely might go away,
and that that's what I'm aiming at. He says, 'Hake Badna Yaki
Habibti. Bravo!': 'That's the spirit, darling!' He's so pleased
I'm talking about and having this positive attitude and
faith. I say, 'You know, my whole perspective on life has
changed!' and he says, 'This is what happens when one
touches death.' I know he's also talking about himself,
because he'd twice almost died during the war in Lebanon.
He's deeply touched when I tell him I've been thinking
about what he himself went through so many times. He
says, 'Habibti: yes, life takes on another dimension.'

5 April 1994

My love is arriving today. How will things be between us? I
feel changed, different. My body is heavy, and I'm tired.
One day, he phones and tells me he's had a horrible dream,
in which I was telling him to take another woman and he
was finding the idea disgusting. In the dream, he screamed,
'It's you I want! I want my Nénette!' He's also suffering
from anguish: it's true that we'd struck a marvellous balance despite each of our families and ages, our distance
from each other, our problems and so on. This illness is
turning everything upside down again. Will it be for the
best? I believe and hope it will.

Yesterday, I have a phone call from Dr IS, a Lebanese doctor who's a friend of some friends and who lives in
Washington, DC. He says that some Lebanese doctors
who've read my cancer report are telling him I should

choose the mastectomy instead of the lumpectomy. I say I don't yet have the choice, because the surgeon has said he can't operate before the mass has shrunk and become self-contained. When doctors talk like that, do they realise what they're saying? It's almost as if they have no feelings about their patients' psychology when the patients are told they're to lose a vital part of their body. Even when the doctors' affirmations are said with good intention, the news is very hard to take. However, I appreciate that Dr IS has taken the time to consult with other doctors and to call me.

Yesterday, because it's Easter time, I phone my family in Lebanon. First, I speak to Adelaide. It's only seven o'clock in the morning, and she's exhausted. She says the family went to church the night before and stayed until 1.30 a.m., and had to go egg hunting early this morning. She's so exhausted she simply wants to drop everything. She's crying. What is it that she thinks is keeping her from changing her life completely? Is she afraid of what people would say? Why are we humans so afraid to break the chains that bind and hurt us? It would be great if Adelaide did break them: she'd be an example of real courage, audacity and vision in the midst of the worst social circumstances: enduring the war, having some unhappy relationships and feeling obliged to take care of our sick parents.

I also phone Théophile. Mother speaks with me, and tells me she's happy that father is now in heaven because he's no longer suffering as he suffered towards the end and he seemed so relaxed and smiling when he died. She asks me whether I still intend to come over in May. I tell her, 'I'm having a treatment for my breast; I don't know yet when I'll be able to come.' She says, 'Is it cancer?' I say, 'Yes, but it's on the right track: the tumour has shrunk.' She says, 'I'm going to pray for you.' She seems very calm, my sweet mother. She seems to know all about it, about me, as if I don't really have to tell her, but I need to anyway. After we've hung up, I wonder whether I should have told her. However, telling her came so naturally, as if she were expecting me to talk about it the way I did. Why should I hide my illness from her?

7 April 1994

My wonderful Alban is back, and I'm so happy to have him here again. Last night, I have a strange dream. We two are in a multi-storey car park that has a lot of parking spaces – perhaps it's the car park in the Convention Center in Mobile, Alabama, the place we dined in, on the balcony overlooking the bay. In the dream, I have to perform all kinds of acrobatics in order to park the car. To get out of the multi-storey car park, we have to slide down poles. When the parking attendants see us sliding down, they ask, 'But why don't you take the elevator?' However, it's already too late: we're on our way down, and for fun, the attendants start rotating the poles so fast that I feel nauseous and as if I'm about to faint. I'm reassured as a result of the dream, in which I'm being told I have enough strength to hold on to something strong that will keep me from falling. Even though my head throbs, my stomach turns and I'm scared out of my wits, I hold on for dear life and manage not to fall off the poles.

It's also a sexual dream. Before, when Alban and I got back together after being separated, we made love passionately: we were so euphoric to rediscover each other after an absence. This time, though, it's difficult. I have an image of my body whereby I'm not incited to make love: a shaven head; a heavy body; a feeling of being tired and bloated as a result of the poisonous drugs I'm being given; my struggling to get rid of the crazy cells; my breasts, which I used to be proud of, along with my hair, but which I'm now frightened by; and a shrunken vagina, dried up as a result of chemotherapy, whereby I've been plunged me into menopause. We two aren't able to 'take the elevator', as we used to, so we resort to playing other games.

Jane: How cinematic and very exciting to visualise these cancer dreams!

Bettina: It's an amusing dream; realistic, too. Even though the chemo made you nauseous – as reflected in the spinning that made you dizzy and sick to your stomach in the dream – you held on and didn't fall!

Manicha: Must we necessarily make love to be well together? Couldn't we just cuddle up together?

Although later and throughout the book I reveal we have this ability to be non-sexually (sexual in the traditional sense because there are many other ways to be sexual) physical, my intimate relationship with Alban was a real letdown that I needed to express and make my readers aware of. The sexual problems that cancer patients often experience as a result of chemo treatment are often not addressed and remain hidden from view.

11 April 1994

My temperature is subnormal. I'm unable to get warm, despite all the care my wonderful Alban is giving me: hot-water bottles, massages, human warmth, and hot drinks! What's worrying me most at present is the swelling I have on my left ankle, because my mother's ulcer is located exactly there in her left ankle. Her ulcer is an effect of a *phlebitis* – an obstruction formed as a result of coagulated blood – she had in her ankle many years ago. The swelling in my ankle hurts.

My body is reacting to all the drugs I'm taking. My breast

is stinging and hurting. The tumour continues to react and diminish. I've learnt some visualisation techniques to help it shrink and hopefully disappear. My wonderful Samira has taught me some techniques, and my friend Cindy has sent some ideas and tapes. One of my favourite techniques is the one in which I imagine I'm inside a light-mauve balloon, feeling secure, and surrounded with light and quiet. I breathe in deeply the sense of harmony that the colour and silence give me, and breathe out all the toxins I continue to carry within me. I do the breathing until I feel that my body has rejected all the poisons in it. I get out of the balloon, and become a bird sitting on the branch of the tree I can see from the couch I'm lying on. I feel free and ready to fly above the clouds.

Do these techniques really work, or are they just wishful thinking? At any rate, I relax more easily when I practise them, and I have the illusion that my will can have an effect on my body, and that I thereby have a measure of control over my disease.

Bettina: This is very important, and not at all an illusion. Willpower can have an enormous effect over the body, and lack of will can have an equally negative effect.

Manicha: Regain control of the body: don't abandon it to doctors, 'destiny', bad luck or God.

Yesterday, I have such nauseous feelings that I can't eat. Alban very elaborately prepares a wonderful fish in a special broth and places corn on the side of the plate. However, the smell of the fish makes my stomach turn, and I can't eat it. I'm able to eat some corn and rice, which Alban, ever attentive, heats up for me. Today, I call Dr JE and explained my condition. She wants to see me tomorrow morning.

17 April 1994

I have lots of ups and downs these days. When I feel that my tumour is diminishing, I feel high, but when I see it's unchanged, I have doubts, anxieties and fears. Usually, my morale is rather good, in spite of it all, mostly because my dear Alban is here taking care of me, pampering me, and remaining attentive to all my needs and moods. I'm so very grateful.

I go and see the doctor with him, and he likes her. She diagnoses that I have an external phlebitis, which has probably been caused by chemotherapy, but sends me to have a more extensive test of my veins. According to the tests, there's no deeper obstruction of the veins. I feel so relieved! I can take care of this kind of phlebitis by wearing special stockings, taking anti-inflammatory drugs such as Ibuprofen, and applying warm-water compresses to it.

Dr JE asks me whether I've had any other problems. When I tell her I'm running a subtemperature, and that Alban has to give me massages and apply hot-water bottles and so on, she says, with her usual humour, 'How nice!' She doesn't seem to be worried about the subtemperature: apparently, it would be more troublesome if I were running a fever.

Last night, I dream I'm going for voice lessons at Beirut's Conservatoire. I'm asked to show the registration card I had when I was an adolescent. After making a considerable effort, the officials are able to find my 1983 card.

However, I wasn't at the Conservatoire in 1983; in fact, years before that, the Conservatoire was destroyed as a result of the Lebanese war. In 1983, when I was 40, I was getting ready to conduct research all over Africa and to teach in Lebanon, having been awarded a prestigious American scholarship called a Fulbright.

I tell myself that at the time, in spite of my goodwill, I haven't really taken the appropriate courses. In the dream, I can't find the names of people from the past, people I would like to have studied under. I ask for Aline Aoun, but am told she's died, and grieve terribly. All the people at the Conservatoire are very young, and I wonder whether Martin – my nephew – is also there. There's a lot of music theory to take, and I know that Martin would be good at it. As for me, I'm not sure I want to take theory.

What does the dream mean? I feel like studying music, and singing again. I'd like to study music in Lebanon, with young people, like the ones at Théophile's place: full of life and hope, even though their dreams have been shattered as a result of the war. I'd like to both bring and receive a renewal, a song, a melody. I'm bored by theory: I like Aline Aoun because she focused on the heart, the emotions and the breathing: her teaching was so beautiful and harmonious. I'd so much like to see her again. I often think of her, and worry that I never hear from her.

18 April 1994

I dream I'm looking for Ibrahima N'Doye, who in real life is one of my students I'm concerned about, to tell him I've found him a job. The setting of the dream is Beirut's Jeanne d'Arc Street, where, on the day before I had the dream, I saw Ibrahima coming out of a 'house of ill-fame' that had a lot of revolving doors; it's a hotel that's been built on the site on which Théophile used to have a shop. In the dream, I then run into another Ibrahima: Ibrahima Wade, who's also one of my students, and who, like Ibrahima N'Doye, is from Senegal. He tells me that N'Doye is inside the hotel. We go in and find him in a room that resembles that of Umm Hassan, in real life one of the women I'd interviewed last year, who lives in one of Cairo's poorest districts; in her room–house, she could barely fit two beds and a cooking stove between them. N'Doye is perched on some furniture near a TV, and is very thankful to me for announcing the job I've found for him. We enter the lobby and encounter a strange crowd, the women in which look like prostitutes, the men like pimps. Ibrahima N'Doye seems happy to be leaving the place. He thanks me effusively … what do all these dreams mean?

Yesterday evening, I'm exhausted by dinner time. Ramin arrives early, before we've finished cooking. He starts drinking, and keeps on drinking all evening. Alban thinks he's euphoric because he's had good news about a job possibility in California. Alban has cooked a delicious salmon meal, but cooking, talking and eating always take time. At eleven o'clock, Ramin is still talking: he seems so happy. However, I'm awfully tired. Fish isn't the easiest food to eat while you're undergoing chemotherapy, and the taste of wine is also hard to take – I'm not exactly a picture-perfect hostess!

Ruth phones to tell me that her presentation about my work has been accepted to be delivered in November at Chicago's MMLA – Midwest Modern Language Association. It's so sweet of her to call. Many of my former students, who are now professors themselves, are doing research into and writing about my work: what better testimony to the interests I have awakened in them?

Manicha: It's good to point out the importance of being appreciated by others – and what's more, to have aroused teaching vocations among your former students!

Gordon also phones, just before midnight, while Alban and Ramin are still talking. I haven't heard from him for ages. Once when he phoned, I got angry with him because he was completely drunk and incoherent, and asked him not to call me any more. He annoys me when he tells his stories about women, children, jobs, money and so on. However, this time he's even worse: when I tell him I have breast cancer, he proceeds to tell me about all the people he knew who'd suffered and died from it, including Jack, his best friend, who died two weeks ago, and Gordon's own mother, who died quite a while back from breast cancer. He talks and talks, and asks me whether I expect to come out of it all. I say, 'Yes, of course: I want to live.' He tells me this wasn't the case with his friend Jack, who didn't especially want to live: he smoked so much that he developed cancer of the throat, lungs and brain; he must have wanted to die.

Why do people phone me to tell me these stories? Do they realise what they're saying? Gordon really gets on my nerves, and at times deeply disturbs me. He also talks to me about his second marriage, to the most beautiful woman in the world, who's lost her mind! He always builds up dramas that exist only in his imagination. However, there's something endearing about his flaws, which is why I befriended him in Beirut when I was teaching there one year, in the middle of the war. He has an amazing capacity to dramatise and to find himself in incredible situations. Because he's audacious, he could be at once a hero, saint and fool. However, I'd rather not have heard from him tonight. Perhaps I should keep my answering machine on all the time – but I'm afraid I'll miss some important calls if I do that.

So, my dreams reflect all the evening's events ... But why do I dream so much these days, and why are the dreams so often about Lebanon; Jeanne d'Arc Street, where I was born and raised; and Beirut's Conservatoire? What does it all mean? Why did I dream I found a job in Beirut for one of my students? It probably has to do with my concern about whether my students will find a job, as in the case of Ramin. During my illness, I'm also being taken me back to the streets of my childhood; to Beirut and its nightlife before the war; to one of the first traumatic experiences I had when I was an adolescent, whereby I was locked in my room because I broke promises I'd made to my father, and through the shutters I could still see the street and have some vision of freedom. I describe these scenes at great length in my first novel, *L'Excisée*.

Bettina: Along with illness, the idea of death is present, even at an unconscious level, because there's a break-off point with normal life and a projection back to the 'first life': the life before the onset of the illness. Childhood also provides a base for the individual, a point of reference for everything that's to follow.

24 April 1994

On Friday the 22nd, I have my third chemotherapy session, and my fourth and last will take place on 13 May, a Friday. I was married on a Friday the 13th: in June 1969, in Beirut. Jay and I chose the date because our parents had been married on a Friday the 13th and been happy in their marriage. For us, though, things didn't work out quite the same way.

I realise I still have many unhealed wounds from my marriage and divorce. The other day, I have a meditation and visualisation session. I do the session by means of following a taped set of instructions. On the tape, the instructor tells you to visualise yourself going to a chest of drawers: it's therapeutic to go to a place such as that because you're thereby enabled to reach events that carry a hidden meaning that you can then unravel, by analysing the events' symbolism and trying to understand why they were major experiences in your life, whether you were hurt or received pleasure as a result of them, and how and why they occurred. Through these exercises, you're able to identify past wounds and seek healing for them: pinpointing what hurts is the first step towards healing.

In my exercise, there's a box I open, and in it is a photo of my wedding. When Jay phones me tonight, I tell him about the visualisation. He asks me whether it's positive or negative, and I reply that it's both, because I'm happy in the photo but my memory of the event is sad.

Bettina: It's positive–negative, like your other compound word: marriage–divorce. I like these words.

Dr JE tells me she thought my tumour would diminish faster than it's diminishing. I'm depressed a lot by her words: why isn't it fading away fast, the same way it came? I hope this third session will be so effective I'll be able to have a lumpectomy rather than a mastectomy.

Today, Mona calls me from Beirut. She tells me that if she were in my shoes, she'd have a mastectomy right away. However, she wouldn't have a choice, just as I don't have a choice. Why do people panic so fast when they hear the word *cancer* whereas actually it can actually be a 'curable' disease, like many other diseases? Anyway, it's good to hear Mona's voice.

Bettina: We also panic because we don't always know how it comes about.

Although I like Bernie Siegel's books, there's a whole angle to them I'm bothered by. In the very individualistic approach that's pushed to the extreme, the disease is made an individual affair rather than a political one, whereby the patient becomes responsible for it. It seems that blame is placed on the victim. However, how can this be so when we know that 80 per cent of what causes cancer is the carcinogenic elements in the environment? Shouldn't that also be dealt with?

Jane: Patients also need to form a united front with reference to the medical establishment. In approaches such as Siegel's, this solidarity, this 'lobby', isn't promoted.

Bettina: Struggling in numbers is easier and more encouraging.

I'd like now to share some thoughts that Séverine later expresses about this subject. She writes the letter when she's experiencing her second bout of cancer. She gives me a copy of it, but never sends it.

To Bernie Siegel, Norman Cousins and other positive thinkers

Thoughts on non-positive thinking

Whenever I see a 'healing yourself' kind of book, I can't resist the urge to take it home and read it. But each time, I end up feeling anxious and angry, stressed by the suggestion that I might be too stressed.

I'm sick and tired of being told to think positively, to be positive. The message I hear is always the same: 'I caused my cancer because I had too much stress in my life, and now I can reverse it by changing my thought pattern.'

I believe that body and soul are intimately connected; I also believe that the timing of my ovarian cancer is related to the fact that I suffered from a severe depression a year before diagnosis. However, my mother died of ovarian cancer at age 39; I'm convinced I would have been diagnosed with ovarian cancer at some point in my life.

I ate my broccoli (I've eaten a balanced, low-fat diet for years!), I visualised my healing, I exercised regularly, and I was still diagnosed with a second primary breast cancer, and then a recurrence of ovarian cancer, a year later.

No, Mr Bernie Siegel: cancer has never been a 'gift' to me. I didn't want it, and I didn't welcome it. It wasn't a wake-up call: I was wide awake.

It has been a painful, frightening disease that I've learnt to live with. I'm coping well, thanks to tremendous, loving support from family and friends.

I didn't chase away every 'negative' thought that came into my mind. I still experience intense fear, sadness and anger, as well as deep satisfaction, profound joy and, at times, an exhilarating feeling of inner peace.

I have a strong will to live, and an indomitable spirit (not always positive), but I want the right to have my feeling – all of them.

I wonder whether it's possible to filter the pain and still be able to feel intense joy.

Séverine Arlabosse, 25 January 1996

How strongly Séverine's words resonate with me. I haven't chosen cancer either, and haven't found it to be a blessing, even if I've learnt things by having it. I also feel angry and resentful a lot of the time. Séverine and I often talk about how we feel. We have a lot in common.

I come back to Bernie Siegel and positive thinkers later.

25 April 1994

I have two nightmares. In the first one, I'm in an Amazonian forest amid magnificent but frightening trees. I'm swimming, and scared of drowning. It's very dark. Fortunately, though, the horizon is clear and sunny, and I know I don't have to stay in the forest for long. Finally, I reach a house. In the second nightmare, I've just been appointed a new professor of Women's Studies. A dog arrives and bites my hand. I tell the person who's appointing me that I can't start work before the dog apologises to me.

I'm suffering anguish about my disease. The dog that bites me is chemotherapy administered via a vein in my hand. It might also be the disease – no, the disease is probably the Amazonian forest, which has frightening shadows, like the shadows of death that brush against me but don't affect me, because the horizon in the background is clear and sunny. I want to take the Women's Studies job only if the dog apologises to me, that is, only if this society, which I believe has given me the disease, regrets having done so and asks for forgiveness: impossible, because a dog doesn't talk, and this society is unwilling to look at the disease's real causes.

Samira thinks it's good for me to be dreaming how I dream, because my subconscious is working and dealing with the shock I've been subjected to at the conscious level.

Bettina: I agree: it's work that has to be done in stages.

Manicha: Why the dog? Expand on the comparison between society and the dog.

I'm afraid of dogs, perhaps because when I was a child I was bitten by a dog. On top of that, the dog isn't a valued animal in Arabo-Islamic societies.

Jane: I believe it's also a question of impurity: a Muslim can't pray after he's touched a dog unless he does his ablutions again – makes me think of your 'unholy' disease.

Samira is truly marvellous, the way she's making me do relaxation exercises listening to her soft voice. And Alban is extraordinary, the way he gives me massages: Alban, so attentive and present.

I have a metallic taste in my mouth, caused by the chemotherapy. It's difficult to bear. It's also difficult to see Petite-Fleur and Diane suffering: one in her own body, the other through her mother's cancer.

Fortunately, I have one of Amel's letters, which I re-read for encouragement. Following are some extracts from it.

La Marsa, 7 April '94

I'm thinking of you all the time. Yesterday, I dreamt of you. You had make-up on: black eyes, with long eyelashes, and tattoos, with harkous [signs, tattoos] on the face, on the chin. Your look was a bit far away, so I hugged you very hard in my arms. My darling friend, how are you? When do you finish your treatment? I'd like so much to be with you, but I'm close to you even from afar ...

I've just finished reading a book: Camille Claudel's A Woman. *It's very powerful: the story of this woman abandoned because she was so extraordinary, a sculptress, unyielding; locked in an insane asylum for 44 years, not so long ago, at the beginning of this century ... It would be so marvelous to go to the desert together, at the end of October, during the date harvest, when the light is so soft ...*

Write to me when you can, to tell me how you are. I know how patient you are. I hope chemotherapy isn't tiring you too much, and that you're getting better, my darling, my sister. Kiss Samira for me: the sweet one I'd so much like to see in Tunisia again; and Diane, the intense one: so intelligent; and all the others. I'm going to write to Cindy: she's a treasure ...

117

26 April 1994

Last night, I have a beautiful dream: Alban and I are walking into a field of flowers, and he's picking a bouquet for me. There's a beautiful sun in the sky, and a few clouds, like big, white wings.

Bettina: Doves; peace; restfulness.

Manicha: Did you dream as much before? I like the very optimistic interpretation you give to your dreams.

No: I never dreamt as much as I did during this illness – or rather, I never remembered my dreams as much as I did during this period.

I wake up happy and confident; thankful that Alban is here; thankful for the way he picks flowers for me all day long, and that he plants flowers and other plants in the garden; and thankful for the way he makes me laugh all the time. We have so much fun together despite my illness – thanks, mostly, to his terrific sense of humour. The 'white wings' I dream are in the sky are promises of peace, freedom and healing.

Tonight, however, my morale isn't as high. A storm is raging, and tornadoes are sweeping through the air. I have strange stinging and burning sensations in my breast – and in a way I like them, because I think the chemotherapy is working: burning the bad cells and flushing them out of my body. I feel nauseous, and my left ankle hurts. I touch my breast, hoping the tumour has miraculously decreased – but it's still as big, even if softer. I have no energy, and lots of anxieties. I think of my father: dead in less than a year, struck down by the same disease.

My body scares me. What if the cancer has spread? But how could it have spread so fast if it's low risk? But if it's low risk, why did the tumour come so fast and grow so large? I keep asking questions that no one seems to have any answers to. Cancer isn't a 'scientific disease'!

I must remain cheerful and not reveal too much of my anxiety to Alban, who worries quite a bit without expressing his anxiety. As for Simone, she's bursting with health, and cultivating her garden.

Bettina: Like Voltaire's *Candide*: to be outside most of the year, taking care of plants and trees, is therapeutic and healing. To see flowers, to contemplate nature, comforts us a little from the negative impression we have of the environment.

To cheer myself up, I'm re-reading some of the letters that have poured in from friends all around the world. Following are some extracts from them.

Suzanne: *Draw, my dear friend, dear sister, from the colours of your faraway lands and the colours of the sea, the energy to re-create what is beautiful in nature, and you will find the same intensity I find in our friendship of these past 20 years.*

Françoise: *I admire your courage a lot, and that you can still be concerned about us when you're suffering so much ... Whatever they take from you, it's recovering your health that matters (plastic surgery does miracles these days, anyway). You know how much we need you, even minus a little piece. Anyway, with age, we lose all kinds of bits and pieces.*

Manicha: The body comes apart with age: hair; teeth; skin. The envelope gets erased, and the 'real self' comes out: more appeasing, more friendly.

Lucien: *We're constantly thinking of you. It's so horrible to be so vulnerable. We feel completely hopeless when disease hits us like that. Perhaps it's also to make us realise how dear you are to us. If only you weren't so far away! If you can't come to Lebanon soon, I'll try to go and visit you.*

Cindy: *I've spoken with my doctor, Dr Wick, about you. She recommends you avoid animal products, because they contain 'growth hormones', and you want to avoid feeding and accelerating your cancer. She recommends you drink at least eight ounces of carrot juice a day; that you take chlorophyll and organic products, as well as whole foods; that you avoid refined sugar and refined flour ... Easter is here; it's the symbolic resurrection of a new season; I'm full of hope.*

Julie, Ed and Sophie: *I'm so sad about the news you gave me yesterday evening. The absence of a father is impossible to fill: it's as if part of our childhood, of ourselves, were going away with him. But the image you carry in your heart is his immortality ... love is sometimes the most immutable element in our lives.*

Gilles: *I feel shattered by your news. But one must face it ... There are two essential factors to take into account, according to what Florence has told me, and to what I've seen in my immediate surroundings. The first one is the treatment. Chemotherapy has made enormous progress in this domain, and I know of one very recent case: one of my sisters-in-law, about your age, was suddenly hit with a very nasty cancerous lymphoma, and was given just the treatment that you should be given; at present, she's completely healed. But it was long and hard. This is where the second factor intervenes. One must have a lot of this active patience called perseverance, and a lot of moral strength, not only to bear with it but to want to heal. Fortunately, you have that strength, beneath an apparent fragility. I also hope that you have friends: it's important, friends who help to ease the repeated shocks of the treatment. But I can well imagine that the death of your father, even if it was genetically foreseeable, is not helping the state of you morale.*

Fortunately, there's also work, and from time to time, some good news, such as about the prize you recently received. Congratulations. Courage, then, and fight the good fight. You know that my heart is with you.

Amel: *La Marsa, April '94: I've just taken Azza to the train station; the sea was very blue and rough; there's a hot wind blowing. I miss you, Evelyne: how are you? How are you bearing up under your chemotherapy? It must be exhausting, but right now you're gathering your strength again, in your house, which I don't know yet. Alban is cooking good meals for you and calling you 'my darling', and you smile at him so sweetly. And you go out walking in the spring light. I try to imagine your days: I'd like them to be as beautiful as possible. April the 17th: I couldn't write. April the 20th: Evelyne, I was so worried, I could write to no one. I started a letter to Cindy. Your phone call, your voice, gave me back my momentum. And this morning, I received your letter: so tender, and so reassuring. Thank you, Evelyne, for all this. These days, I think a lot about what was written in May '68, on the walls of the Latin Quarter, in Paris: 'Society is a carnivorous flower' for sensitive people, enamoured with sincerity, beings who haven't forged an armour around themselves. When I met Farida, I understood better the connection between armour and the system, and success in the thick of the system. Evelyne, my darling, how I understand better with distance the wounds you suffered at a time when you were fragile, wounded by the war in your country. Fortunately, you wrote that book [Wounding Words]. It's a way to not let yourself be undervalued; to lift your head; to be alive, on the side of life. You know, right now, a lot of people are reading your book, which they're finding interesting. It's touching, what this Lebanese cultural attaché wrote to you ... I'm so happy that our plans for a trip in the desert are making you dream, and are making Samira dream. Before leaving, Angelo told me it would be good for all of us. I receive it as a gift to share with you; a hope made of all the colours of the desert, steeped in its silence, its serenity; a dream of meeting, of time for us, together ... Thank you, Evelyne, for starting to compose again, to write and to sing. I miss your voice and our laughter ... Thank you, Evelyne, for healing so well. Kiss Alban for me. I often think of him, and I thank him for being the love of your life. It's beautiful. I see your smile. Thank you for Cindy's smile.*

29 April 1994

For most people around me, life doesn't seem to have changed: it remains normal. My life, however, has stopped: I've lost control, and I'm afraid.

How can I know the disease hasn't spread? What are the doctors waiting for in order to do the tests – bone and liver scans – that Anaïs, my niece, is telling me should be done? I must be more assertive; ask more questions; not let myself become passive. I must act, and take things into my own hands! But I feel so tired.

Manicha: It's true that Evelyne is all smiles, sweetness and tenderness, the spring of beneficial warmth or freshness for everyone who approaches her. But how to face aggression non-violently? Life's instinct commands counter-violence. When we're confronted with killing power, we must kill faster.

There's also active non-violence, as developed by people such as Mahatma Gandhi, Martin Luther King and Jesus Christ. See my book *Sexuality and War* for more analysis of this phenomenon.

Alban is pampering me, and it makes me feel good. At the same time, though, I've become too passive, as if I were very ill. However, I refuse this disease; I reject it, and want to overcome it!

This morning, Souad phones. She and Pierre are in Bretagne, with Mona. They want to wish me well, and to tell me they're thinking of me. I'm not awake, and I barely speak. I fall asleep again. I dream I've awakened, and tell myself I should call Souad. I phone, and reach Pierre, who puts me in touch with her. Then I'm in a big house that's full of people who are Souad and Pierre's guests, including Dalal Bizri. I feel obliged to invite everyone to a good French restaurant, but wonder how I'd be able to afford the food at one of Paris's most expensive restaurants.

I'm so lucky to have all these friends phoning me and writing to me from various places around the world in order to let me know they're thinking about me. Even when I'm sleeping or feeling dizzy, I'm uplifted to know they're concerned. I want them to know that they're instrumental in helping me heal.

30 April 1994

I finally muster the courage to tell Dr JE that I want to have a bone scan. She tells me she doesn't believe it's necessary at this stage of my disease and treatment. I insist, and repeat what Anaïs has told me. The doctor mumbles something about how expensive I am, but orders a scan for me anyway.

I go to have the scan done with my sweet Alban. He encourages me to ask questions and be daring. He doesn't always follow what's being said in English, and Dr JE's mumbling about cost escapes him. When I tell him about it, he finds it outrageous.

Manicha: I didn't like this JE from the beginning: didn't she also, after VZ, give you the wrong treatment for the wrong diagnosis?

During the scan, I have a radioactive substance injected into one of my veins, and then have to wait a few hours for it to reach my bones, before I can return to the clinic to be scanned. I'm then put under a machine that moves slowly, millimetre by millimetre, over my body, and in which an image of my skeleton is sent to a screen. A picture of my whole bone structure is thereby created, and a specialist can analyse it and look for abnormalities.

The process seems to take forever, and I ask for Alban to be there. He tells me he can't see anything abnormal. I hope the radiologist will tell me something, but unlike in France, in which you get the results immediately, in America they make you wait for your doctor to tell you by either phone or letter, and that's a nerve-wracking way of letting you know.

In my case, it's exasperating because days go by on which Dr JE doesn't phone me. I finally phone her myself and ask for the results. I'm told that someone will phone me back immediately. I wait and wait. My fate seems suspended during the minutes and hours I spend watching the clock, the hands of which seem to move as slowly as the scanning machine moved over my body. I keep thinking, *What if the cancer has reached my bones? They're not calling me back because it has, and they don't know how to tell me – my whole treatment will have to be modified now!* Finally, unable to stand it any longer, I call again, in tears, and ask for Dr JE's nurse, who's always been very nice to me. She goes to get my results, and in a daze, I hear her voice over the phone: 'You're clean: there's nothing in your bones!' However, I can barely hear her because I'm crying so much.

Fortunately, that day, a letter and package arrive from my wonderful friend Cindy, and the package contains all kinds of herbs and music tapes. Following is an extract from Cindy's letter.

This evening, with my meditation group, we did a 'healing circle', in which we visualise someone we want healed. I put your name in. I hope you felt it, this love and light of the group projected on to you! I'm in a hurry to finish the translation [she's translating my third novel]. *I thought – I don't know why – that if I could finish the translation before your operation, it would be like a gift, something finished, and you'd feel lighter. At any rate, I'm working on it eight hours and more every day, and I put all my heart into it, thinking of you and of Amel ... I feel as if I'm living your experience through fiction, in translating you ... The birds in this picture remind me of you. Free; free; fly away!*

Of course I felt your healing touch, Cindy, through your thoughts, your letters, your little gifts, and the big gift you gave me by translating my novel. It's thanks to friends like you I was able to overcome, dry my tears and heal. I'll never forget!

Manicha: I didn't know that friendship lavished in this way could be so necessary during an illness such as this. I feel bad, now, for having neglected friends when they were ill, for having excused myself by thinking that fatigue and pain were overpowering them, and that I shouldn't go and catch them in such a poor state. I myself prefer to be in top shape when I have friends over!

I'm glad that Manicha has expressed what many people must often wonder about cancer patients. Even though each case is different, and not all people react in the same way, I've found out, from most cancer patients I've talked to, how important it is to have your friends' support. Many times, although you feel quite good physically, morally you feel so overwhelmingly anxious that a friend's touch, phone call or letter are, I'd say, absolutely vital!

On average, breast cancer robs the woman it kills of twenty years of life. This means that in the United States, nearly one million years of women's lives are lost each year. In 1964, Rachel Carson died at age fifty-six – twenty years short of the average life expectancy for the US woman at that time. (Steingraber: 1997: 20)

Just diagnosed for a second time with a rare cancer of the spinal cord, Jeannie is in between surgery and radiation treatments. She is recovering quickly – getting well in preparation for becoming sick in an attempt to get well ... Although our friendship is a recent one, the many parallels in our lives promote intense conversations whenever we are together. Both of us are writers in our thirties. Both of us became cancer patients in our twenties. Both of us grew up in communities with documented environmental contamination, high cancer rates, and suspicions that these two factors are related to each other (I was adopted; Jeannie's mother was adopted), and we each have a keen curiosity about the interplay between heredity and environment in our lives. And we have spoken at length about all of these topics. We have talked about what it means to have cancer as young women and about the relative significance of genealogy and ecology in that context. We have discussed our relationship with our doctors, our families, our hometown, our writing, our bodies. (Steingraber: 1997: 19)

What my friend and I do not choose to talk about this afternoon are the dark days that lie ahead for her. Days of lying under the crosshairs of a proton-beam cyclotron. Fatigue, vomiting, blood tests. Continuously handing one's body over to technicians and doctors in a process that we call becoming medicalized. (Steingraber: 1997: 20)

Neither of us can believe what we have just heard. After eight miserable weeks of radiation treatments to the tumor in her lower back, the original tumor in her neck – successfully removed and treated six years ago – has returned. 'Massive recurrence,' to quote the neurologist who had just received the scans from the radiologist ... 'Massive recurrence.' I struggled with my buttons, my scarf, the zipper to my book bag. My hands refused to work correctly. It had become my job in these settings to serve as the scribe and, as such, to provide complete documentation of conversations between patient and doctor. (Steingraber: 1997: 22)

It is rare that the media explain how intimately we depend on plant life for our existence, how we are necessarily children of the plant kingdom. And yet we do nothing to protect plant life on a world scale; we behave instead as if we were plant parasites, destroyers of plant life. What's more, given that everything gets exchanged and very little breaks down, otherwise it would be polluting, every time you contaminate a field with insecticide or herbicide in order to enhance production, you are polluting a hamburger or a steak. And it follows that you then pollute a human body, and we die a slow death, for our bodies are never really finished physically: our intestine, for instance, renews itself about every six months; our bodies are perpetual substance-relay stations. Few children will have really understood that by the time they leave school, even future biologists who arrive at university. (Séralini: 1997: 211)

4

CANCERS, DISEASES, SUFFERING ALL ROUND

LIFE, DROP BY DROP

I looked at myself in my bedroom mirror: there I am, about whom Simon once said, when I was younger: 'Lola without her long hair is like Réaumur without Sébastopol.' I then rubbed my eyebrows: they were disappearing too. I pulled on my eyelashes: no more eyelashes either. The hair on my legs, armpits, my pubic hair; all gone. I started having a laughing fit. Just then, my sweet mother entered the room, with Mira, her daughter Noémi and my Aunt Rivke. Of course, Rivke says:
– So, you're off to the gas chambers, are you?
And we both were doubled over laughing. My aunt couldn't stop rocking back and forth; she was almost crying.
– If you could have seen us at Auschwitz, when we were all together, naked, shaven, tatooed. There were some who started crying, but Tsiporka and I, we began to laugh, and I mean laugh! Oï! Mir hobn gelakht! (We did laugh so much!)
(Francos: 1983: 134)

Urbana, 4 May 1994

I'm paying the price of living in this civilisation. It's become a *leitmotif*, this so-called progress: we're polluting the earth so much that the environment has become a source of disease. Everything we eat, breathe and drink contaminates our body.

And what of me in all of this? Would I have had this disease if I'd stayed in Lebanon? How could I now know? The whole world is contaminated, but there's more contamination and more cancer in this part of the world: the industrialised nations.

Cheris offers me a book by Sandra Butler and Barbara Rosenblum, entitled *Cancer in Two Voices* (Butler and Rosenblum: 1991). It's a dialogue between two women, one of whom dies of breast cancer because she's poorly diagnosed. During the year, her mammography isn't read correctly, and in less than a year, the cancer has spread throughout her whole body. I can't continue reading the book after I learn these few facts: I can't stand reading that type of material at present. I have to have uplifting thoughts so my morale remains boosted – thoughts such as the ones expressed by Caryl, who lives in Alabama, or the ones expressed in some of the letters I'm continuing to receive from my friends all over the world. I include some extracts from these friends' precious letters as follows.

Souad and Pierre: *The trial you're going through is unfair, gratuitous. It knocked on the wrong door, because you have so many wonderful things to do and to live: you don't have time to deal with this burden. But there it is, and we're sure that your strength, so soft; your will, so tenacious; and your joy of living, so intense, will tame and overcome it ... You and Mona cultivate friendship similarly to how the Yemenites fish for pearls, by singing beautiful songs to the oysters.*

Noureddine Aba: *There is between us a secret link: what we feel for you and what you feel for us. I saw many signs of it in the past, signs that have been recently confirmed. Two weeks ago, I dreamt of you. When I woke up, I told my dream to Mady. You looked very sad, but there was tenderness in your eyes. You looked like the 'little fairy whipped up like frothy egg-whites'* [an expression that Aba used for me: *'la petite fée battue en neige'*], *who's retreated into her magic cave, enclosed in her loneliness and her secret treasures. Mady, who knows my dreams, wondered what this sadness would announce, and then your letter arrived. So the father is no longer there, and he left just when you are finding out that your body is failing you. It's a double death, and you have to face it. You'll succeed, I'm sure, in confronting this ordeal with dignity. You have so many resources in you through which you're filled with riches, even in the worst of sorrows. You live to give to others, to be available to help, and there are so many who need you and are expecting you to be there still: tomorrow, always, beautiful and brave, as only a fairy knows how to be. Warmest regards. Hold on! Hold on, Evelyne!*

Bruce: *The news in your last card really stunned me. I've wanted to write sooner, but to be honest, I just couldn't find words to express my profound shock, sadness and regret; to be honest, I still haven't. I remember well the passing of my father, and know how hard it must have been for you. I hope the chemotherapy is going well … and that your wonderful, lovely hair will return with time … Compared to what you've been and are going through, any news of my recent activities will certainly seem slight, so I won't bore you with the details … I hope you received the plant I sent. I meant it as a symbol of life, to be nourished and to grow. I hope it brought and continues to bring you some small degree of happiness.*

Diane: *It was so wonderful to spend those days with you when Anaïs was here. So many of my fears and insecurities dissipated, and I was able to simply love and be loved … You're in my thoughts. Knowing you brings me closer to myself, and to the creative life energy that brings beauty to this world.*

Monique Fecteau: *Evelyne, I had a thought for you while I was reading this funny article: 'I'm collecting for cancer,' said the woman at my door. 'Thanks,' I replied, 'but we already have it.' 'That isn't funny,' she informed me. 'Then the joke's on me,' I replied ... And one of my doctors, a young resident who's so inexperienced that he still speaks candidly, said, 'You all get the same treatment, basically – it's all we've got; then we pray.' ... Is it something about women, or is it just me? My friends and family hung examples before me, like so many banners, and exhorted me to be stronger; deny harder; keep the sunny side up. Why? They said it was for my own good ... The chemotherapy ended. One of the doctors said, 'You look good – but you never know. The best thing is to get on with your life: put this behind you, and forget about it.' Do they give a course in clichés in medical school? I wanted to put it behind me – you bet – but forget about it? 'Forget about it!' I did get on with my life, of course. What were the options? I revived. Home alone on a quiet evening, I was stitching away at my 'crazy quilt' of medical bills and insurance-claim forms, slowly realising I could never fit the pieces together. The billed amount exceeds our allowance for this procedure. I chuckled, because I plan to try that line on the insurance company when my next premium payment falls due ... Signed, Marilyn Greenberg*

7 May 1994

I've been invited for dinner tonight. Usually, I'm better at tolerating the small talk I encounter at these dinners. However, since I've become ill, it's been almost as if I'm reverting to the time I couldn't stand superficial conversations, in which what people are saying seems so trivial compared with life's vital issues. I leave the dinner early – I have a good excuse to now! But why should you have to have an excuse to leave when you're bored or you believe you're wasting time, or you simply want to get back to doing your work or reading a good book?

I'm surrounded with cancer problems at present. I'm feeling anxious about Séverine, who's just discovered a lump in her breast. This morning, she comes to take back some books about cancer, which she'd loaned me. I ask her to show me where her lump is. I feel it: it's hard. She feels mine also. We both laugh about the fact we're touching each other's breasts in order to find out about cancer, and we talk about the misery involved in our mutual illness – it's good we can laugh about it.

Tonight, however, I feel anguish mainly because I have to sit through this vacuous dinner conversation. I manage to slip away early, because it's so dull having to listen to people talk about subjects such as their house, garden, vacation and insurance when I'm surrounded with cancer and finding out that every year, about 165,000 American women are contracting the disease. I'm paying the price for living in a civilisation I've never chosen, nor ever loved.

Bettina: We didn't have the choice.

Yes, of course: it's much more complex; however, at the time, that's how I felt about it and needed to express it!

Cindy arrives tonight, and is to sleep here. I'm so happy to see her. She shows me a letter she's received from Amel – how much that dear friend is suffering about what's happened to me! I wish I could have spared her the anguish. In her letter to Cindy, which I include as follows, she writes about the seismic effect my news had on her, as well as about the suffering that Alban must be feeling. What a dear friend she is: I'm so anxious to see her and reassure her.

Amel: *Evelyne, ma chérie, I learnt of your disease bluntly* [I'd tried to call her to tell her, but I hadn't been able to reach her], *and I'm unable to overcome the shock. I felt the earth quake under my feet. Since your phone call a week ago, I've been feeling better.*

Yesterday, I went to see my doctor for my yearly check-up. I showed him the paper you'd sent me [it was Dr JE's prognosis and the lab's pathology report]. *He told me you would heal. My darling, do you remember how every time we part I'm stoic? But to know you're suffering makes separation unbearable, absurd. And I feel terrible being away from you, Evelyne. It reassures me to know you have women surrounding you: Diane, Samira.*

Before, it was hard to even write to you. It's hard to know you hurt in your body, but you're so full of patience, of wisdom. Chemotherapy is a stage towards healing, and so is surgery. My Hayat [which in Arabic means 'life': the name I use for myself in some of my novels], *so loved, I know you're stronger than the disease. It's a difficult trial; you'll come out of it more in love with life. Forgive me for talking so much about your disease. I know that right now, in two days, you start your treatment. You must be tired, wanting to talk about something else. The love of your life is near you, and so are your friends. And in a few months, you'll come to this warm land, with its birds that are drunk from the sun, and you'll take your shower after going to the sea ...*

Do you remember the translucent water that makes one's skin more beautiful? We walked to the dunes, and had tea at that café-marabout [in Islam and the African religions, a marabout is either the tomb of a saint or the saint himself or herself]; *we had our feet in the sand, facing the sea – Sidi El Bahri. On the road, we bought fresh fruits and vegetables; tabouna bread; and coral-coloured, black-eyed fish. I thought of you so much, about your joy in plunging into the Mediterranean: so blue and placid. The whole month of March has been beautiful.*

The next day, I went to sing. It gave me strength to celebrate my fiftieth birthday … Azza has been adorable. She offered me a bouquet of mauve flowers, and wrote on the card, 'Mauve should remind you of your dear Evelyne. Happy birthday, Mother.' Isn't that cute? I feel her so close to me right now, so attentive. I was telling you in that note I sent with Fedwa – by the way, did you receive it? did she call you? [No, Amel, I never received the note] *– about the work we did with Angelo … Angelo asked me to tell you to be careful with your nutrition, and to do meditation …*

Here's the diet given to me by Choi Sun Ja, the Chinese doctor I consulted in Rome: (1) Breakfast: soy milk (one unsweetened glass); unsweetened, diluted coffee; bread (whole wheat if possible); pine nuts. (2) Lunch: fish or meat; pasta or rice; green vegetables. (3) Dinner: fresh vegetables: squash, carrots, tomatoes and cabbage; rice or potatoes; pine nuts. Have bread only in the morning, and cut sugar out altogether. Since I've been following this diet – more or less – I've been feeling better, in greater shape. And since my fiftieth birthday, I've been doing yoga every morning, and meditation.

My darling, I could go on writing. Give me news when you can. Don't worry about me.

Alban leaves yesterday. He has a very hard time leaving, and I'm extremely sad to see him go. He'll be back soon, in about a month. We used to like having these separations, because the future joy of being reunited was implied in them. Now, however, things are different: there's our fear caused by the disease, and our anxiety about not being together at a difficult time when the closeness of love is so important.

8 May 1994

It's Petite-Fleur's birthday. I'm tired and don't feel like going out, but I go anyway, to see a film with her: *House of the Spirits*, which has been adapted from Isabel Allende's novel about the Chilean revolution. It's a very beautiful and powerful film, in which the characters speak for the revolution and against hatred. I cry many times during it. I've always been very sensitive, but I'm now hypersensitive. When we're leaving the theatre, Petite-Fleur starts having pain in her legs, and has to sit down. She's in tears, holding her medicine in her hands; wanting to take it but unable to; grinding her teeth from the pain. It hurts me to see her in so much pain.

Petite-Fleur had an auto-immune disease called poly-arthritis nodosa, which I discuss later in the book.

I'm surrounded with suffering. Things have always been like this, but even more so now, or so it seems to me: Séverine has a lump; Salwa has a cyst on her ovary; Margaret, who's my age and a colleague of Cindy, and who I met last year, has breast cancer; and everyone telling me about people who have cancer.

Françoise Collin phones me from Paris. I tell her to contact Alban there: I'm worried about him, because he has no one to talk to about my illness, and I think it isn't good for him to have to keep things inside the way he does. He gets rid of his anxiety by pampering me and sometimes being overprotective of me: my sweet Alban, the love of my life.

9 May 1994

I receive a copy of *The New Our Bodies, Ourselves in the '90s*, and when I read the breast-cancer statistics; about the casualties and deaths that result from the cancer; and that, contrary to what the media tell us, hardly any progress has been made, I'm completely depressed. And this is when Alban calls me. He immediately knows, from my voice, that I'm upset. I wish he didn't feel my moods so quickly, and that I could hide them from him, because I know he worries when I have mood changes. How can I prevent him from suffering, especially when he's so far away and can't talk to anyone about me?

Later, he told that if he didn't talk to people, it was because he wanted it that way: he thought it was inappropriate to talk about so grave a matter, especially because it was to do with me and my disease. He thought that were he to speak about the situation, he'd trivialise it. However, it worries me that he often had to get through the situation alone.

Manicha: Is it true that the rates of healing have remained more or less the same over the previous decades? I can't believe that's the case. Most cancers are found in time *[in France]*, at least for breast or uterine tumours, thanks to a relatively widespread screening campaign *[which is paid for through social security]*.

Yes, it's unfortunately true. Despite the fact that medical advances have been made in all the industrialised countries, the number of breast cancers is increasing and the healing rate in relation to the detected cancers has remained the same. In the United States, a quarter of all women hit with the disease die from it, and in France, the figure rises to a third! Later in the book, I examine the reasons for this phenomenon.

After I've talked to Alban, I go swimming at my local pool. I see Ramin and tell him about my worries. He tries to cheer me up, but has his own problems to do with matters such as conducting his research, looking for a job and finishing his thesis. I also see Belden, and thank him for phoning me one day, on which I couldn't take his call. He says he often thinks about me. He's spoken with Resa, who's a graduate student who accompanied me to Africa when I travelled there, in 1983; in 1985, she was also diagnosed as having breast cancer. I say, 'I now realise how much she suffered: what she had to go through.' Belden says that Resa knew how to take things well and remain optimistic in the midst of the worst storm. I almost say, 'Yes – even a bit too non-chalantly at times, such as when she was doing the work she'd been hired and paid to do for me.' However, I abstain, and think I should call Resa to find out how she's doing. Belden adds, learnedly, 'A positive attitude is very important!'

People who are constantly telling me to maintain a positive attitude are starting to get on my nerves! It's a very American way of thinking: to be positive at any cost! I do have the feeling I'll come out of this disease, especially because the tumour came so suddenly and, I contend, was provoked as a result of the estrogen-replacement therapy I was given. However, I become furious and unhappy when I think about all the women dying from breast cancer who are in terrible pain, and who are blinded by this civilisation as well as by doctors who are promising their patients both a miracle and a long, healthy and blissful life! All these ideas are actually myths being forced on patients in order for them to feel good and remain falsely optimistic – but we're all being misled!

Tonight's support group is good. I'm uplifted to be there and to hear the stories of people who either have or have had cancer and are who either continue to struggle or have come out of it. One man has suffered from having a brain tumour, which he describes to us in his own, very moving, way; another man also speaks, and we all feel for him very much. It's mainly male participants tonight, whereas it's usually mostly female, and the leader, Dr Alex Sorkin, is often the only male. He always makes us laugh!

I'm with my dear Séverine, who worries me so much! She finally tells me why she drifted away from me for many years: it was because of Dalila. One evening, Séverine was at a party at my place. Lots of people were there, and she said, in front of some other people, that Dalila's students were complaining that she was always arriving late for the classes she was teaching. It seems I wasn't happy about Séverine's accusations, and that I took sides with Dalila, thereby letting Séverine know I wasn't supporting her. I now tell Séverine how sorry I am, especially because she was absolutely right in making her assessment: Dalila is irresponsible; she claims to have finished her thesis when she's neither corrected it nor deposited it, as she's supposed to have done; and she hasn't responded to the letter that the head of our department has sent her about the matter. I'm glad we're able to talk about all this and to clear the air. I'm glad that Séverine feels she can talk to me the way she does, and that we can be open with each other. I've always admired her for being frank. Why didn't I believe her back then? Why was I so blinded by and protective of Dalila? I could've avoided many mistakes if I'd been more vigilant.

I have lunch with Juanita, who's a friend born in New York, and who has a Calabrian (Italian) mother and a Guyanese father. She's adopted a little Indian girl, named Laxsmi, who's adorable. Juanita's mother had breast cancer, and her father died of lung cancer. She tells me that on Long Island, in New York State, 65 per cent of the female inhabitants have breast cancer; that when you have a shower in a public place, you can see lots of women who don't have their breasts any more. I find Juanita's attitude very uplifting. She's funny and strong, laughs about life's miseries and sees everybody's weaknesses.

An epidemic on this scale simply must have an environmental cause. I believe that the data included in *The New Our Bodies, Ourselves in the '90s* are correct, so I firmly believe we should say no to estrogen-replacement therapy. Let's stop promoting and accepting it: according to the book, prescribing it is one of the reasons there's been so great a rise in the incidence of breast cancer. Let women become conscious of their body, and of the fact that their health is being manipulated in order to create and maintain a market for all the legal pharmaceuticals we're being served and encouraged to consume. In the United States, a mixture of estrogen and progesterone is apparently the number-two drug, right after the anti-depressant Prozac. We women have to become aware of the people who are trying to fool us, and mustn't let our voice remain passive! Long Island, for example, is also marred by the presence of many nuclear reactors, as well as chemical leaks and other scandals we'll probably never hear about. All this environmental contamination is probably also the source of the cancer epidemic that's plaguing the world's industrialised countries.

I'm phoned by Nawal El Saadawi, the well-known Egyptian feminist novelist, activist and doctor. She's called to tell me she's concerned about me and my health. Her concern is obvious, and I'm overwhelmed that someone who has her hectic schedule cares so much and phones me. I hope to see her and her husband, Sherif, again soon.

Tonight, when I speak during the support-group session, I evoke torture: it's truly a torture I'm living through, and what I and other cancer patients have to endure. And the torture will continue to increase. During this session, it's mostly the men who speak; Séverine and I are the only women. I realise that men need to speak just as much as women do, and that they suffer in the same way when they lose their hair and undergo other bodily changes. It's moving to hear the story of the man who suffered a brain tumour: he speaks about his weakness, his anxieties, the subnormal temperature he ran – just like I did – and his hospital stay.

13 May 1994

My body is changing, and I have no control over it. I'm blowing up, my stomach is getting big, and I've lost almost all my pubic hair and all the hair on my head; even my eyelashes are starting to fall out. I feel different, and I don't like what I see; therefore, I'm starting to use all kinds of tricks to look pretty, such as wearing a wig, a scarf, make-up and attractive clothes. I'm a good magician: many people think I'm in great shape – if only they could see what's under it all and how I feel! However, it's helpful to have people pay me compliments about my 'good looks', because I'm finding it hard to deal with the aggression and breakdown that my body is suffering, and with how terrible I think I actually look.

This morning, I go for my final chemo session. Dr JE tells me she thinks the tumour should have shrunk more by now. However, like me, she thinks that perhaps the mass we're still feeling could be not only cancer but fibrosis: development of excessive fibrous tissue. She calls my surgeon, Dr Yoto, who says he still hopes to be able to do a lumpectomy – breast-conserving surgery – rather than a mastectomy; I, too, hope I can have the former operation. I like the attitude of these two doctors: cancer seems less threatening when you're being treated by doctors who have a realistic but positive attitude. I still don't understand what could have caused the tumour – other than the estrogen – and through what treatment it could be removed completely. I believe its cells have now stopped proliferating.

This is an extremely difficult period of my life. Alban phones me – that sweet, soft voice that's always impressed me. Since the very start of our relationship, I've been attracted by the way he talks: the timbre of his voice. Amy, the nurse who takes care of me and administers the chemotherapy, notices how sweet Alban is with me, and how dismayed we are when she tells us we can't kiss because he has a slightly sore throat. I like it when people like my Alban. After the final chemo session, before I leave, I give her a hug, a copy of my book *The Excised* (Accad: 1994), and some chocolate. Fortunately, there are still people like her in the medical profession: through them, I'm given hope for this world.

I won't be operated on before the end of the first week in June, because my blood and bone marrow have to be replenished.

15 May 1994

Using my hands, I've been measuring the tumour several times a day. I'd so much like it to disappear. What's it doing there in my body anyway? Foreign cells; mad cells, invading me, trying to invade me, now under control.

I feel weak, and have a metallic taste in my mouth. During these past two nights, I've been feeling my heart beating like crazy. I'm worried by it, especially because I'm told that the heart muscle is weakened in response to administration of the chemo drug Adriamycin. But no: my heart is beating; sending out all the toxins – sending them to the places that have to receive them in order for me to fight the bad cells located in my breast.

Last night, I dream about Stan. In the dream, I go into his house: a palace that has a beautiful garden, somewhat like the Cochrans' residence – where Ireland's consul to Lebanon lives. Stan has to correct one of my works, but has only the first draft of it, which is poorly written and barely readable. I tell him I have a good copy of it on my computer, if he wants it, but he says it isn't necessary to give him this other copy. Loraine, his wife, takes me to their basement, in which there's a huge dining room. Their daughter is there, at the end of the dining table. She's very beautiful. They tell me she has skin cancer, and that everyone has one type of cancer or another. Stan is scared, because he's found blood in his urine.

What does the dream mean? It's a mixture of my anxieties about both my work and my health. I described the house in the dream to Jim last night: I often dream about things I've talked or thought about during the previous day or evening. I'd have to have Freud's patience, evident in his *Interpretation of Dreams* (Freud: 1955), to understand and explain all that the dream means.

I know I'm in for 10 difficult days now, having had all the chemotherapy I was prescribed: during these 10 days, the 'poison' has its strongest effect, whereby it attacks the bad as well as the good cells, and the blood and bone marrow are thereby weakened. After these 10 days, your blood starts to reconstitute itself, and the cancer cells that haven't been eliminated are liable to start proliferating again. I'll feel weak, have a backache, have a bad taste in my mouth and so on. However, the symptoms will go away. What operation should I have? Do I have a choice? Will I be able to accept having a mastectomy, psychologically as well as physically? If only my cancer cells could be eliminated once and for all.

16 May 1994

I go to the office, feeling nauseous. Denise Koglin and Julia Diliberti bring me a can of 7-Up, which I drink and feel better after having. I go home and go to bed. Séverine phones: although she won't have her cancer-test results until Thursday, she's been told her tumour looks 'suspicious'. I can neither believe nor accept this assessment: why should she have to go through a trial such as this again? I feel hurt when I think about it. I was already feeling bad before she called, and now I feel terrible, as if my life is being bound up with cancer stories being told all around me.

Manicha: It does seem that the number of cancers keeps increasing, but could it also be that before, youth preserved us from the awareness of all these diseases, the mounting problem?

Youenn's woman friend has also been struck again: her cervical cancer has returned. And yesterday, Margaret, Cindy's colleague and friend, calls me to talk about her breast cancer.

Is my breast full of cancer? How could a low-risk cancer have developed so fast? I wish I could understand what's happening to me. I'm aching – aching all over, for both me and Séverine. Why does my friend have to go through that again? Why should she suffer again? It seems so unfair! There's no justice on this earth; is there any elsewhere? Is there an elsewhere?

Fortunately, one of Cindy's letters arrives, and I'm uplifted again. I include an extract from it as follows.

Evelyne, you are a star that will continue shining – even if you're sick for a certain time. You're beautiful inside, and everybody notices it immediately. This treatment can change some things superficially for a certain time. I'm sure you must feel a little beyond yourself, but the essential remains always as brilliant as ever – and will transform you later. We manifest who we are through our gaze – and yours has no equal ... Rest well. Know that I'm thinking of you every day, sending you many smiles!

Manicha: She's right: beauty is light, and light transcends appearance.

19 May 1994

Yesterday, Emile, the head of my department, informs me that my student Nnennaya has died of a cerebral hemorrhage. Poor Nnennaya: I'm stunned when I receive the news. I'm sure she was terribly stressed and unhappy because she hadn't finished her thesis. I feel so sad for her.

Ann, one of the department's secretaries, comes into the room in which I'm printing after I've spoken to Emile. I burst into tears and express my indignation at life's injustices. Ann says she believes that every human being has his or her time already inscribed at birth. I think of the maktoub that Arabs believe in, which literally means 'written up in heaven' and is what some people call fate or destiny; however, I don't tell Ann, because I believe she wouldn't have understood. She says that sometimes it's better to leave this world, especially when life's problems become unbearable – is she talking about herself, or about Nnennaya, who she liked? I look at her. I don't think she's very happy about her life, especially not right now, what with all the problems she's facing. As for me, I used to be very happy before all this happened, but I was undoubtedly too stressed. I have to admit it so I don't repeat the kind of life I was leading. I'll definitely go about my life differently when this ordeal is over.

Manicha: Ah, the promises of hard times that one doesn't keep!

However, I'm keeping my promises as much as I possibly can; for example, I took leave of absence without pay in order to finish this book.

Bettina: It's so important to emphasise how important lifestyle is. It's better to become aware of it early, before the onset of disease.

20 May 1994

I can't believe it: Séverine's cancer has come back. This tumour is ovarian cancer, and is feared to be a metastasis. I remain in shock at receiving this horrible news.

Life, drop by drop,
like chemo, drop by drop.
Viscous red colour of Adriamycin:
scarlet poppies in the bushes.
Nausea turning my stomach;
heart-ache;
fear, hung up on barbed wire;
revolt of the ruins.
I am trembling all over for my little sister Séverine.
Injustice of a world spreading its decay,
man controlling nature and illnesses,
producing other illnesses.
Is life but a winter?

Alban thinks the process can't be stopped: that the chain of events unravelling the earth will continue and lead to an increasing incidence of cancers in ever younger people, and that doctors will continue to use radical treatments that lead to other cancers and illnesses – what a happy prospect!

Fortunately, Juanita makes me laugh today, by describing the disastrous habit of one of our colleagues in the Comparative Literature department: putting his hands on women's buttocks.

Juanita: No! Correction: he used to kiss women on their neck.

He passed away not long ago.

Juanita thinks he's the biggest harasser in town. However, she doesn't know the harasser we have in our department. I remember that Europeans – especially the French – treat the subject of sexual harassment almost as a joke when they're discussing it, because they view it as being an 'American phenomenon', and that Americans are obsessed with the idea of harassment. I like Juanita: she's beautiful and strong. She's thinking of adopting another child from India. She also feels she's at risk of contracting cancer because the disease runs in her family.

I don't know what got into me to phone my younger brother Pierrot tonight; I should have known better. He hasn't been phoning me recently because he's having financial problems again and couldn't afford the calls. He's angry with father for not leaving him any money. I tell him that father has left us better things than money, and that he's left us properties in Lebanon anyway. Why doesn't he consider that, and why doesn't he feel angry for having persecuted father at the end of his life? I believe that if he and Adelaide are feeling bad at present, it could be because they're feeling guilty for having made father suffer at the end of his life: my poor father. However, I desist from raising my thoughts with him, and limit the conversation.

Manicha: Money has a way of dividing brothers and sisters, and parents and children, even on their death bed.

21 May 1994

I intend to lead a life that's more peaceful and in which I'm less stressed: fewer professional engagements and more outings for fun; fewer people to see, and only the people I really like or feel like seeing; more time to myself, to write and do the meaningful things I really want to do.

Séverine leaves a message on my answering machine, telling me she's had a chemotherapy session in which she was administered a very strong, relatively new drug called Taxol. I phone her back. She tells me she has to go to Chicago in order to have a bone-marrow transplant, and that I'm not to worry about her – that I should think of myself first. What an incredible little sister! She's going through hell, but tells me to think of myself!

Why has her cancer come back? She didn't feel anything in particular before she discovered the tumour in her breast: how can I not think of her?

Twice today, I swim in the pool, under a beautiful sky. What a gorgeous day! I can't help thinking about my youth and adolescence – how carefree it all seems in retrospect! I look at Ramin, who's laughing with a group of young people, plunging and swimming, and having a good time. He seems carefree, as I used to be. I wish I could go back to that time, before my breast was stung by a scorpion; long, long before this illness. How I wish I could protect my little sister Séverine: she chose her husband Charles to protect her from the world. Why does she have to be poisoned by this cruel venom?

22 May 1994

Séverine phones, and I go to see her this morning. She received four hours' worth of Taxol yesterday, and her oncologist is considering sending her to Chicago to decide whether she should have a bone-marrow transplant. It's a process whereby the patient's bone marrow is removed in order to administer to him or her intensive chemotherapy that attacks all the cancerous cells in the body. When the process is finished, the bone marrow is re-injected. It's a dangerous process, and just thinking about it makes me shiver.

Poor Séverine, who's already had to put up with so much. I remember when she was a student and I a young professor: she was so pretty and delicate. We were both young and pretty. How much we've changed, now both of us are swollen from the chemo and losing our hair. Today, I bring along a colourful scarf and show her how to tie it. She says it makes her look like a pirate – she hasn't lost her sense of humour! – and we both laugh.

Then Charles arrives. I kiss him, and we hug. The three of

us have tears in our eyes. Laura, their daughter, also arrives, on roller skates and with a friend. She's pretty and delicate, like Séverine used to be. She seems shaken by what's going on. I feel so terribly sad!

Later, and fortunately, I see Juanita and Zohreh at Zorba's, the village's Greek restaurant. We have a Greek-style sandwich that reminds me of the Lebanese shawarma. I'm overwhelmed by Juanita's personality: she's very impressive, a remarkable woman who talks with much passion and humour. Because I have her as company, I come out of my sadness. We four then go to the pool with Juanita, her daughter Laxsmi and Petite-Fleur, who's just had her hair braided, African style. It seems it costs a lot to have someone do your hair in this way, and I wonder whether it's worth it, although I must admit the style looks charming on Petite-Fleur.

27 May 1994

I phone Monique to wish her a happy birthday, and I feel her love for me. Eva's arriving tonight, and I'm a bit apprehensive: I'm concerned that too many memories might be stirred up. I've been hurt as a result of the attitude that she and Milo have expressed towards Alban. They haven't understood my love for him. I can't forget this misunderstanding, and feel awkward that Milo died before we could clear the air by having a frank discussion. Alban has taken such a huge place in my life: he's truly the most wonderful man on this earth, and the people who don't see it's so can no longer be my friends. They aren't true friends if they don't understand our relationship. Some people tell me it's jealousy and normal for friends to feel protective and critical about each other's partner. According to my concept of friendship, though, it isn't normal: real friends aren't jealous that their friends are happy; they're happy too.

Bettina: I couldn't agree more!

Manicha: But love is blind!

I'm having lots of ups and downs at present, but more downs than ups: anxiety about what lies ahead when I have the operation, and anxiety in the face of an illness through which it's possible that your life will be thrown into disarray.

Yesterday, I go and see Juanita. She's just had a breast biopsy. Her mother, who's had a double mastectomy, was there from New York. It's very moving to see Juanita's mother: flat chested, and talking very vivaciously, a bit like Juanita. She kisses me very warmly, and starts telling me her cancer stories, including that in New Jersey, where she lives, breast cancer has become very common. When you cross cancer's space, it's a different time zone; a different space; a different place. Lots of local women have lost one or two breasts, and many have lost their hair as a result of chemotherapy treatment.

This space of illness is painful and hard to accept – an uneasy place to be living. I have lots of books to read at present. Sometimes I don't feel like reading books about illness any more, especially this illness. It's all so utterly depressing. However, there are some excellent books, such as Susan Sontag's *Illness as Metaphor* (Sontag: 1977), in which the author compares tuberculosis with cancer and discusses the metaphors that have been invented to describe the illnesses. Tuberculosis was a more romantic and soft disease, and people who had it were sent to a good climate and instructed to eat good food in order to recuperate. Cancer, on the other hand, is associated with violent images and metaphors for war: the body is attacked with poison, radiation, knives (wielded by surgeons), and all the other 'weapons of warfare'. The war association must be one of the reasons I hate the disease so much! How I wish there were softer cures.

Sontag (1977: 63) writes,

Cancer is described in images that sum up the negative behavior of twentieth-century homo economicus: abnormal growth, repression of energy, that is, refusal to consume or spend.

She describes cancer as follows (1977: 63).

Cells without inhibitions, cancer cells will continue to grow and extrude in 'chaotic' fashion, destroying the body's normal cells, architecture, and functions.

She also writes (1977: 71),

Tuberculosis was associated with pollution ... and now cancer is thought of as a disease of the contamination of the whole world. TB was the 'white plague.' With awareness of environmental pollution, people have started saying that there is an 'epidemic' or 'plague' of cancer.

I also read Sontag's book about AIDS, entitled *The Way We Live Now* (Sontag: 1991), which is a very poetic and analytical story in which the author shows that we're all caught up in this dreadful disease and nobody's spared.

I also find Audre Lorde's book *The Cancer Journals* (Lorde: 1980) fascinating, but find it painful to read because the author suffers so much. Lorde thinks that women who've had a mastectomy should refuse to have their breast/s reconstructed, because if all the women who've been subjected to this mutilation were to march on Washington's Capitol Hill, bare breasted and asking for radical changes in the way the environment is being poisoned, as well as demanding more funding for cancer research, people would become more aware and changes would take place. She's so right!

Her description of the Reach to Recovery nurse who comes to Lorde's hospital room after she's had the mastectomy, in order to show her how to hide her missing breast, is incredible. She describes how women such as the nurse are trained to be upbeat, and come in bearing clothes through which their breast implant is emphasised and the whole tragedy is hidden under the veneer of normalisation: if you seem normal, you are normal, and everything's okay! I enjoy engaging with her because she's politically aware of the disease and raises the issues to the political level. We must work on raising people's consciousness in order to transform society and this decaying world.

All this is so revolting. It really is 'the end of time', says Adelaide, who last night feels my need to hear her voice, and phones me. I, however, don't view the disease as being the result of losing your religion, a cause–effect relationship inscribed in biblical prophecies – no, it's we humans' irresponsibility that's caused our own downfall.

I turn to my sweet Amel's letter for encouragement, and include an extract from it as follows.

Thank you for reassuring me; only you know how much I need it. Thank you for writing to me despite your fatigue. You speak of torture performed on your body, and you say 'sometimes'. How I know your modesty, your patience: I imagine how hard chemo must have been. It hurts me to think about it, but it's finished now, as of the 13th of May, and the operation will surely be less painful. Today, your niece is with you. I'd so much like to know her, and in a few days your 'love' will be there. What is good in the United States is that they tell people everything about the disease. Here, nobody talks about it: it's hidden, and it hurts everybody ... I'm also glad you're in the United States for the quality of the treatment. Soon, you'll be healed, and you'll pursue your path, more conscious, more relaxed, more in love with life, with people, closer to yourself.

29 May 1994

Eva arrives, and we have a wonderful day. We're able to speak very openly and deeply, and we connect just as we connected in the good old days, despite the wounds we inflicted on each other.

The day she arrives, a student is going from door to door bearing a petition for people to sign and collecting money. On the petition are the sentences 'Let's get rid of cancer-causing pesticides in our foods. No one has the right to give you cancer.' I'm thrilled to see this young woman going from door to door. I notice that Jeanie, my neighbour and feminist friend, has signed the petition. Are feminists more concerned about these problems? The world's getting more dangerous every day; whereas before I knew it in an abstract way, I now know it in my flesh.

Eva is debating what to do about estrogen-replacement therapy. She's terrified of going through menopause and of ageing, and is reading a lot about both subjects. She's inspired to think because of what's happened to me. I wish I'd been more careful. Why did I let myself be persuaded to take hormones? Why didn't I read more about ERT? I was under the influence of Alain and of all my women friends who also have it: Mona; Monique and her sister; Karen; Zohreh; even my own sister. It's difficult to fight a whole system, especially when a doctor's telling you that in order to prevent the osteoporosis that's afflicting your mother, you must have ERT now – not later – and at a high dose.

A high dose is what American doctors call a megadose, and French doctors told me that a dose of that strength was much too strong for me.

This morning, Juanita comes by. She and her mother are furious with my doctor and her nurse for not taking more seriously my visit to them on Friday. They're disgusted I was treated as if I were a hysterical woman in need of consolation.

I return to that incident later in the book.

I think I'm accepting my age better than are many of my close friends, thanks to the excellent relationship I have with Alban. I feel secure in the relationship and that I have his love, so I feel good about myself. I hope he lives many more years, and I with him. Tonight, I have a nightmare about him. He's talking to his children, and I'm there, wearing a scarf on my head. I think that Patsy, one of his daughters, is going to say something to me. However, because she doesn't speak, I catch her attention. She says to me, 'I hope what you have isn't contagious, like scabies or something.' I say, 'It's worse: I have cancer.' She barely reacts. Her brother, Alban's son, doesn't say anything, but seems to understand everything.

From Séverine, we learn that her cancer 'return' isn't a metastasis of her ovarian cancer but is, in fact, breast cancer. When she receives this news in the pathology report, she calls all her friends to let them know about it, and is exuberant with joy! Someone from 'outside' would think she's crazy to be jubilant about having breast cancer: only a cancer patient could understand the extent of her relief! She's gone down a few notches on the 'Richter Scale' of this killer disease – my sweet little Séverine, who's already gone through so much pain. How much can a person endure in his or her lifetime? She'll now have to have her lymph nodes under her arm removed, followed by radiation, and possibly more chemotherapy.

In my dreams these days, I'm constantly returning to the same space in various houses that in reality I've never even seen. Sometimes this recurrence is reassuring, sometimes it isn't at all. It's strange and mysterious, and I'm trying to understand what it means. It's like a space in my childhood in which there are many rooms, and there's a specific enclosed place I'm trying to escape from. It comes back every night in my dreams, with greater or less intensity, and with more or less identifiable elements. I've read that it's important to untie the knot in our past – the dilemma from which the disease nourishes itself – if we want to heal completely. I seem to be untying the knot in my dreams. How many more closed rooms do I need to open? Will I be able to run free and exalted as a result of going through this process? Once I've revisited these stifling places of my life, recognised them, identified them and gotten rid of them thanks to the demystifying work I'm doing, will I be better able to recover my physical and moral health?

The sick person – and here I am talking about those who know they are afflicted with a possibly fatal disease – if he has not already thrown in the towel, can prove to be wonderfully enriching company. This is perhaps because he senses he now has to live a shortened form of his life, because he knows that time, which for him is ticking away in a more precise fashion, fills him with an intensity that is often lacking among the insipidly healthy folk who, spoiled or jaded, are unaware of how precious this existence that they are squandering really is; they're alive but not living; or perhaps another reason is that since they now refuse any form of lying, they wish to confront their own truth (and in doing so, provide the mirror for us to gaze at our own). For all these reasons, and many others, intimate and particular, the person who senses the threat of death weighing upon him has countless things to teach us. (Lambrichs: 1995: 10)

Of course, it is only when forced to do so that we will renounce the three-car garage, the insult to third-world nations that is the profusion of food in our supermarkets. But all this progress might very well come to a stop all by itself, if it is the human species that ceases to thrive. It is not completely outlandish to raise that possibility. Between 5 and 40 billion species have lived on the Earth since life first appeared, some 3.8 to 3.6 billion years ago; not a one has lasted without undergoing some kind of transformation, and 99.9% of them have completely disappeared. By virtue of what, therefore, would we humans constitute an exception, if not by dint of our consciousness that distinguishes us from other animals, of the felicity of knowing how to develop our capacity to wisely manage this world? (Séralini: 1997: 31)

5

LYMPH NODES

MY BREAST OFFERED IN SACRIFICE

Granted, mutilations against women do not take place solely within the context of this disease, but cancer treatment provides the surgeon with all the necessary alibis. Misogyny is rampant in this field, where there are practically no female cancer specialists of note.

How long must we wait before there is a commission of inquiry into female mutilations, and not only the excision of young girls, that poster child of cultural difference, but an enquiry into the whole range of mutilations inflicted upon females, excision in the name of custom, mastectomy in the name of cancer, and on-the-off-chance hysterectomies! (Hyvrard: 1987: 168)

Urbana, 2 June 1994

I'm facing a difficult choice: I saw the surgeon today, and he now doesn't know whether he'll be able to do a lumpectomy instead of a mastectomy. If the tumour is well contained and the margins are negative, he'll be able to remove the lump only; otherwise, he'll have to remove the whole breast. Therefore, I don't really have a choice, although I could've told him to remove the breast right away. This is what I believed that my niece Anaïs, who's arrived, thought

I should tell him. Although she didn't voice this opinion, I could sense that she thought it would be safer for me to have a mastectomy. However, I couldn't resign myself to having it: if my breast could be saved, why not save it? I value it, even more now it's been sick. It's almost the way I used to feel about Lebanon: loving it more because it was being torn apart through a war it had no control over. My poor breast also has no control over these mad cells invading it and trying to kill it.

Manicha: We love more what we're about to lose – we regret it already: this 'something' that was, what we used to be.

I'm feeling anxious about all this. Fortunately, my sweet love is arriving this Sunday, and I'm so excited about it. It's so wonderful when he's here. It's also good to have Anaïs here at present, although she's very anxious this time. She doesn't seem to be doing very well. She saw Emma today, and told her right away what she thought: that it was a duty rather than a pleasure to see her. She refused to pray with Emma. My Anaïs is so honest and courageous, and at the same time can badly hurt people she loves, because when her feelings are very intense, she doesn't know how to say things tactfully. I love her dearly. I hope she finds what's right for her and won't be anxious any more. I accept her, however she chooses to be. I think she's wonderful, sweet, beautiful, intense, serious and full of humour. At the same time, I wonder why she thought she had to hurt Emma, who she doesn't see very often; no doubt, she must still feel very strongly about Emma and what she means in her life, to be hurting her in this way. She could face Emma and their past relationship more serenely only if she were indifferent to her.

Emma is an undeclared lesbian. Although no one has ever told me she is – not even Anaïs – I assume it's so because of the way she lives, and because of her relationship with Anaïs. It could also be that she's bi-sexual, like most people, or asexual, as Christ is portrayed as being. Whatever the case may be, she overcame what traditional moralists consider to be 'bad tendencies', thanks to her faith and beliefs, and helped Anaïs, at one especially difficult point in Anaïs's life: when her parents forced her to return with them to Lebanon in the hope they'd be able to reform her. Later, when she was 'cured', they sent her back to the States – the country they called the 'centre of evil and decadence. Emma was instrumental in getting Anaïs 'back on the right track' by accompanying her to church, talking with her, encouraging her, and developing a strong friendship with her on a professional level – Emma, like Anaïs, is a scientific researcher – as well as on a personal one. They have a 'non-sexual' relationship, which is therefore a non-threatening one and is accepted by the traditional religious dogmatists.

I rewrote this section two years later, after I discovered that Emma had also been hit by this 'un-nameable' disease. Poor Emma: at the time, we didn't know she'd have to go through this hell, and neither did she. To the family, she wrote a very moving letter that she's allowed me to share as follows. I include a few extracts from it in order to show how differently each person deals with the disease.

14 June 1995

Last July, my mammogram revealed a lesion. Due to some circumstances with the surgeon, I chose to delay the biopsy and have another mammogram this past January. The lesion was still there, so I chose a different surgeon ... The excisional biopsy – actually a lumpectomy – was performed on the 10th of February. I chose IV [intravenous] sedation so I could 'chat' with the surgeon – must be the veterinarian in me. Even though he normally prefers his patients to be unconscious, he was responsive to my questions, and even laughed during some humorous comments – yep: I found several things amusing during the procedure.

A week later, he told me it was cancer – less than 1 centimetre in diameter – and that he'd excised it completely. God's Hands were all over this episode, because 90 per cent of these lesions are benign, and cancer – let alone breast cancer – hasn't occurred in my family on either side. Also, the cancer cells had hormone – estrogen and progesterone – receptors: a very rare thing for a pre-menopausal woman such as me. That means these cells have been bathed in these stimulating hormones for at least 10 months; yet the Lord kept the lesion the same size between the July and the January mammograms – it just doesn't make any logical sense. God was definitely starting to confound my intellect – put it to death so that He can restore it under its proper authority. We just can't figure things out apart from His wisdom.

The next step was axial dissection, on the 22nd of February, to remove the draining lymph nodes to determine whether the cancer had spread. The surgeon removed only 12 instead of the normal 24 – thankfully a more conservative approach, because recovery from this procedure is painful enough. Although the Lord kept telling me and others in my fellowship that it'd be all right, the prospect of what could happen hit me hard, and I was undone. On the Sunday before surgery, He had the people in the fellowship inter-cede in the Spirit for me – some were weeping louder than I was. I didn't seem to fear death, but feared the possibility of IV chemotherapy – I knew I wouldn't be able to choose that treat-ment, and that God would have to physically manifest Himself to tell me to go down that path. I didn't think I'd have the pathology report until that Friday, but God was merciful to let me know 36 hours after surgery that all the nodes were normal. I was joyful! And I realised how merciful He is, because what I went through was intense yet very mild compared to what other people have experienced. The second surgery resulted in about 60 per cent loss of arm function. After the surgery, I saw the oncologist. There were pre-cancerous cells present in the normal tissue of the biopsy, so they scheduled me for radiation therapy. The treatment should bring about a 90 per cent cure rate – nothing is 100 per cent. How very merciful of the Lord to limit my need to make a decision to just this!

The radiation therapy began on the 17th of March, for 30 'zappings' – five days a week for six weeks. The major side effect, besides skin changes, was extreme fatigue, due to the radiation damage to the tissue – radiation releases all sorts of chemicals from the damaged cells. I was surprised by the level of exhaustion I experienced, and also how much my mind was befuddled as a result. The radiologist told me to just take a 10 minute nap during the day: not very conducive at the office setting, as a means to handle the fatigue – he obviously never experienced this treatment! It took a good two weeks after the last treatment to get some energy back, and for my mind to clear up so I could think and concentrate once again. During it all, I continued to appear at the office, and got some deep-muscle massages to keep my arms, especially the affected shoulder, in some sort of condition; both really helped to quickly bring my arm function back to near normal – 95 per cent after only 3.5 months 'post-op'. So, now I'm starting to do some exercises to build up stamina and lose some of the weight I gained during my inactivity – radiation treatments don't affect the appetite.

He told me years ago that if He were in the process, I needn't fear the outcome. In all that I've faced over the years, He's constantly fulfilled that promise. I've begun to understand that we're here at His pleasure and that for each of us He's numbered our days. He didn't spare His own Son, so He won't spare our life when it comes to issues that have eternal significance. The momentary discomforts of this body aren't that important when compared with healing the soul – putting the old nature to death so we can experience the resurrection of Christ while we're still here. In that light, cancer wasn't the issue; rather, it was my intellect that was out of place. The intellect, from the rational masculine side, was in authority within me. He's started to put this aspect to death so He can restore it in its proper position, under the authority of the Holy Spirit, through the feminine (intuitive) nature so His wisdom and understanding will be manifested to me ... Never a dull moment during this adventure of understanding the ways of the Lord and knowing Him! ...

Indeed, Emma's is quite a different way of dealing with cancer. She seems to have found an inner peace, and you can only be happy for her if through her faith she found strength and courage in the worst adversity. I remember having similar reflections about the war in Lebanon: I noticed that people who had faith were able to face the war more serenely. They were strong in their serenity, and maintained a peaceful yet actively resistant attitude in the midst of terrible violence. I could understand their faith: it's only when it's transformed into proselytism, and into rigid dogmas about right and wrong, which have to be imposed on other people, that I find it repulsive.

Manicha: Faith and God's company are what the cane is to the one who limps: necessary and beneficial, more than a friend. Atheists are lacking in this respect: rationality doesn't replace faith.

When I wake up from the anesthesia, on the 13th of June, will I still have my two breasts? I'm anxious, because I don't know what lies ahead or what they'll find in my lymph nodes. I've been reading that the future prospects of follow-up treatment are determined according to whether the nodes are positive or negative. I'm really going through some of the most difficult moments in my life. At the same time, and probably because of the difficulty, I'm finding out who the people are who really count in my life: the ones who really mean a lot to me.

4 June 1994

I dream that my left knee – the one that was operated on when I was an adolescent – has gotten out of joint again, and that blood is gushing because of the disconnection. In the dream, I go to Dr JE to tell her they have to re-set it, and stop my pain and the bleeding. She reacts by singing in a very melodic voice, and doing nothing to help save my knee. I'm happy to hear her sing, but extremely frustrated not to receive her care.

I feel anguish at the prospect of having the operation. My anguish is reflected in the dream, and also reflected is how I feel about the medical establishment: doctors' irresponsibility, and the big, infernal machine that's geared towards making money rather than healing people.

Also, my dream comes after I have the experience of going to the clinic on Friday afternoon. Juanita and her mother urge me to go because I tell them about the pain I'm feeling in various parts of my body, especially my arm. They advise me to go before the end of the week, because I won't be able to see anyone on the weekend. When I go to see Dr JE, her response is to tell me I need a hug, which I actually find sweet; however, Juanita and her mother are infuriated when I tell them, and say it's unbelievable that the doctor so easily dismissed my pains, as if I were sick in the head! Also reflected in my dream is my need to hear music, even from 'scientific' people: the need to find different, more harmonious, responses to and cures for the disease.

I'm reading a book by Eric Siegel (Siegel: 1986), who writes about these alternative ways of dealing with diseases, even with surgery. He explains that when he operates, he plays soft, harmonious music – often classical. He's convinced that music has an effect on his surgery patients; that they're reassured and calmed when they hear it; that they can hear it even under anesthesia; and that they better react to having had the operation. Siegel himself needs to hear music in order to better wield the scalpel and go right to the lesion. He also says it's important the surgeon talk to the patient before he or she operates, and that if the patient is to recover from the disease, it's essential there be a good relationship between the patient, the doctor and the surgeon.

Bettina: In fact, it's vital!

Manicha: For me, as for many other people, in order for the doctor and patient to face the disease together, there has to be the kind of confidence that can spring only from having the fullest and most open explanation of the disease.

5 June 1994

Alban is arriving today. Tonight, Anaïs and I must call Adelaide and wish her a happy birthday; we must also tell her to keep the baby she's found abandoned and in need of parents. Anaïs and I view the baby's arrival as being a gift; a ray of hope; a sign; a good omen; sunshine in the existing gloom, in all the news about illness and death, which are all around us. I also think the baby is a gift when I'm thinking I should've been in Lebanon at the time Adelaide discovered her, and when I'm thinking that Adelaide told me I could've registered her in my name, on the spot, and that no one would've known she wasn't mine. I also think this baby is a gift when I'm recalling how long I've been wanting to have a baby to care for, and thinking that now would've been the perfect – perhaps a unique – opportunity, if only I hadn't gotten sick. Why did I have to get sick? Also, I promised father I'd go and take care of mother and him in the Aïn Saadé house he loved so much. Now he's dead and I'm sick!

This morning, I see Nina. She shows me her mutilated breast, or rather the place her breast once was. I'm neither frightened nor anguished to see it; on the contrary, I'm able to 'de-dramatise' the fear I have about having the operation, and I'm thankful to Nina for sharing her experience with me. She's so likeable, sympathetic and serene – a truly great woman! She believes that the statisticians skew the 'stats' about breast and other types of cancer, and that the women who die from breast cancer are mostly much older than we're made to believe. Her reasoning is aligned with Youenn's: that things aren't really getting worse, as some people would have us believe; they've always been hard. As for me, I'm not so sure. I believe that the world is getting worse. It's suffering from an accumulation of damaging effects that people everywhere are feeling. How could anyone not see these effects? We have a world population that will double in a few years; the ozone layer continues to be depleted and pierced; we live with unbearable pollution, in 'un-liveable' cities that have become what a sociologist has termed 'anti-cities'; and drug addiction, AIDS and cancers are rife. Even though cancer has existed for a long time, it's manifesting differently and more aggressively, reaching epidemic proportions, and hitting younger and younger people. And what of other forms of disease, such as the one that Petite-Fleur is suffering from – diseases that are difficult to diagnose and cure, illnesses that are attacking humans' immune system in strange ways that were unheard of before? No, I don't think all this existed before.

Nazik: Other diseases existed before: ones that have been eliminated thanks to medical discoveries. Because people are living longer, they're more exposed to all kinds of disease.

I'm not sure that people are being more exposed to disease than ever before; I'm inclined to think we're having to deal with more diseases than we had to deal with in the past. My conviction has been reinforced through my reading of Laurie Garrett's *The Coming Plague: Newly Emerging Diseases in a World Out of Balance.* According to Garrett (1995: 619–20),

Time is short. As the Homo Sapiens population swells, surging past the 6 billion mark at the millennium, the opportunities for pathogenic microbes multiply. If, as some have predicted, 100 million of those people might then be infected with HIV, the microbes will have an enormous pool of walking immune-deficient petri dishes in which to thrive, swap genes, and undergo endless evolutionary experiments. 'We are in an internal competition. We have beaten out virtually every other species to the point where we may now talk about protecting our former predators,' Joshua Lederberg told a 1994 Manhattan gathering of investment bankers. 'But we're not alone at the top of the food chain.' Our microbe predators are adapting, changing, evolving, he warned. 'And any more rapid change would be at the cost of human devastation.' The human world was a very optimistic place on September 12, 1978, when the nation's representatives signed the Declaration of Alma Ata. By the year 2000 all of humanity was supposed to be immunized against most infectious diseases; basic health care was to be available to every man, woman, and child regardless of their economic class, race, religion, or place of birth. But as the world approaches the millennium, it seems, from the microbes' point of view, as if the entire planet, occupied by nearly 6 billion mostly impoverished Homo Sapiens, is like the city of Rome in 5 BC. 'The world really is just one village. Our tolerance of disease in any place in the world is at our own peril,' Lederberg said. 'Are we better off today than we were a century ago? In most respects, we are worse off. We have been neglectful of the microbes, and that is a recurring theme that is coming back to haunt us.

Manicha: Warrior aggression, especially from the United States, finds expression in research towards 'massive chemical effectiveness' or the so-called selective surgical strike. Have Dr Strangelove–like experiments leaked out of the Pentagon labs and spread all over? All-out economic victory is like an all-out military victory. Is AIDS a naturally occurring disease, or was it concocted by the US military, who 'let' it slip into the wild? The jury remains out ...

Yesterday, I take Anaïs, Petite-Fleur and Diane to the New Orleans restaurant located inside Champaign's train station, to celebrate Anaïs's birthday. Later, we go to hear some blues at the bar. While trains travelling to Chicago and New Orleans are passing above our heads, I write the following poem.

> My body, filled with the poison of chemo,
> is heavy and tired.
> The guitar weeps on the pulses of stars.
> A train passes above our heads,
> going where I shall meet the love of my life.
> Will this season pass?
> Can I be renewed?
> How many more crosses for my little sister?
> She cries out she does not want to be
> just a statistic on a doctor's desk,
> and I scream out my anger with her.
> A sparrow has landed on my breast:
> hope of a flying away beyond the dark clouds.
> In the night, red roses grew.

Diane has made a beautiful vegan cake – it contains no animal derivatives at all – for Anaïs's birthday, and brings it to the restaurant, so we can eat it in the midst of the other people attending the concert. I think, *Only in the US is this done: singing 'Happy Birthday', taking photos and celebrating in the middle of a crowd.* I'm reminded of Simone de Beauvoir's journal of her travels throughout the United States, in which she recalls how people sang 'Happy Birthday' no matter which place she was in. Juanita joins us, and we laugh a lot, share the cake with the diners at the neighbouring table, and have a good time forgetting our miseries for a while.

Manicha: It's true that a strong 'nationalist' feeling exists in the United States, but is it due to the herd mentality; to the 'pioneering' roots of its people; to its hospitality, which is more evident than it is in 'Old Europe'?

10 June 1994

I'm entering a new phase: on Monday, I'm to have surgery. The surgeon can't tell me what kind of operation it'll be: a lumpectomy or a mastectomy. It'll depend on what he finds when he opens up my chest. If it's a self-contained tumour, he'll be able to remove it and only the surrounding tissues. If the tumour has positive margins, it'll mean that cancerous cells are going elsewhere, and he'll have to remove the breast. At any rate, he'll also have to remove the lymph nodes under my arm in order to find out whether they're infected. The doctors have no other way to know except through removing the nodes, and once they the nodes are removed, there's no way they can be put back. I find the practice barbaric, but there's nothing I can say. When I've had the operation, I'll be sent home, and a nurse will come every day for about a week in order to empty the lymph drains that'll be connected to me, under my arm.

A few days ago, I feel very anguished about all this; now, though, I'm relatively calm, and I tell myself that whichever operation is performed, everything will be all right. I don't have a choice anyway, and trust my doctors, especially my surgeon: they're all very competent. I must say I'll be happy when this stage of my trial is over. I see Alban suffering from it all, and I'm hurt. He tells me how barbaric he thinks the procedures are, and he's is so right: for centuries to come, the people of the various societies will probably look back on our society and say, 'How barbaric they were! How horrible were their ways of practising medicine!'

16 June 1994

It's been three days since I had the operation, and I'm trying to remember what's happened. It's the first day I feel strong enough to write. I'm sent home the day after the operation, and I almost pass out when the nurse first comes to change my dressings and empty the lymph drains. Hospitals send people home very early in order to reduce the insurance companies' costs, but is this a good thing when the patient is still very weak? It's good I have my sweet Alban with me, but what of the people who don't have someone to take care of them?

I'm trying to remember the details of what's happened: I'm in the operating room, in the surgical unit, just before the operation, and I'm still awake. I hear music, and make some comments about it. The anesthesiologist tells me he sings, and I tell him I'm also a singer. Then I fall asleep. I wake up in the operating room, and put my hand on my breast. I immediately know it's gone. Strangely, I feel at peace, and go back to sleep. In the recovery room, I wake up slowly, and talk with the nurse, who's checking me by taking my pulse and seeing how I'm doing. She doesn't know much about my condition, or about what's been done to me. She tells me that my doctor will tell me everything.

Later, I learn that Dr Yoto, my surgeon, tried to do a lumpectomy. However, when he sent the tumour to the lab and was told there were too many positive tissues around it, he had to make the decision. He took into consideration that he'd already removed a quarter of my breast anyway, closed the incision and performed the mastectomy. From now on, then, I belong to all my sisters who've been breast mutilated: Amazons crossing Amazonia; one breast cut off, the other flowing freely in the wind.

After the operation, I wake up in a lot of pain. I'm given tranquillisers, which in the United States they call painkillers. It's amazing how, in the context of illness, everything is charged with war connotations. Chemotherapy was discovered during World War 2 as a result of use of nerve gas. During the war, nitrogen mustard gas exploded aboard a submarine, and the sailors who'd been exposed to it became ill and were found to have had most of their white blood cells destroyed. Because leukemia is characterised by an over-abundance of white blood cells, doctors wondered whether nitrogen gas could stop unwanted white blood cells from proliferating, and that's how chemotherapy was invented.

I wish that different, milder cures for cancer existed. My whole self – body, mind and spirit – rebels against this 'war' aspect of the disease, as well as against other aspects of it, but especially against this one, because I'm a pacifist and can't condone violence.

After the operation, I'm taken all the way to the hospital's eighth floor, to the pediatric ward, with the children. The room features an armchair that can be made into a bed, which Alban will be able to sleep in. Jim arrives. He explains that Dr Yoto has said the operation went well: the mastectomy was well performed; no tumour was found elsewhere; the tumour's margins were clean, and the nodes looked clear; however, the doctors couldn't know for sure until they'd had the lab examine the nodes more closely.

I receive a beautiful bouquet of flowers, from the French department of my university. I'm alone in the room, with Alban. Several people come to visit us. Juanita, who Alban and I have nicknamed Dolorès, comes and makes us laugh by telling her funny stories, in one of which she describes a bed that 'pops up' when you open it – only America could have a gadget such as that! Ramin and Petite-Fleur follow, and they're more solemn: they have a tender look that's filled with complicity. Dr JE also visits me for a few minutes, to see how I'm doing; later, I notice she's billed me $60 for the visit. I thought the visit wasn't really necessary: I'd rather have seen my surgeon.

In the night, a child is screaming, and I wonder what he's suffering from. I start feeling pain in my stomach as well as in various parts of my body. I worry about the antibiotics the doctors have given me: is it the drug that in the past gave me bad pains, followed by tests through which it was revealed I had diverticulitis – a problem to do with veins in the colon? I ring for a nurse, who comes and gives me an injection – probably some other painkiller, which sends me back to sleep. I'm glad I have Alban with me: my sweet love, sleeping on the couch in the same room.

The next morning, Diane comes to take us home from the Share clinic. I'm sent home in a wheelchair, as a precautionary measure so the clinic can't be accused of neglect if I were to pass out while I was leaving the premises – after all, I'm still on the clinic's territory! Once I step out of that territory, I do so at my own risk. The staff members give me cute balloons 'to cheer me up' and let me know they 'care'. The balloons are tied with a string; one of them is in the shape of a heart, and the other is inscribed with the message

'At Share, We Care' – again, to boost my morale, to demon-strate the clinic staff's great concern, even though by casting me back out into the world they're demonstrating the exact opposite!

Madeleine: What a mentality! It's a perfectly aberrant and ridicu-lous combination of commercialism and childish 'dumbing down'!

I give the balloons to Diane. I think that rather than give them to me, it would've been better if the clinic staff had kept me there an extra day and made sure I was all right – but, of course, staying would've been more expensive! And we're in America.

Manicha: Incredible: publicity balloons, like the ones you used to get when you bought a pair of Bata shoes! Because you're a liv-ing ad, maybe you should go around bare breasted; that way, your 'product' would have more effect on future 'consumers'.

Today, we have a surrealistic day: Diane brings us a macro-biotic soup that contains melon, strawberries, cucumbers and mint, and it tastes insipid. The only thing that has some taste in it is the mint. 'They haven't succeeded in changing the taste of mint yet,' notices Alban, who's always able to say something humorous and sarcastic in these situations. I adore this man, and I love it when he gets excited and talks about things volubly, especially when he's discussing some-thing with Waïl. Alban is very Mediterranean.

In the afternoon, the nurse returns. She came the day after my operation, and I almost passed out when she was emp-tying my drains. She didn't seem to know what she was doing, she didn't have the necessary equipment, and we even had to look into Alban's little pharmaceutical kit to find some ointment and bandages. And because I felt so weak and helpless, and she was so unconfident, slow and hesitant, my 'post-op' state was only exacerbated, to the point that I fainted. Today, she comes at the same time as does the Reach to Recovery nurse. The two women have a lot to talk about, and seem happy to be meeting around me.

The Reach to Recovery nurse brings me, compliments of the American Cancer Society, a floral-print bag, which she tells me has been sewn by volunteers. In it, there's a small cushion made out of a fabric printed with little blue flowers, which, the nurse tells me, is 'to use when you lie down, and place where the breast used to be.' She also gives me a little ball that's hanging on a string, for me to use to exercise my arm and prevent it from becoming numb as a result of the lymph nodes' removal. Finally, she gives me some little pockets, which I'm to fill with some sort of cotton wool and pin in my bra. *Pitiful!* I think, but don't say, to this woman, whose good intentions I find touching; instead, I thank her, and ask her about herself, because I know that hospital volunteers such as she are women who've had a mastectomy or lumpectomy themselves.

The volunteer tells me she underwent her mastectomy when she was 48, and that her sister underwent one when she was 50. When I say I think there's a breast-cancer epidemic, she responds in the same way that most people respond around here reason: that we notice the cancer more because it's detected earlier! However, this kind of reasoning doesn't make any sense. If the cancer is detected earlier, why do so many mastectomies have to be done, and why, despite the fact that breast cancer is being detected ever earlier, has the death rate from it remained unchanged?

The question we could also ask is *Why does society want to hide the truth about the epidemic proportions of today's cancer rates?* Naturally, we have the authority of the practitioners within the medical establishment, but why aren't they telling us the truth? Don't they know it? It's very likely they aren't even aware of what's going on – there are so many bureaucrats among them. However, it could also be that they want to hide the truth about the death rate, so they don't worry their patients or seem to be critical of society. In that mindset, it's very important to belong to the group, not to distinguish yourself from it and not to 'rock the boat', whereby if practitioners were to speak out, the bureaucrats – in the insurance companies, hospitals and other institutions – might marginalise them.

What we're dealing with is the American cult of consensus, in which the bureaucracy is just as terroristic as that of the former USSR, and its non-conformists are deprived of work. People are permitted to have their individual fantasies but are forbidden to question society: the two things are dialectically linked. In the end, the doctors are accomplices; for example, the only question they ask a patient might be whether cancer antecedents exist within his or her family, whereas we know that the percentage of hereditary cancers is very small. They should also ask the person about his or her diet, hormones and lifestyle, and study any environmental factors. When they don't consider these factors, they're conspiring to remain silent: accomplices in covering up what's necessary for the social good. In World War 2, the German people knew about the gas chambers but kept quiet. Of course, the conditions back then were much more difficult; however, it remains a striking analogy.

Manicha: It isn't a heresy to draw a parallel between the forming of a consensus between, on one side, doctors and our consumer society, and on the other, and the German people with Nazism. Of course, to rise against Hitler meant death, whereas I believe that to rise against today's anti-human system costs you your social status and profession: the 'order of doctors' is watching!

I think to myself, *Would I be able to mobilise women such as these two hospital staffers to take political action?* At the time,

I think not: they're too caught up in the system to want to change it; however, when I think about it more, I'm not so sure. At any rate, there's something about this big, Midwestern woman who works at the hospital that I find oddly touching. She boasts that she hasn't had to stop any of her activities because of her breast cancer; in fact, since she's recovered, she's been engaging in them as never before. She's even doing extra work, such as her volunteering to help other women who've had a mastectomy as a result of having breast cancer. Her activity in this area is effectively pointless and ridiculous, and yet poignant. In what other society could you ever see something like it? Considered in the context of the country's fabulously huge hospital budgets and the hospitals' outrageously inflated charges, these knick-knacks made by volunteers, which are unworthy of even the 'junkiest' airport gift shop, are simply pathetic! What I find so revolting is this colossal deception of a community of simple people who fail to understand what's happening to them at the hands of the techno-scientists, who continue to shamelessly make use of trivial symbols of solidarity in order to 'dull down' and daze their fellow citizens. This hospital worker's negation of the epidemic and of society's responsibility is organically linked to the social structure.

Jane: You're so right to stress this point: all this 'feel good' silliness, meant to take our minds off the root causes, must be denounced.

Manicha: And what about the NGOs *[non-government organisations]* for development or humanitarian emergency, which are meant to nurse the gaping wounds of Kapital by administering public charity!

I give both the nurses a copy of my first novel, *The Excised* (Accad: 1994), and thank them for their help. I wonder

174

whether they'll read it and what they'll think about it: two middle-class women from the Midwest, both exploited by the system – they receive a miserable salary: barely $US1000 a month, I'm told – but not questioning it or wanting to change it. One of them does extra volunteer work, and all of this takes place juxtaposed with the institutional opulence, the doctors' wealth and the American medical establishment, in which mega-millions of dollars are generated. In some of the bills I'm receiving, the doctors are charging as much as $US225 for a consultation during which they did hardly anything except order some tests – for a nurse, $225 is a quarter of his or her monthly salary. It's simply outrageous! I must write about all this: testify, and bring these injustices to light. I call for more and more people to write, denounce and revolt!

Jane: This is the real scandal of the health system in the United States. The same hierarchy is reflected in large American companies in which the CEO's salary is so disproportionate to the rest of the staff's. The discrepancy is by far the largest of all the industrialised countries'. Something akin to this discrepancy is probably reflected in the medical establishment.

18 June 1994

Yesterday, I learn that my lymph nodes were negative, and I'm so happy about the news. For a while, I've been wondering whether cancer has been in me for a long time. Now I know it isn't so, and that the hypothesis I made at the beginning of my 'journey' is probably correct: my cancer was activated, if not created, as a result of the additional artificial estrogen I was prescribed.

My breast has been offered in sacrifice to the gods of modern civilisation. Dr Yoto tried in vain to save it: unsuccessful! failed operation! Admirable surgeon does his best, and is willing to listen and talk; he tries to provide answers, but admits when he doesn't know them! However, seen from my end of the scalpel, he's no more than an especially expert butcher, or one of those ancient high priests who sacrificed their victims according to specific rites.

Today, Cybel and Greg come over with little daughter Daisy. Alban and I are overwhelmed by their thoughtfulness. They bring all kinds of little presents. I recall how they were when their baby was born prematurely and was saved; it was a very intense time. Yet, I couldn't help thinking to myself, *Big medical money can save premature babies in this country, while thousands of malnourished ones are dying all over Africa and the so-called Developing World.* Why shouldn't other infants in the world benefit from all the marvels that medicine has been able to achieve? All children are precious to their parents, but the world is organised so that thousands are being sacrificed. However, why do I have to have these morose thoughts, mixed with my happiness, rather than rejoice with my wonderful friends? Why am I always concerned about the rest of the world? Will my friends be upset with me if and when they read this section of the book?

Because I'm concerned about the world and carry its burden on my shoulders, have I become ill, as someone has suggested to me? I don't believe so, and am revolted at these thoughts. People who say these things to me are highly individualistic and often selfish, or have been disappointed in their struggle and political commitment, and have now done an about-face. They're unable to see that things are complex and involve all kinds of layers, and that the personal is mixed with the political, whereby the two are intertwined in a multiplicity of causes.

Where do I fit in all this? Would this cancer have manifested itself had I lived elsewhere, in another country? How could I know? Had I stayed in Lebanon, would I have experienced it? From what a doctor there told me, the epidemic has reached huge proportions in Lebanon as well. During the war in that country, some militias allowed nuclear and other highly toxic chemical wastes to be buried in the south in exchange for money to buy weapons. The Lebanese people are now paying the price for this sell-out. Even embryos are being attacked with cancer in their mother's womb!

Nazik: Nuclear waste was dumped not only in the south but all over Lebanon!

Manicha: Thanks to the 'senders': France? The US? The West, without a doubt!

19 June 1994

I don't have much energy. I'm half sitting, half lying down on the living-room couch, looking at the trees on the avenue: beautiful trees, swaying at the approach of a storm. I'm re-reading some of the letters and cards that have come in, and admiring the many bouquets and plants of all kinds. I include some letter extracts as follows.

Amel: *Evelyne, my dear one, a week has gone by. Last Sunday, I lived through a day of anxiety. I couldn't move out of bed. Rachida called me in the evening, and decided to call you. What a relief! The following day, there was your letter, telling me your surgery was scheduled for the 13th: exactly the same day and month I became ill. I don't know why, but I knew everything would go well. It must have been hard to live through. In your eyes, there's sadness, but what makes them shine is hope, with the acceptance of suffering. I find your expression much more relaxed. You're very beautiful, Evelyne. You abandon yourself, and the light shows through your smile, your look. Thank you for sending me these pictures; I needed them. Thanks also to Eva* [the photographer] *and to her extraordinary eye. You have such a green garden. It suits you ...*

Watching all the TV shows on Lebanon, I've been thinking of you so much. I saw Andrée Chedid. I liked her. She said she was always impressed by the vivaciousness, the stamina of the Lebanese, their capacity to hope. She quoted a saying: 'Drown a Lebanese in the sea: he'll come out with a fish in his mouth.' I also liked Amin Maalouf a lot. To the cumbersome questions of Pivot [the host of a French literary-talk show] *about exile, he answered, 'It's in one's head that one is exiled, but I never left Lebanon in my head.' He said that the Lebanese had always been travellers. He cited Alyssa, who left with the people from Tyre, to found Carthage. 'I have cousins all over the world,' he said. 'What unites us is belonging to an ideal of planetary community.' He compared Lebanon to 'a sick brother one wants to see healed'. What moved me is this strong attachment to Lebanon from all the participants on the shows, which went on for several days, and also their will to rebuild 'the Lebanon of all communities'. I thought about the multiculturalism conference we attended at Purdue University. It remains a fundamental question: 'How to save plurality when one group tries to dominate the other?' We have a lot to learn from people who aren't subjected to monotheisms ...*

I heard sister Marie Kayrouz sing the gospel according to Saint Matthew. It was beautiful, and this woman is beautiful. Feyrouz also sang in the ruins of Baalback. It was so moving. You were present in all of these meetings ...

Yesterday, after singing at the Club Tahar Haddad, there was a reception organised by the journalists of Amnesty International, for the Palestinians. I spoke with a writer, Liena, who wrote The Stars of Ariha *a year ago. She affected me greatly. She's from Jericho, and I read in her voice, in her look, her joy to be returning there, even for a short time. It's such a strong will, to feel the earth one belongs to under one's feet. I thought of*

Husni a lot. He, also, would like to know Palestine. I have no news from him …

Evelyne, my darling, it will be so wonderful to discover Lebanon, which you've taught me to love before breathing its air … Sometimes I worry about tiring you with all my talking … I send you much warmth, much light …

Françoise: *I didn't expect to hear your voice: so courageous, coming out of the operation. I learnt through Alban that the surgeon had opted for the most radical procedure. I can imagine how hard it must be. But for a writer, what matters is to be able to continue to write, to think – to love and to be loved (and plastic surgery does miracles). But I didn't know, when we left each other this winter, that you'd have to go down such a road. I think of you. I know it's hard. I would have liked to call you sooner from Brazil, where I'd gone for a colloquium in Rio, but I hadn't brought my address book. In spite of its 25 degrees Celsius winter and the beauty of its landscape, Rio distressed me, with its contrast between wealth and misery, which borders on barbarism: apolitical and amoral misery, where unforeseeable violence reigns.*

Marcel: *Let me know about how your recovery is coming along, if you're able to, of course, because I do realise how helpless one can feel sometimes in these circumstances. Above all, know that even after these years of silence, of distance, I've regularly continued thinking of you … and this is what counts: this presence across time.*

David Bruner: *I don't know much what to say or do. I do understand the rage one feels with the evils and betrayals, etc., and I'm even more in admiration of you for your continuing efforts. I played a few moments of the interview we taped back in 1991 for Nawal El Saadawi, just to let her see and hear you. It was a bittersweet moment for her, and for Charlotte and me of course, and therefore we kept it brief.*

179

I feel calm now that the cancerous tumour has been removed and the lymph nodes were negative. I've been very scared; I couldn't understand anything any more. I'll have to watch the other breast.

Séverine has also had her lymph nodes operated on, and is in pain. She comes over the day before her operation, to see me and talk. Alban asked her to stay with me while he was doing something over on campus. I feel very close to Séverine. On this day, we share our memories of our early days in the university department: SJ screwing in his office in the evening – Séverine was so fed up with the noise, because her office was next to his, she asked him to take a hotel room; and FL and TG and their orgies. What crazy years: difficult for both of us new and inexperienced women, entering a highly competitive system and being in the early days of working out our identity!

I have four questions to ask the doctors tomorrow: (1) 'Is radiation necessary?' (2) 'If it is, why?' (3) 'What are the studies about it?' (4) 'Can reconstruction be done after radiation?' (5) 'If it can be done, how long after?'

Petite-Fleur isn't doing well. She comes with Ramin, who's talking about his love affairs. He tells us that he's been accused of raping someone, although according to him, it was the woman who was the aggressor. Petite-Fleur tries to explain the reasoning that a woman could have about being forced into having sex. Alban thinks she's accusing Ramin, and gets upset. I find it amazing that Alban can get into such a rage about this. He tells me he doesn't like it when people are accused unjustly, and that he's exasperated at the way Petite-Fleur has gone about accusing him. According to Alban, what she's actually saying is, 'You aren't guilty according to the facts; nonetheless, you're guilty according to feminine subjectivity.' Her ways remind him too much of Stalin's methods, and it's the spectre of that dictator that infuriates him. You can't judge if there aren't positive elements, or positive acts; nor can you make your judgement based on subjective content, even if someone such as Ramin completely recognises its importance. However, Ramin doesn't seem to be upset by the discussion; he even acts rather amused, and happily answers Petite-Fleur's questions. My sweet Alban leaves the room, and Ramin and Petite-Fleur say goodbye. Everyone's on edge at present, and tired, on top of it all.

Petite-Fleur still doesn't know what's wrong with her health: she's been told it could be leprosy, tuberculosis, lupus or even some kind of myco-bacterial infection. She's already been sent to many places: the Nesbitt Clinic and another clinic, located in Indianapolis; now they want to send her to Chicago. She perceives that some of her doctors are genuinely racist towards her because she comes from 'over there': the so-called Developing World, even though she's lived almost all her life in Belgium. They treat her as if she's stricken by plague. I find it ironic that the real plague of this century, cancer, is being manufactured mainly in the States – as well as in the other industrialised countries – and yet the medical profession considers the people of the Developing World to be the producers of plagues and epidemics, against which the West must protect itself by taking all kinds of control measure at its borders.

Jane: To a lesser extent, men feel the same way about women: they view them as being more 'prone' to disease, and as being 'carriers' of infection.

22 June 1994

I often wake up feeling anxious. Fortunately, my love is by my side. His smile, warmth and presence are so comforting. Last night, I dream I'm trying to get into my Paris apartment, on Rue Ganneron, but that Jean and Marie are telling me there's still someone there, and that anyway, it isn't easily accessible at the moment. As for them, they've moved to the first floor, into a 40 square metre apartment. I tell them it's much bigger than my apartment; Marie, however, argues that it isn't – that they've measured both apartments. She's grading some papers, and Jean is waiting behind the door and telling us about his anxieties. Their apartment is very well arranged and sunny, whereas mine is dark and seems inaccessible.

I must be depressed about not being in my apartment. Usually, at this time of the year, I'm in my little apartment overlooking Paris's Montmartre Cemetery, and writing.

26 June 1994

We have dinner at the Rbeizes'. Their daughter, Nathalie, who's pregnant, is finishing a thesis about treating cancerous tumours by way of administering a new type of chemotherapy, a sort of pesticide her father has discovered. He and his colleagues are able to inject it into the tumours of mice, and when the injected mice are placed under a light, their tumours disappear. It's a photodynamic process: malignant cells absorb more of the product than do normal ones, and are destroyed as a result of the photodynamic effect. Nathalie tells me that the Canadians have started using the product to treat cancer, but that in the States, it'd take about 10 years for the FDA (the Food and Drugs Administration) to approve the product. At tonight's dinner, we all think that if Nathalie has already found such a remedy, there must be many other possibilities for dealing with the disease: solutions other than the usual 'Poison, cut and burn'. If more research were conducted via more funding, and more researchers were committed to finding solutions, we'd see a glimpse of hope.

Later, as I'm doing more research into cancer, I read (*Cancernet*: last modified in September 1993) that this treatment, which is also called PDT (photodynamic therapy),

... is often combined with laser surgery. Lasers can be used in two ways to treat cancer: by shrinking or destroying a tumor with heat, or by activating a chemical – known as a photosensitizing agent – that destroys cancer cells. In PDT, a photosensitizing agent is retained in cancer cells and can be stimulated by light to cause a reaction that kills cancer cells ... Lasers are used to treat several kinds of cancer ... for breast cancer, it is becoming more common and may result in a shorter hospital stay and less pain for the patient ... The photosensitizing agent injected into the body is absorbed by all cells. The agent remains in or around tumor cells for a longer time than it does in normal tissues. When treated cancer cells are exposed to red light from a laser, the light is absorbed by the photosensitizing agent. This light absorption causes a chemical reaction that destroys the tumor cells. There are several promising features of PDT: cancer cells can be selectively destroyed while most normal cells are spared, the damaging effect of the photosensitizing agent occurs only when the substance is exposed to light, and the side effects are relatively mild ... Researchers are looking at different laser types and at new photosensitizers to increase effectiveness ... As more cancer surgeons become trained in laser use and the technology improves, lasers may make increasing contributions to cancer treatment.

I can't help but wonder how things might've been if only they'd tried this treatment on my breast. I have a feeling it might have been saved, and I wouldn't have suffered so terrible a torture.

Today, I call Dr WI, the Milwaukee doctor who treated Théophile, and the doctor who told me I should have a double mastectomy. I ask him what he thinks about the treatment I'm having. He says that it seems excellent to him, and that it's the way that breast cancer is being treated nowadays, starting with chemotherapy. He thinks I should have radiation because of the size of my tumour, because the risks of a return is thereby reduced. He also tells me that estrogen must surely have accelerated my tumour's growth and inflamed the tumour. Referring to his believing in the afterlife, he adds that we're lucky we have the hope of meeting 'up there' some day.

When I tell Jay and John, who are visiting Alban and me, that in the twenty-first century, people will view today's procedures as being barbaric, Jay says I'm being optimistic: he doesn't believe things will be that much better in the future.

At one point, when I'm talking to Jay, I become sad when he tells me he's looking forward to death as being a great rest. It isn't that he wants to die or that he's thinking about committing suicide; rather, it's that he isn't scared at the thought of dying, and even yearns for it, because he's often tired by existence. Alban and I later conclude that Jay isn't really happy.

Manicha: The 'neither sad nor happy' state – without stirring passion – leads to a 'fatigue' about living. Repetition dulls one's taste for things. If one looks outside of oneself and gets interested in the world, there's little else but unresolved conflicts, of 'race', of class, between countries and so on. It's discouraging to see things getting repeated ... There's no progress.

I'm always slightly saddened to see Jay whenever we've visited since we divorced. He's gained weight, and he's no longer the attractive young man I knew in my adolescence. Although he still has bright, shining eyes and a wonderful, quick sense of humour, he moves slowly, and I worry about his health, because his father died of a heart attack when he was only slightly older than Jay is now. Jay tells me about the time he drank, before Alcoholics Anonymous helped him overcome his addiction. In those days, he got up in the morning and started by downing a Screwdriver or Bloody Mary in order to get back into shape from the previous evening; he then spent the whole day drinking, and continued into the evening, after which he passed out. Sometimes, he woke up in places he couldn't remember he went to.

I'm saddened when I think that Jay isn't happier in his life. I'd much prefer so see him accomplished and fulfilled. He tells me he's happy now, that he's stopped drinking completely: he doesn't even have a drop of alcohol on special occasions. He tells me this is what excessive people have to do: quit completely; otherwise, they fall back into the habit. I've always thought that if Jay had put his madness, his crazy excesses, into his art, he'd have become one of the twentieth century's great artists. All his teachers and professors agree about this. Because of his talent, his imagination, his fantasies, his humour and his patience for creating tiny details, he produced incredible paintings and drawings. What could have happened? What is it that cracked within him to convince him he was doomed to fail?

And why is it that in Tunis several years before, during my group-therapy session with Angelo, it was because I was remembering my relationship with Jay that I cried so much that I couldn't stop? I remember that the other group participants surrounded me with their comforting touch and feelings of concern that I be able to express my pain at having lost a friend, partner and husband. It was as if I'd never been able to express the pain I'd been feeling over the years. It was as if, all of a sudden, Angelo, who senses people's problems in an amazing way, was challenging me to express them. Is this knot in my past one of the places I visit in my dreams? Must I untie it in order to heal completely? Do we ever overcome our past wounds completely? Do we ever heal completely?

All types combined, the incidence of cancer in the United States rose 49.3 percent between 1950 and 1991. This is the longest reliable view we have available. If lung cancer is excluded, overall incidence still rose by 35 percent. Or, to express these figures in another way: at mid-century a cancer diagnosis was the expected fate of about 25 percent of Americans – a ratio Carson found so shocking that it inspired the title of one of her chapters – while today, about 40 percent of us (38.3 percent of women and 48.2 percent of men) will contract the disease some time within our lifespan. Cancer is now the second leading cause of death overall, and the leading cause of death among Americans aged thirty-five to sixty-four. (Steingraber: 1997: 40)

Many of the cancers now exhibiting swift rates of increase – cancers of the brain, bone marrow, lymph nodes, skin, and testicles, for example – are not related to smoking. Testicular cancer is now the most common cancer to strike men in their twenties and thirties. Among young men both here and in Europe, it has doubled in frequency during the past two decades. These increases cannot be attributed to improved diagnostic pratices. Brain cancer rates have risen particularly among the elderly. Between 1973 and 1991, brain cancers among all Americans rose 25 percent. Those over sixty-five suffered a 54 percent rise. (Steingraber: 1997: 41)

There are eight cancers whose incidence and mortality are both on the decline: those of the stomach, pancreas, larynx, mouth and pharynx, cervix, and uterus, as well as Hodgkin's disease and leukemia. (Steingraber: 1997: 41)

We have undoubtedly consumed more, polluted more and depleted more of our natural resources in the last fifty years than in the previous ten thousand centuries. Misery has grown in proportion to the population on many points of the globe. (Séralini: 1997: 219)

6

RADIATION

MY BODY LIKE A BATTLEFIELD

They abandoned me in that darkened room, lit only by the reddish ray of the lasar that split my body and the glow of the multicolored buttons as they blinked on and off. I knew that radiation was painless, yet I was totally terror-stricken. They were going to forget about me. They would find nothing but a little pile of radioactive ashes ... The story that Rivke had told the night before in a burst of laughter suddenly came back to me: 'I saw Sonia last week. She thanked me once again: "Thanks to you, in Auschwitz, I was really lucky. Thanks to the solidarity of your Communist friends, you found me a good job in 'Canada', in a warehouse next to the gas chambers where I sorted, washed and ironed the clothes of Jews who were arriving from all the cities of Europe, straight from the train to the gas chamber. Then the clothes were distributed among the Germans. As for us, we stole, we bartered, we organized, we ate a little. Thanks to you, Rivke, I survived ..."'
(Francos: 1983: 98)

Urbana, 1 July 1994

I feel that the worst has passed. I'm getting back on my feet slowly, despite the pain in my arm and my chest wall. I'm an

188

Amazon, and I'm wearing the warrior marks. I'm already looking forward to leaving for Paris.

Yesterday, I have a dream that mother let herself die because she missed father too much. I also miss father a lot. In time, we'd learnt to trust each other. We could discuss many things about our past misunderstandings, and in the end we communicated well. I learnt a lot from him. He advised me about how to invest the small amount of money I'd saved over the years, and it's thanks to him that I purchased real estate. Like many Middle Eastern people, my father was convinced it was best to invest in things that couldn't be destroyed through war: things such as land and gold. Poor father, though: due to the war in Lebanon, many of the houses he'd built by the sweat of his brow – he had very few means – were destroyed. However, I never saw him shed tears at losing the houses, whereas my uncle who'd invested with him did. Father believed that they were only material things, and that the real riches where to be found in heaven. Nevertheless, when he was on this earth, he invested in it. Mother was less materialistic, and would gladly have given up all her possessions if father had allowed her to. Father was convinced that the other best thing to invest in was education, because no one could take it away from you. I remember that when he came to visit me at the University of Illinois, he was very impressed with the main library. His whole face glowed as he ventured into the rows of books stacked on the shelves, and he told me he wished he'd had the opportunity in his life to study in an environment like that. I wish I could've helped him meet his wish! In the end, he suffered so much as a result of this awful disease, which was eating away at his bones. It hurts me to think about it.

I must tell the story about some of my life-insurance agents, who I won't name but I hope will recognise themselves.

Alban: They'll recognise themselves, because they're all the same!

So-called life insurance is really about death, and should therefore be called death insurance. Some insurance agents are treating me in a disgusting and racist way. One of them says, 'You're at greater risk because you travel to the Third World, so we have to raise your premium.' I respond that people who live in New York face just as many risks. The other day, a pair of agents visit me in order to sell me more insurance, on top of the policy I already hold with the university. When they learn I've been operated on – the secretary's told them! – they ask me what kind of surgery I've undergone. I tell them it was for breast cancer, and that I had a mastectomy. They quickly change their mind about wanting to sell me insurance. *So much the better*, I think. Why do they waste my time? And why, many other times, have I been duped and persuaded to buy extra coverage that I subsequently lost because I didn't agree with the companies' policy and ways of tricking me? *Good riddance*, I think. I must warn other people not to be taken in by these 'good talkers', who are interested in only taking money and not giving back what they promise they'll give.

Cindy: You have to be more specific in order to help your readers understand this point.

Originally, I buy a policy whereby I'm given excellent coverage through an agent I believe I can trust. The following year, the agent leaves the company and is replaced by another man, who contacts me about changing my policy in order to enhance my retirement benefits. My premiums are raised, and in the event I die, my benefits are lowered. At the time, I'm not cunning and careful enough to realise I'm being tricked and losing money. Several years later, I'm contacted again, by yet another agent from that company. At that point, I should question the seriousness of a company the agents for which change so often; however, I don't know enough about business to understand I'm being tricked.

When I realise I've lost money by changing so many times, and am fed up as a result of the previous agent's racism, I want to cancel my policy completely. However, if I decide to do that, I lose all the money I've invested up to that time: about $2000, which would be non-refundable and therefore a means through which the company keeps its clients bound to it. Also, one agent tells me that life-insurance companies managed to 'pull through' in the midst of the Great Depression of the 1930s, and were 'safer' than other investments, because many families never claimed the benefits they were entitled to. Sounds familiar, doesn't it? – similar to the story of the Swiss banks and the heirs of the Holocaust victims. I'm therefore warning you, my readers, to be extra careful when an insurance agent is presenting you with a policy you think might not be *bona fide*. Trust your feelings and instincts!

Manicha: Things being what they are, who can tell whether, in the future, these insurance outfits will still be here to pay out their policy holders? Perhaps they'll be absorbed and gone, like other retirement policies that people thought would be eternal: nothing is sure, and everything's in flux!

6 July 1994

I'm flying between Chicago and Seattle, along with my sweet love. It's one of our thousands of honeymoons.

Yesterday, I receive some markings in preparation for having radiation at the Share clinic. The technicians don't let Alban into the room to be with me, even though having the markings isn't the 'real thing': radiation, during which 'healthy' people are at an increased risk of becoming decidedly unhealthy. I'm upset as a result, and at least five times ask the technicians to let Alban come in. My radiologist, Dr LE, is the first person to tell me that a support person isn't allowed in during the procedure because it's like being in an operating room. The technicians then tell me the same thing. I feel as if I've entered a different world, which consists of high-tech machines used for measuring me, taking films of my 'hot spots', and showing images that are a bit like the ones that in the early 1990s were beamed to TV screens during the Gulf War in order to reveal where the 'smart' bombs were falling.

Jane: The people who invent medical terms borrow words that are associated with war, such as painkillers, and the people who invent war terms borrow words from medicine; for example, in the so-called surgical strikes that the Israelis made in Lebanon, only the intended target was meant to be killed, and collateral damage was meant to be avoided! In cancer-related medicine, the intended target is the tumour; however, we know that much collateral damage – both physical and psychological – is involved.

Manicha: And what about the trauma?

I feel all this precision high technology being laid on me, and am not reassured; on the contrary, I remember reading Ivan Illich, who remarks that although the cost of medical technology has risen to billions of dollars, people's health hasn't been especially improved. I feel as if I'm a prisoner of the whole system, despite the fact that the technicians and other people around me are being very kind.

I notice that there are differences between the chemo room and the radiation room. The chemo room has an aquarium that's full of fish; armchairs that could be opened out to be beds; friendly nurses; ugly IV drips in which the 'health' poisons slowly descend; and wounded and hurt human beings sitting around, looking at each other compassionately and in commiseration. Somehow, I find the scene less threatening. The radiation room, on the other hand, has huge machines; pop music blaring out; and an overly made-up female technician and a contemporary-looking male technician measuring, photographing, and working with high-tech computers. I have the feeling I'm in a spaceship filled with scary nuclear weapons.

At one point, one of the technicians becomes angry with me. He's left the room for what seems like ages. I feel claustrophobic, revolted at being attached to and measured by machines, and have to go to the toilet. I decide I want to see Alban, so, with all the tubes still glued to me, I sit up and climb down from the table I've been placed on. The technician comes in as I'm about to 'cut loose' and tells me that what I'm doing is dangerous. He therefore helps me get down. Because the toilets are in the other room, I'm able to see my Alban.

The session then starts all over again. It's difficult, because I have to keep my arm bent above my head: the arm that still hurts a lot as a result of the mastectomy and removal of the lymph nodes. The technicians tell me they have to 'mark' me with little tattoos that won't wash away, because in about a week I'll be coming back to have the radiation treatment.

I don't like having these little, blue ink dots on my skin: together with my mutilated chest, they're a constant reminder of the disease I have. Perhaps I could accept them better if they were mauve and heart shaped!

Dr LE tells me he hasn't seen such a large tumour in four years! This is just what I didn't want to hear – especially because now I've had the chemo, the tumour should've shrunk more! When I ask him what he thinks could have caused the tumour to be so big, he doesn't reply. I ask him whether he thinks that blood has entered and fed the tumour from the inside. I've been reading that tumours grow more quickly when they're nourished by blood, and in my pathology report, I read that my breast has a blood clot in it. Also, when I was taking the estrogen, I hemorrhaged a lot. I immediately think, *The estrogen is the origin of all my problems*: *growth of the tumour, hemorrhaging, and cancer*. However, Dr LE doesn't say anything about that.

Fortunately, when I've had the markings, Alban and I see my surgeon, Dr Yoto. Compared with my other doctors, he's much more reassuring and frank. He's pleased with the scar, and says 'It's healing well.' He's happy that my lymph nodes were negative. I tell him that Dr JE has said that the reason could be that because I've had chemo, the already existing cancer could've been destroyed, and that we can't be sure the nodes were totally negative because I was subjected to chemo before they were removed in order to check them. He says that if some cancer had been present, the doctors would have observed it and mentioned it in their pathology report. Even though malignant cells were being destroyed as a result of chemo, traces of their destruction would be evident. According to Dr Yoto, my lymph nodes were clean, and contained no traces of cancer infection. He expresses his surprise at seeing a tumour having come so quickly and growing so fast. He explains that when he operated, he noticed that the cancer was located in many places rather than one well-defined tumour. He says it was a *multi-focal tumour*, and that he had to perform a mastectomy in order to ensure he removed all the malignant tissue. He also tells us he noticed that my breast contained a lot of fibrocystic tissue. He says that after the operation, my margins were clear of any cancer, and tells me he's confident he removed all the malignancy.

10 July 1994

We're flying between Seattle and Chicago, returning from our honeymoon. My love has a headache, and we're complaining to the flight attendant that we didn't get the seats we'd hoped for: in a window aisle, so we could look at the landscape below as well as at Mount Rainier, Seattle's unusual mountain that looks like Mount Fuji. The attendant explains that we missed out because the plane was fully booked.

However, our stay with Anaïs is delightful. She lives in a romantic little house located near a lake that's peppered with ducks, geese, seagulls, boats and sailors. Her housemate, Jessica, is about my age and has a daughter who's about Anaïs's age. Jessica has spells of depression and is on one of the anti-depressant drugs from the Prozac family – the United States' number-one pharmaceutical, which is closely followed by the estrogen–progesterone cocktail – I'll call it the EPC – I was given, after which my catastrophe commenced. When people are on Prozac, they feel 'high', but when they stop taking it, they enter a big depression. In the States, the drug is now widely used to treat people for depression; according to Anaïs, even the pastor of her former church is on it.

Prozac comprises fluoxetin, an active molecule that works on serotonin, which is one of the brain's major mood neuro-mediators. Depression is often associated with serotonin deficiency, which the medication is used to redress. Many people now view Prozac as being the 'happiness pill'. The reason they do is because fluoxetin is the first commercialised anti-depressant to work by way of only one pill a day, and people who take it suffer very few side effects such as nausea and weight gain. In some cases, it even acts as an appetite suppressant and therefore a weight reducer. Also, the risk that the patient will overdose is almost zero, and this is an important factor when we consider that the drug is often prescribed for very depressed people.

Prozac is now the 'yuppie' drug. Having 'been there and done' the individualistic adventures of the 1960s, we're now witnessing a quest for risk-free happiness and peaceful management of our human drives. Prozac isn't only a molecule that 'chases the blues away': in some cases, the patient's true personality is revealed. People who've never been very happy, who have a 'controlled' personality, who are often altruistic and who function through guilt might become depressed. One day, they break down and become truly depressed. When they take an anti-depressant, they discover they're happy and experience a feeling of fullness of life that they've never before known. For the first time in their life, they feel as if they're 'themselves'. On Prozac, they find a life they never thought they could have – it's almost as if they've been wearing dark glasses that are suddenly removed. Because the drug was revealed to have these effects, it took on a magical aura. Its effects were proliferated as a result of its commercial success, and probably also via the American media machine.

Later, I read that when people take these *psycho-tropes* over a long period of time, cancer can be provoked.

Two years ago, Jessica's partner left her, at a time when her research also wasn't going well; it was just beginning to improve when she was fired. She now wants to change her life completely, because she believes she's failed. Will she be able to 'change gears' and make her life have meaning? At 69, her mother died from having a type of skin cancer through which people die very quickly. Jessica's daughter lives with a woman who has advanced breast cancer that she's been battling with for four years. The woman has a four-year-old child, and probably contracted the disease while she was pregnant. Now she's dying, and she's only 29! How sad it all is: I feel as if I'm surrounded with cancer.

I could've become sad due to many things on this trip if I hadn't been with my wonderful Alban, and visiting sweet Anaïs. One instance of sadness is when we visit Gerald, who's aged so much I barely recognise him. Thirty years ago, at Beirut University College, he taught me theology. He has prostate cancer now, but hopes it's under control. Not long ago, he had to have his testicles removed because his blood's tumour markers – PSA: Prostate Specific Antigen – were high, whereby it was indicated that the cancer was climbing. We tell Gerald and his wife, Amalia, that my father died of the same kind of cancer, which metastasised to his bones. We share our memories.

Our visit to Melanie, Anaïs's 'lab chief', is equally sad. We wonder why she's invited us, and I think it's probably because at the lab, Anaïs is valued because she's an excellent researcher. During the visit, Melanie's husband is making passes at a female guest, who's also the chief of a lab, which Anaïs might be joining. Alban, with his usual humour, describes him as being someone 'whose only virtue is to let mosquitoes into the house, so we end up having some entertainment'. I'm worried about the radiation treatment I'll be having, and ask the researchers whether I might not contract other types of cancer as a result. Some cancer researchers responded by saying I might, but only in 20 or 30 years' time. I think to myself, *What a prospect: some consolation!*

The next day, with my sweet Alban, we take a trip to Bainbridge, which is a somewhat dismal little island; however, the boat trip there is wonderful: the view of Seattle; the skyscrapers in the distance; and a host of slow-drifting, multi-coloured balloons.

One day, I read some of my work and sing at Seattle's Elliott Bay Bookstore. Anaïs is there with all her friends;

even Susan, her future boss and lab director, has come along. I'm touched. We visit the city's market. Alban and I laugh: we're in love. He buys me a big bouquet of magnificent, sweet-smelling sweet peas. For a present for Anaïs, we choose a good bottle of Bourgogne wine, some Reblochon cheese and a kind of salmon mousse.

In the evening, with the people from Anaïs's lab, we talk about estrogen, radiation, cancer and tumours. These scientific people put it to me this way: 'It's difficult to say whether estrogen really caused your cancer, even if it seems quite obvious and the most probable factor … And we can't know for sure whether radiation will give you another cancer in 20 to 30 years' time!' All these contingencies and doubts seem to be the condition of this civilisation in our post-modern world. The title of the course that Alban and I are planning to deliver next time is Post-modernity, Literature and Society.

Sitting on this plane, I wonder how I'll commence my book, and whether, for its genre, I should choose the novel or the diary, plain and simple. I contemplate, for example, commencing the novel by paraphrasing the words of my doctor and Alban something like as follows.

The doctor says, 'You were chosen as a victim of this civilisation: someone has to pay the price for its madness. You're its scapegoat, its sacrificial lamb. You have cancer, and you're to receive twentieth-century torture: chemotherapy, surgery and radiation. I've made appointments for you with various doctors. You aren't crying, are you?'

The friend responds, 'I can't believe it; it can' be true: not my love – she was in excellent health; she took good care of herself; we took good care of each other. We ate well, exercised, and had an excellent love and sex life. It must be a mistake. She can't be infected with this disease; it can't be cancer. And anyway, how can you prove it? What makes you say it's cancer?'

The doctor replies, 'It's my opinion.'
The friend asks, 'But an opinion should be based on something, shouldn't it?'

However, when I reconsider this beginning, I find it too shallow: it doesn't reflect the disease's urgency and immediacy. If I choose to write about my experience in fiction form, will my readers find it real enough? How can I convey to the world my anxieties and my message? If I use my diary as the basis for my writing, what if people recognise themselves and get upset with me for talking about them? However, haven't I gotten upset enough to win the right to scream out my pain and suffering, to tell the truth as it is and to shout it to the world as it happened, without censoring myself? Why are people so afraid of hearing and reading the truth? If I write my story as fiction, wouldn't people recognise themselves anyway? What if I use the diary form but change people's names? Why should these dilemmas matter anyway when we're all being confronted with this fatal disease? Aren't I in the United States, the so-called centre of democracy, in which censorship isn't the issue it is in the other countries I've lived and worked in: Lebanon, Egypt and Tunisia? Why should I worry about how and why I write, and most of all about whether people will accept my story? In a 'free' country, why should I have to censor myself?

Jane: Because your freedom ends where other people's rights begin; that's the whole battle in this country, and why lawyers are so damn rich!

13 July 1994

We're back in Urbana, and ever since we've returned, I've been wanting to write. First, Monique arrived with Cindy,

199

and it's wonderful to see them. I'm touched that Monique has travelled all the way from Paris just to be with me during these difficult times, and that Cindy is so kind to have driven her from Chicago to Urbana. I feel as if I'm surrounded with love.

In the afternoon, Alban accompanies me to the radiotherapy session. Someone's substituting for my radiologist, Dr LE, who's on vacation. We ask the replacement radiologist lots of questions. He's accompanied by an intern: a young 'pubescent nitwit' is how Alban puts it. I tell the radiologist that my niece, who works at the Hutchinson Cancer Research Institute, has explained to me that radiation can cause DNA to be destroyed, and that later, other *oncogenes* – cells that produce a tumour – can be provoked as a result of the radiation I'm about to receive. He replies that this explanation isn't completely accurate: when a person has had radiation, a chemical reaction is produced in the cells, and in very rare cases, the result can be a very destructive and usually fatal type of cancer called a *sarcoma*, which is located in the connective tissue of the skin. He adds, however, that this type of malignant tumour is very rare!

He shows me a textbook diagram of the type of radiation I'm to receive. The diagram includes several rays, one of which will slightly graze my lung. However, he doesn't show me a diagram of the final treatment I'm to have at the end of each day's session: an electron beam, aimed at the middle of my chest, that's to penetrate to a depth of 2.5 centimetres. When the doctors have left the room, I turn towards Alban and see that his eyes are red. I ask him what's wrong, and he replies, 'I don't like people touching my love.' I'm upset to see him this way, especially because later he'll have to wait outside again while they keep me for an hour and a half in order to measure me again and redo the markings on my chest wall, which the rays will be aimed at.

I'm lying down, looking at the machines positioned above me. My body's like a battlefield being prepared for bombardment by rays: a dismembered body. I consider the geography of my wounded body, which is to be subjected to rays of both life and death. I wonder how long it will be before other cures for this terrible disease have been discovered. In this cruel civilisation, I'm being poisoned as the earth's being poisoned; we're both being subjected to death and destruction. Poor, fractured, wounded earth.

During the night after this first session, I can't sleep. I'm worried because Alban's departing tomorrow and because I'm haunted by the images of radiation. I'm afraid of the 2.5 centimetres of radiation that are to penetrate my body every day, and afraid that as a result of the radiation, I'll contract other types of cancer that are more terrible than this one. I'm supposed to be being cured but I could end up having a cancer that's more fatal. During this sleepless night, Alban prepares me some chamomile tea to relax me. He shares my sorrow, fears and anxiety, and doesn't want to leave. Cindy, who the next day is to drive him to Chicago's O'Hare Airport, later tells me she didn't know how to pull him out of his sadness.

I go for my second session, and ask to speak to the radiologist again. When I tell him about my fears, he replies that for the moment, this is the best treatment they have: 'Perhaps, in several years, they'll have found better treatments, but right now, it's the best treatment we have.' Monique comes with me. She looks quite upset to be witnessing my physical pain; I've rarely seen her face look so tortured. Even during our most difficult days, when, in our twenties in Indiana, we were struggling with personal and monetary problems, we managed to pull each other out of our depression by making fun of events and places and the people around us. This time, though, we found it hard to laugh.

I tell Monique that I appreciate her coming with me, but

that there's no need for her to come another time and be subjected to my torture. It's enough that one of us has to go
through it, and anyway, she isn't even allowed to enter the
radiation room; instead, she has to wait outside. I'm touched
that she's come to visit me, as I am in the case of all the
friends who've come to be with me during my treatment.
They've been part of my recovery, and I'll never forget the
love, care and friendship they've been showering on me.

15 July 1994

I take Cindy, Monique and Samira to 'happy hour' at the
New Orleans bar. I'm having many anxious moments this
week because I'm having the radiation treatment and failing
to have my questions answered. I'm worrying about
Séverine, who has to have tests done on her colon in order
to find out whether cancer has spread to it. Yesterday, when
I have dinner at Severine's place, Séverine feels nauseous.
She walks me back to my house, which is close by. She
'doesn't want to know' when Salwa is depressed: she can't
do anything about the depression, because she's undergoing therapy with Salwa as her therapist. Tonight, I'm being
soothed: I'm out with my friends – listening to music, sitting
beneath the whistling train rushing to New Orleans, enjoying the jazz rhythms of the music, and being comforted
when I see my friends smiling and laughing. I almost forget
I'm in the middle of a horrendous treatment.

16 July 1994

At the swimming pool today, I see a young woman I've
noticed before who has a prosthesis in place of one of her
legs – she has to remove it in order to swim or to take a
shower. I remember her from before my illness, when I was
shocked at seeing her removable leg. I think, *What courage*

this woman has! Today, it's she who looks at me and my mutilated breast. I feel like talking to her and asking her whether she's lost her leg to cancer, as I've lost my breast to it. However, I don't dare. I look at her for a long time as she's swimming. She seems to be happy and free in the water. I wonder whether I'll become as joyous and serene as she is despite my loss.

18 July 1994

Today, I see Dr JE and ask her about the blood clot in my tumour, which is mentioned in the pathology report. Was the clot what caused the tumour to grow so fast? However, she hasn't even seen the report yet – therefore I show it to her. She says, 'I wish I had an answer: I know you'd like to have rational answers to all your questions.' I tell her that my surgeon, Dr Yoto, has said that if my lymph nodes were infected before the chemo, traces of the infection would have been evident even if the nodes were negative. She responds that the only way the doctors could have known whether the nodes were positive would have been to remove them before I had the chemo treatment and to then 'put them back in' for the treatment, and that this would have been an impossible procedure. However, doctors don't agree about this assessment. I wish they could agree on at least something that seems quite simple. If it's so simple, though, why haven't they found ways to detect lymph-node infection without engaging in the barbaric practice of removing the nodes and leaving the patient mutilated and vulnerable to infection, pain and swelling for the rest of her life?

Dr JE hadn't read my report. She didn't know that the second report, about the 'hormone receptors', was again negative. She seems to be more interested in my intention to write about cancer than in answering my questions. I'm irritated.

Madeleine: What good is this Dr JE if she doesn't even read her patients' records?

For our next consultation, the doctor orders a mammogram of my other breast and a blood test. At the reception desk, when I ask whether the blood test will include detection of cancer, I'm told that it won't. 'Why?' I ask. 'Is there no such thing?' *There must be,* I think to myself.

Madeleine: Of course there is!

'Why not do it, then?' I ask. The receptionist tells me I should wait for Dr JE to come out of her room in order to ask her to add cancer detection to my order for a blood test. I then have to wait 20 minutes to see the doctor again, and to have her approve my request and add cancer detection to the test order. I can't believe I'm having to be 'on my toes' so much: checking everything and having to insist on having procedures. What about the women and men who let themselves go, completely trust their doctor and don't watch what's being done to them, as I completely trusted mine, before I took the estrogen and got cancer?

Fortunately, during Séverine's tests, cancer of the colon hasn't been revealed – only ulcers that'll have to be checked by way of biopsies. She tells me she cried when she heard the word 'biopsies' because the nightmare of cancer came back into her mind. People who haven't gone through the horrors of the disease can't ever understand.

21 July 1994

Today, I see my radiologist, Dr LE, because some of my ribs hurt in the place in which I've been exposed to radiation, and I'm worried that the pain might be as a result of the large amount of radiation I'm receiving. Dr LE tells me that the painful area isn't in the 'field' of my radiation, and that I should take paracetamol to alleviate the discomfort. I think he's taking my complaints too lightly, and am worried. I decide to phone Tracy's father, who specialises in cancer treatments, in order to put my questions to him. When I phone Eva to tell her about my worries, I'm very thankful to her when she suggests I phone him. He apparently specialises in treating cancer by using both the traditional methods – chemo and radiation – and the non-traditional methods of vitamin supplements, improved nutrition and relaxation. He works for one of the Midwest's biggest centres for cancer treatment. When I phone him, he's very kind, and he reassures me by answering my questions very thoroughly. I'm glad I decided to phone him.

I talk with Alban by phone. I wish I didn't cry with him over the phone, and regret that I also cried with Zohreh when I phoned her. However, sometimes it's very difficult to go through my trial alone. I let myself get into 'catastrophic thinking', whereby I get all kinds of notions that I then build on. For better or worse, I have an overly fertile imagination.

The difficult thing about radiation is that it's relentless: I'm having to receive it every day. I can never stop thinking about it; it's always at the front of my mind, no matter what I'm doing. Every day, I have to go under those machines, one of which makes a grilling noise, as if it's burning my skin. Today, I cry my eyes out; I don't even know why, and when I see my mutilated breast, I cry even harder.

While I'm receiving the treatment, I think of the male technicians looking at my chest. I'm not even androgynous, because I don't have a nipple: I have a chest that's been mutilated as a result of 'civilisation'. I think, *Here's a chest that's had its sexuality excised, a chest in which the element of desire has been removed.* Sometimes it's very difficult being so 'hyper-aware' of all this. I yearn for some release, to be able to not dwell on my situation all the time, and to be more trusting of doctors and medicine.

I'm glad that father is no longer here: he would've suffered a lot if he'd known what I'm going through. He taught me, and gave me so much. Augustus and Pierrot didn't understand him. However, it's natural for boys to measure themselves against their father: it's the Oedipus complex at work.

24 July 1994

It's Sunday. Tomorrow, I start having radiation again, and I'm worrying about it. I get only two days off for the treatment: Saturday and Sunday. On Friday morning, I wake up with an unusually sore throat. When I try to swallow my vitamins, some of them get stuck in my throat, and I panic because I'm alone and worried I'll choke. I think I might have a sore throat and be in the early stage of a flu, and because my blood count is down due to the radiation, I decide I'll warn the technician who's supposed to administer the treatment that I could be getting sick. When I tell him, he says that having a sore throat can be one of the side effects of radiation. *So, why haven't I been warned about it?* I think, but I keep the thought to myself. The technician tells me I'd better see Dr LE before I start having the treatment.

After I wait a while for Dr LE, he has me go into his office. He's obviously just come back from lunch. He tells me I'm probably having a reaction to the radiation I'm receiving on the upper lymph nodes, under my collarbone. He prescribes a medicine to numb my throat so I'll be able to swallow. I ask him whether I should be concerned about this reaction. He says, 'No,' and proceeds to show me diagrams of where the rays could be hitting and to explain why my esophagus could have become affected as a result. I should've asked him whether that area can be avoided; however, I'm always intimidated by doctors, and think about what I should've said only after I've seen them.

Manicha: It's intolerable that the overwhelming majority of doctors take patients for idiots: they treat them as their professional 'terrains', and as more or less interesting 'cases'. But it's mainly their training that must be incriminated, like all training of elites: the world of power is a secretive one, in which the practitioners don't share their knowledge – and most of all not with the concerned patient!

When my radiation session is finished, I go to the pharmacist to fill the prescription. The pharmacist, a woman, tells me to take it easy with this medication because it has definite side effects. When I ask her what the side effects are, she replies, 'It can slow down the heart.' *Why*, I wonder, *aren't we told about all these 'side effects' that are so central?* I'm happy that this pharmacist is conscientious enough to tell me. However, I'm extremely depressed as a result of going through all this.

As soon as she hears I'm suffering, Séverine comes to see me, and we cry and cry together: about our fate of contracting cancer, and about the torture we're living. Never, never would I have understood Séverine and other cancer victims if I hadn't gone through this. Séverine asks me whether we've become better people as a result of having cancer. I believe we have – I want to believe we have – and in several ways, we must have. My dear little sister, Séverine: how precious she is, and how much I love her.

Eva arrives, and it's wonderful to have her here. We talk and talk. She especially needs to talk, and I'm happy to listen and thereby get away from my own worries. She tells me about the man she's involved with. She's afraid of the relationship, and has good reason to be. He tries to manipulate her and tell her what to do. The head of their department, Photography, doesn't want her to direct the department any more. He must've guessed that something was going on between the two of them – in fact, Eva is responsible for hiring her new lover. The head, who used to like Eva a lot, is probably jealous of the new love in her life, because he used to like Milo, her deceased husband, and feels protective towards her. The man who Eva is involved with is the opposite of Milo: he antagonises people because he's extremely frank and aggressive. Milo was someone everybody liked, and encouraged the people around him. He remained optimistic in spite of the terrible health problems he developed. I know I wouldn't be where I am academically if it hadn't been for him.

Although Eva's worried about this new relationship, she's very much in love with the man. She grieved so much for Milo that for a while, I worried she'd never emerge from the depression she'd fallen into. Milo and she had been so close and so much in love for many years. I'm glad the new love has snapped her out of her depression; however, I wish it could be someone who was able to give her the confidence in herself she so badly needs.

We spend some wonderful moments together. Eva takes some amazingly sensitive and powerful photos of my mutilated chest, my wound, the scar that's healing, the radiation markings, and my whole self as it's expressing the Calvary I'm going through. It's extremely therapeutic to have her photograph me, and to share with her the statement I'm trying to make through revealing my wounded body, my bleeding soul, my fears about this body that I don't recognise, and my desire to have the world know about it, about what this civilisation does to people, especially to women.

Being photographed is a way of dominating my anxieties and fears, for me to say, 'Look at me: I'm here. This is what you did to me, how your poisoned civilisation poisoned my breast – invaded my whole body with its mad cells.' I think of all the women: Eva's aunt; the dean of her university – so many of them have one or both arms disabled because of breast cancer. It's horrible, the way their arms have swelled. It's horrible that Eva's aunt has lost the use of one of hers and now has to use her other arm to move the disabled arm around, to lift it, to carry it and to change its position. I'd never heard about this phenomenon before. Why are women so quiet about their suffering? I'm discovering a whole world I'd never known before: a world of pain and silent suffering; a world of tears well hidden; a disease that continues to kill a quarter of its victims; unchanged statistics despite all the claims that progress has been made in the area of cancer.

Manicha: Butchery: chemotherapy and radiation are very hard. However, in France, the real ordeal starts later, when you have to make the department of social security recognise you're 50, 70, 80 or 90 per cent incapacitated. Social-security doctors control, skimp, and lower the rates so that patients' rights to be paid benefits in compensation for being forced into unemployment are infringed on. This is especially the case for less skilled tradespeople.

25 July 1994

Eva leaves, and I'm very sad when she's gone. Last night, I sleep very poorly: I think about all the women who are suffering. I take the book about cancer that Alban brought me from France, and start to read about the side effects of radiation: bruises on the arms, cardio-vascular and lung problems, and possibly other radiation-induced cancers. I decide I'll talk to my doctors and try to either modify my treatment or stop it completely. Poor Eva: I wake her up, and she listens to me. We cry together. She encourages me to talk to my doctors and/or stop the treatment, and to trust my gut feelings. I have to take a sleeping pill in order to get back to sleep. When Eva departs the next morning, I'm devastated.

Then, I go for my treatment, after which I see Dr LE. I bring my book about cancer, which is written in French, and ask him lots of questions. He takes time to explain things to me. He says I don't have to worry about getting a swelling, 'fat', arm because the radiation of my lymph nodes is going not under my arm but under my collarbone. Part of my lung might get scarred, but then again, it mightn't. He tells me he's asked the technician to have me turn my head a specific way in order to prevent the ray from hitting my neck, because that action was apparently what caused my sore throat. He gives me an article and a book to read. The article is the report of a study conducted into the effect of radiation on patients who've undergone a mastectomy. After that operation, the chances that cancer will recur on the patient's chest wall are considerably reduced. I feel reassured to have been able to talk to Dr LE. *What power doctors have over us!* I think.

Now I've received the treatment having had my head in the new turned position, I'm no longer suffering from having a sore throat. I'm thinking that if the symptom could've been avoided, why wasn't it avoided from the beginning? Why weren't the technicians more careful? Why didn't they tell me to turn my head? How many other things have I been missing because, being ignorant, I didn't know the technicians were hurting me and that they weren't being as careful as they should be?

Madeleine: Because they work like brainless robots, without thinking, and as long as they don't get the disease, they couldn't care less. It's selfishness: pure and simple.

26 July 1994

I'm feeling that some of the people who are asking me how I am aren't sincere, even when they're telling me they're thinking about me all the time and they know I'll be okay – unlike their assessment of the other people they know who are dying of cancer or other diseases. Their words and tone of voice ring false. Also, why should I feel reassured when other people are dying from this horrible disease? What kind of consolation is that? It's amazing how sensitive I've become to the way people are speaking, and how good I've become at detecting sincerity or lack of it.

When Eva tells me that her doctor wants to surgically remove the cyst on her ovary, I'm revolted. He wants to completely remove her ovary, through a process called *oophorectomy* or *ovariectomy*, which is really female castration.

I first wrote the word 'historectomy', which is wrong, not only in its spelling – it should be 'hysterectomy' – but because in that procedure, both the ovaries and the uterus are removed.

Jane: 'Historectomy' would also mean surgical removal of your story, your history! You definitely must use it some time in one of your poems or novels!

When Eva asks her doctor, 'What if the cyst isn't cancerous: how are you going to put it back in?' he answers, 'You told me you were having pain, didn't you?' To this, she counters, 'I can live with pain, but can I live without my ovaries? I'd like a second opinion: can you suggest someone?' He tells her to ask her friends, and slams the door as he leaves the room. When she tells me the story, I say to her, 'Thank God you didn't go to see someone *he* would've recommended, because most doctors tend to stick together about some issues, and form "little mafias".' She decides to see a doctor in Columbus who, as in Monique's case, tells her that the cysts are functional cysts that come and go according to the menstrual cycle.

I fear that Hadia has been operated on for nothing. Her doctors have removed her ovaries because she too had

211

cysts. She let herself be persuaded to have her ovaries removed because she was afraid. It's a terrible thing to 'go under the knife' just because a doctor says it's necessary. I find it revolting, what some doctors do to women.

Madeleine: For them, it generates money: period! 'Profit' is the operative word here – pun intended.

I'm disgusted with modern medicine.

Later, I read that these operations are performed too often in the States – more than in any other industrialised nation – and that more than half of them are unnecessary. On 17 February 1997, I read (*New York Times*: 10) that in this culture of hysterectomies, many people are questioning whether they're necessary:

Hippocrates thought the uterus wandered and so drove women to hysteria, but in that belief he was the mad one ... The debate over hysterectomy is one of quiet fury. Nobody bombs surgical suites in protest, but for years critics have assailed what they call the hysterectomy industry ... Each year, about 560,000 women in the United States undergo a hysterectomy, a rate that is among the world's highest ... Ms. Coffey, director of Hysterectomy Education Resources and Services, a nonprofit counseling and information organization, contends that the effects of a hysterectomy are profound and that women must be warned of them in detail before undergoing the operation ... She and many others strongly oppose the practice of removing the ovaries along with the uterus, an additional bit of surgery that occurs in the majority of hysterectomies even when the ovaries are perfectly healthy and are still carrying out their endocrinological tasks.

Jane: I heard on the radio that in a new study, the 'benefits' of estrogen-replacement therapy for a youthful skin had been proven! How Faustian the choice is: to exchange your health for eternal youth. Once again, this is America in denial of death!

Today, I hurt and am enraged. Cancer is reaching younger and younger people, but few people are reacting to the news. There's a conspiracy of silence in the face of this disease.

Madeleine: Of course, there's a kind of conspiracy of silence with reference to cancer. And fear has a lot to do with it: don't we still hear, in France today, people spouting euphemisms such as 'He passed away after a protracted illness'? It's just so they don't have to use the 'C' word.

Today, after my radiation session, I'm still very worried, so I decide to try to see my surgeon, Dr Yoto, without having an appointment. I take the elevator to his fourth-floor suite, and ask to speak to his nurse. I ask her whether there's any chance I can see him between two of his appointments. She says she'll try, and she did manage to squeeze me in. I don't have to wait very long. As usual, Yoto is very upbeat and jovial. I tell him I'm worried about the radiation and the many effects it could cause. I ask him whether he thinks it's absolutely necessary for me to continue with the treatment: could I not simply stop the treatment at this stage, because all the cancer's gone?

He tells me he understands that I'm concerned. He doesn't think I'll get a 'fat' arm, because he's performed the operation by making a horizontal cut rather than a vertical or oblique one; surgeons used to make the latter types of cut when 'they didn't know better'. Of course, one can never be sure, but he doesn't think I'll get the 'fat' arm, because I'm healing so well. He prefers me to finish the radiation treatment, 'just in case some cancer cells have escaped on my skin'. Even though he's sure he's gotten rid of all the cancer in my muscles, some cells might've escaped on my skin – he can't tell, because they'd be microscopic. I thank him for taking his time, during his busy day, to speak with me. He's been operating all morning. I notice that he doesn't bill me for these words of wisdom and comfort. I decide to follow his advice and continue the treatment; after all, he was the one who saw, with his own eyes, the precise state of my disease, when I was on the operating table. I also decide to make an appointment to see Dr Land, an oncologist at the Share clinic. One of my friends, Janie, tells me he's also a good communicator, that he takes his time, and that he listens and tries to give answers.

Manicha: One can imagine the state of neglect that cancer patients face when they must 'decide' – or get advice from friends – to see such-and-such a specialist in order to find someone who at last will talk and explain! What an obstacle course! And to think this is the most common disease in the world! What loneliness!

27 July 1994

Miriam arrives tonight, and how marvellous it is to have her here! I feel we're building strong links outside of academia. We've already begun to build them a bit, but the essential elements of friendship are now being brought out through illness; for example, we're able to speak, in depth, about our families as we've never done before, and as a result of the urgency of the moment, and of moments we want to capture and keep in our memory.

29 July 1994

Having Miriam with me, as with Eva, is very stimulating. Both women have their 'eyes wide open' to the contemporary scene and are leaving their mark. My conversations with them are always very intense.

Tonight, Yvette arrives for dinner bearing a delicious African fish dish, and Fadia, out for the first time since having her operation, also arrives. Miriam and I are to dine with them, and I'm overwhelmed by each woman's sensitivity and strength – I feel so close to them during these moments of pain and suffering. Cindy then arrives with her partner, Richard, and brings the translation of my novel *Blessures des mots: Journal de Tunisie* (Accad: 1993) that she's redone, as well as a letter from my publisher, Heinemann, in which the company expresses interest in publishing the translation. What a gift! I feel surrounded with love.

During her stay, Miriam insists on accompanying me to the radiation treatment, and I find it very comforting to have her with me. Even though her face reflects the same pain and anxiety as Monique's, she seems more at ease, talking with the technicians, coming into the radiation room when she's allowed to and entertaining me by telling me stories about her life. I'm stretched out under the machines, waiting for the rays to start. She holds my hand. She tells me that she lived through similar experiences when both her parents had cancer. She leaves the room, and the grilling starts ... When it stops, she comes back in, I cheer up when I see her smile, and her expressions of concern and love: I'm not alone.

Miriam wants to organise a conference at Duke University, at which she teaches on the theme of war, sexuality and cancer. I understand how much cancer is present in her life when she tells me about the death of her parents, both of whom died of cancer. She's haunted by the illness, and believes she'll be hit by it one day.

She tells me that Séverine's visit and illness has affected her a lot – more than my illness has affected her. I know that my little sister Séverine looks very fragile and vulnerable at present. I'm upset to hear Miriam's words, because I worry a lot about Séverine, and her situation has deeply affected other people as well as me. I'm afraid for her: in a strange way, I sense she's an 'easy target' in the 'cancer industry'. I very much want to have some photos taken with Séverine, and this is something that Eva has promised to do when she returns.

30 July 1994

I feel distraught when Miriam departs. It's been so wonderful to talk with her about the many interests we share, from Middle Eastern literature to women's roles, and issues about violence, sexuality and war. We also connect at a deep emotional level; we talk about our fears, joys and experiences. She finds Eva's photos of me to be very powerful. It's true that they have an odalisque quality, because the viewer is confronted with images that are reminiscent of Eastern female slaves. Eva's photos are reminiscent of African masks, and are also highly symbolic statements. Miriam cooks a delicious chicken Marsala, and we have many lunches under the trees in my garden, surrounded by the beautiful flowers that my neighbour Rod's been planting to cheer me up.

Jane: How many people going through this experience have any outlet, any way to talk about it? As a writer and poet, you naturally must talk. But what about the people who have no words? This is why I think you should edit an anthology of poems, or short statements, from people you know who have the words to talk about the disease, in order to let other people out of their horrible silence.

I hope to be able to produce this anthology with Eva: she'll allow the women to express themselves through the photos she takes, and I'll record their stories in interviews, poems and other narrative forms.

When Miriam departs, I'm left feeling disoriented and lost. It's strange how when you have a disease, you're dependent on other people, especially when they're close friends who nurture you and surround you with love. I'm re-reading some of the letters that keep coming in so I stay distracted from the loneliness I'm feeling. Following are two extracts from them.

Rachida: *We're thinking of you a lot, of the precious friendship that links us from one continent to the next, of the energy we communicate to each other, and of the strength that we all – and you in particular – have in order to overcome evil, to turn our back on hatred and destruction.* With Fatima Mernissi [a well-known feminist researcher], *who also got the same disease way back – some 15 years ago, I believe – we spoke a lot about you, and she was categorical in saying that no disease can resist the strength of life and of love that inhabits you, and that inhabits us. She spoke about you in very beautiful and true terms, and it pleased me and made me feel even more proud of our friendship. In Morocco, still, I met by chance Khadija Boutni, because I'd just missed my flight, and it gave us a chance to spend a very beautiful afternoon together in Casablanca, during which she had me listen to a tape of your songs. This is where I discovered she'd known you for quite a long time, and that she'd received from you a copy of* Blessures des mots [*Wounding Words*]. *How small and close the world is!* ... *For the workshop about violence, we'll see when you come to Tunis, for a convenient date. At present, I'm working on a text in which I'm trying to analyse the relationship between women's rights and democracy in the Maghrebian* [northern African] *context. The exchange of reflections by women from all over the world, especially from India, at a conference in Germany, has stimulated me a lot. It gave me the desire to know more about those feminist experiences* ... *I want, most of all, to tell you that I'm thinking of you a lot, and wishing you a speedy recovery so we'll continue sowing together the seeds of love and friendship* ...

The instinct for life must win, and life is love; it's beauty, it's also your guitar and your beautiful voice, your way of being ... [In French, which is the language in which Rachida wrote the original letter, *voix*, which means *voice*, and *voie*, which means *way*, are pronounced the same.]

Amel: *Bochum, Germany, July '94. Here, the weather's very hot, and there's no sea. I've tried to cycle near the river, and fallen twice. I'm black and blue all over, and my knees are bruised. I see you smiling, and I'm laughing, my darling friend: how I miss you! I hope the radiation isn't too exhausting; as you say so courageously, my Evelyne, it'll soon be over and done with, and you'll travel again, at the beginning of September* ... *It's so important for me to see you soon – please give me some dates* ... *See you soon, my Evelyne. Be well, and preserve the light you have in you, my beautiful one. Kiss Monique, Cindy, Alban and Samira for me.*

There is nothing unique or even unusual about Tazewell County, Illinois. As true everywhere else, its agricultural and industrial practices – from weed control to degreasing parts – were transformed by chemical technologies introduced after World War II. As true everywhere else, these chemicals, many of them carcinogens, have found their way into the general envrionment ... There is nothing special or unusual about the toxic release inventories for Tazewell and Peoria Counties. Of seventy-eight regions in Illinois, the Pekin–Peoria area ranks only thirteenth in TRI emissions. Nonetheless, I cried when I first read through these emissions for area industries during the years since 1987, when this information was first compiled. In 1991, for example, large manufacturers in Peoria and Tazewell Counties legally released 11.1 million pounds of toxic chemicals into the air, water, and land. Among the known and suspected carcinogens released were benzene chromium, formaldehyde, nickel, ethylene, acrylonitrile, butyraldehyde, lindane, and captan. Captan is a carcinogenic fungicide prohibited for many domestic uses in 1989. In 1987, according to the TRI, 250 pounds of captan ended up in the Pekin sewer system. In 1992, 321 pounds were released into the air. (Steingraber: 1997: 107)

7

BUREAUCRATIC DOCTORS
BUT WHO'D WANT TO LIVE ANYWHERE ELSE?

There I was, naked on a board in a huge, darkened room, surrounded by several young women who, under the orders of Patricia Milhaud, and by virtue of some complex system allowing them to take aim at my vertebrae and ovaries, set about marking in indelible ink the outline, in the form of a barb wire fence, around the field of radiation. My belly looked like a camp. Dr. Milhaud made them do the outline over again.

– Don't burn my cunt, I said, trying hard to be jovial. One fewer breast, that'll pass, but a cunt …

I remembered Marise who, after radiation sessions on her rectum, two months before her death, gave me a call: 'The worst was when they burned my cunt. I can't screw anymore. They're all bastards. All male doctors are jerks. They should do an article in the 'Ideas' section of *Le Monde* entitled: 'Cancer specialists: the New Nazis.' (Francos: 1983: 96)

Urbana, 1 August 1994

I'm having a hard time getting back to writing my manuscript. The radiation is starting to affect me. I'm tired today, and one of the technicians notices. My skin's starting to turn lobster red. When I'm under the first machine, I see these two eyes looking at me: two red eyes in the middle of a cross, lights from which lightning bolts are struck into my mutilated body. Before, I was proud of my body, but now I'm seeing it being mutilated, stitched up and mended. In the other room, the machine is making grilling noises, as the electrons penetrate my body, grill my skin and make me grind my teeth.

Tonight, Alban seems very sad when he phones. His mother, who's about 102, called out during the night, but no one wanted to hear her. Alban went to her bedside, to reassure her until early the next morning, when the other people in the house would rise. One of his sisters takes care of her, as Adelaide takes care of my mother and used to also take care of my father. Adelaide, however, is a more attentive carer: during the night, she rises many times to make sure that mother's all right, and even if there's only a slight noise, she's on hand to reassure her.

In contrast, the people around Alban's mother refuse to be disturbed, and Alban is worried. He tells me, 'It's over these past two years that I've gotten attached to my mother and that I've learnt to appreciate her – and now she's 100 years old!' I reply, 'How wonderful!' I'm looking forward to putting my head in the nest of his shoulder when he returns.

Andrée Chedid phones me, at 3 a.m. her time, in Paris. She can't sleep because it's too hot, and is thinking of me. Séverine also phones, from Turkey Run, an Indiana resort spot she's holidaying in with her husband Charles and their daughter Laura. I'm very touched that she thinks of phoning me while she's having some fun, and tears well in my eyes. It's really helping me to have all these phone calls from my loved ones.

4 August 1994

I have a bad night: there's a storm, and I can't sleep. I've just read Reynolds Price's book about cancer, entitled *A Whole New Life* (Price: 1994). When the author is writing about radiation, it's frightening, and because I'm going through radiation myself, I shouldn't be reading disturbing descriptions of it, especially before I go to bed; in fact, I've learnt not to read anything about cancer before I go to sleep – it's too upsetting. Otherwise, the book is uplifting, and very well written. Price is an English professor at Duke University who'd already made a name for himself as a creative writer before he became ill. At age 56, he was diagnosed as having a cancerous tumour on his spinal cord. He became paralysed, but rather than become melancholic about his disease, he decided to learn things from it and to grow in a different direction. He became more spiritual through discovering faith and 'a whole new life'. His creativity increased in spite of the fact that he was feeling cruel and unceasing pain in his back, and during the years of illness that he describes, he wrote a greater number of meaningful books than he'd written during his entire earlier career. He strengthened his relationships with the people who counted in his life, and was able to express, at a very deep level, the important, relevant issues we all have to confront. He's indeed an inspiration. However, this evening, I shouldn't have read about how he mistrusts the medical establishment, or about his lack of faith in radiation, a treatment that he believes did him more harm than good. The next morning, I wake up with a headache.

Perhaps I'm also in this mood because I go to hear Dr JE, my oncologist, at the Cancer Center of Urbana, accompanied by my friend Nina, who several years ago was also treated for breast cancer. She comes to pick me up in her convertible, wearing a dress that has a Monet-flower print. She amuses me when she says, as many other people do, that there are more cancers today because people are living longer. However, her explanation just doesn't make sense to me: if it were valid, why are younger and younger people being hit by cancer?

Dr JE is conducting a conference about women's cancers. She starts by showing us the statistics: among women, breast cancer is the most prevalent type of cancer but is also the most treatable. Each year in the United States, 182,000 new cases of breast cancer are diagnosed, and each year from the year 2000 onwards, it's estimated that one million new cases will be diagnosed. Even though the doctor tells us all this very matter-of-factly, I'm shocked and appalled.

How can we accept these statistics so 'coldly'? Of the 182,000 women who contract breast cancer, 49,000 will die – more victims than as a result of road accidents, a fact that no one's talking about or doing anything about! To prevent road accidents, people are told to wear a seatbelt, and have to by law. Speed limits are enforced. What, though, is being done about breast cancer? Nothing! And in the States, only 5 per cent of all funding for cancer research is allocated to breast cancer, a statistic I learn not by listening to Dr JE's lecture but by viewing a TV show about breast cancer.

I've since found out that funding for breast-cancer research has increased many-fold and is continuing to increase.

I'm very depressed. Dr JE is now speaking about the risks involved in having cancer. She says that women who live in North America and Europe are at greater risk, and adds, 'Yes, but the quality of life is so superior here: who'd want to live anywhere else?' I'm really taken aback by that one. I quietly whisper to myself, *What quality of life, if breast and other kinds of cancer are on the rise? What quality of life, if women have to undergo treatment that I consider to be 'twentieth-century torture'?*

Alban: People who think that living anywhere else isn't as good as living in the States are people who've obviously never lived anywhere else.

223

Manicha: How can one trust a doctor like JE, who's so arrogant and self-assured – not even in herself but about her country and its systems? When one knows about the US, it makes one shiver … It's the same imperialistic, conquering ideology the original pioneers had: they undertook genocide of the Indians, and that was the founding act of the same country that waged war against Vietnam, Iraq and so on. However, Western Europe is following in the Americans' footsteps.

The notion of 'twentieth-century torture' might come across as being too emphatic, but I did experience it as such. The twentieth century has been marked by so many tortures! Nevertheless, as was the case with the Holocaust, the two world wars, the colonial wars and so on, whereby modernity was 'put on trial' and the events are the origin of a rethinking about modernity, cancer and its treatments are forming the basis of criticism of modernity and its so-called progress. Each year, in the United States alone, 50,000 women die from breast cancer, and hundreds of thousands of women are mutilated. How many more women will die or be mutilated in 20 years' time? These figures are the equivalent of a very widespread and protracted war. When a few Americans get killed in a 'modern' war, the public is immediately outraged; however, the torture that the 'developed world' inflicts on *itself* counts for nothing. This indifference is scandalous, and is bureaucratic in origin.

Although the thought might be considered scandalous, I can't help but draw an analogy between the bureaucratic attitude of some modern-day doctors and the bureaucratic attitude of the doctors employed in the Nazi regime.

Manicha: The analogy seems correct to me: on both sides, there's the will to ignore whatever the causes and consequences are, and the Hippocratic oath is violated – but whoever is making the analogy had better watch out for the guardians of the 'Shoah and Co.' sanctuary'!

Of course, today's bureaucratic doctors want to heal their patients.

Madeleine: And make sizeable profits in healing those patients!

However, their indifference to the illness's origins is criminal.

When Louis Pasteur 'discovered' microbiology, he was trying to prevent specific diseases – especially smallpox, from which thousands of children were dying. The bureaucratic attitude evident among modern-day doctors is a return to the pre-Pasteur days: in reality, it's an attitude that's both obscurantist and anti-modern.

Madeleine: But Pasteur had to fight fiercely against the members of the medical establishment, whose wrong-headed certainties he was calling into question!

This is why, when I read Elie Wiesel's *Memoirs* (Wiesel: 1995: 339), I identify with what the author is writing about and with the Holocaust survivors:

In truth, my major concern has always been the survivors. It was for them that my first works were meant … I strove to make them speak … With my books and articles I tried to convince them of the need to testify: 'Do as I do,' I told them. 'Tell your stories, even if you have to invent a language. Communicate your memories, your doubts, even if no one wants to hear them.' I shared with them my conviction that it is incumbent upon the survivors not only to remember every detail but to record it, even the silence. I urged them to celebrate the memory of silence, but to reject the silence of memory.

On a different scale, this is precisely how I feel about breast cancer and the women who survive it, and why I write and urge other people to write and testify.

Manicha: I wish that Elie Wiesel would confine himself to the fault-less memory of the Holocaust victims, and of all the other genocides and massacres, past and present, and not bring out the Shoah in order to cover up the disgrace of the Zionist state of Israel. The victims of the Shoah share a grave with three million Poles and 20 million Russians, all massacred by the Nazis. What's the difference? The ghosts of these dead all demand the same thing: 'Never again'!

When I repeat, to some of my friends, Dr JE's statement about not wanting to live anywhere else in the world, my friends tell me she must've been saying it ironically, that she couldn't have been serious. But no: she was serious – even the friend who accompanied me to the conference agrees she was serious! For most Americans, America is the best country in the world, and they aren't willing to change their way of life, even when they can see it's responsible for destruction of the environment and creation of all kinds of disease that before were unheard of.

Madeleine: Like a good sorcerer's apprentice, and in order to get the maximum gain, the United States does all it can to export to the rest of the world its sensational trans-genetic manipulations, before working out what the long-term consequences might be. It's all about 'pseudo-science' and big bucks!

Jane: The wages of affluence! People accept the evil of breast cancer in order to enjoy material goods.

I'm worn out from all this thinking, and from the radiation.
 Last night, I have many confusing dreams. In one dream,

I dream that Mary Lee Sargent is the daughter my friends the Francescatos and is receiving a prize for all the good she's done for her community. In the dream, the Francescatos have gone to New Mexico to live, so I'm mixing them up with two of my other friends, Denise and David, who in real life have moved to New Mexico; in the dream, the Francescatos are inviting me to visit them there.

This morning, I have a headache. My friend Maalouf phones, and has just learnt that I've had the operation. When I hear his voice, many memories come rushing back, and I feel like crying. I remember that when I knew Maalouf, I was 30, and Jay had just left me. Some afternoons, I rode my bike to visit Maalouf in his apartment, in Champaign. It was a wonderful period of youth and folly, which is why I'm crying now.

At present, the 'road' is long and hard. My deepest wish is to see Alban so I can rest my head in the hollow of his shoulder and stay there without moving, surrounded by his tenderness and love. I phone Resa today. In 1986, she was treated for breast cancer, and underwent surgery, chemo, radiation and yet more chemo. She's since had a mastectomy and reconstruction, and she's doing fine. She thinks that we women should undergo reconstruction because it's the best way for us to recover completely and to forget the trauma of having lost a breast. It's something she couldn't have done without.

I'm rewriting this section two years later, while Resa is struggling with a recurrence of breast cancer. After 10 years of surviving without having cancer, she's been hit with the disease again, this time in the bones of her chest wall. Poor Resa: she'd returned to the States because she couldn't stay in Paris any more. She didn't have health insurance in the States, and no insurance company wanted to take her if she had a pre-existing condition such as cancer. She was careless about having follow-up tests, because of the costs involved and because she thought that after 10 years, the likelihood that the cancer would recur was only very slight. In Paris, she'd had all the treatments and follow-up tests free of charge: in France, cancer is one of the diseases that's treated for free, and because Resa was a student at the time of her early treatment, she could benefit from not having to pay. How I wish that every country had France's health policy: wouldn't the world be a much more humane place if we could live in a universal environment in which everyone cared for the suffering and ill? And how I wish that Resa didn't have to go through that living hell again!

Manicha: In France, cancer treatment is completely refunded by social security; however, when it comes to indemnifying unemployment as a result of illness or disability, social security is much more stingy, and Dickensian images are conjured up when one considers the bad faith evident in its policies. Does an organisation exist to protect cancer patients in their wrestling with social security? They have to be able to live after they've had the treatment!

7 August 1994

According to René Char, 'the essential is always threatened by the insignificant.' Milo often quotes the saying, and it seems like an appropriate one to include at this point in my diary.

I spend a very intense weekend with Eva, during which we bury parts of Milo's ashes. I take his blue napkin into my hands, open it and let his ashes flow through my fingers, like seashells. Eva and I cry and cry when we find little pieces of iron in the ashes: the remnants of some operations our poor Milo had to undergo and endure. Eva digs a hole under the small, bushy tree standing near the room in which Alban usually works, and I, with my bare hands, put the ashes into the hole. We cover the hole, then go to Farmer's Market in order to buy some herbs to plant. We choose the herbs that Milo would've loved – he loved to cook! – as well as some flowers.

At the market, I notice a young woman in a wheelchair, wearing a funny-looking hat. She stops me to tell me she thinks I'm wearing an interesting hat – it's the African one that Eva has given me – and when we speak, I understand why we recognised each other: she had a cancerous brain tumour, for which she had radiation treatment. She's taken up painting, and today we buy one of her watercolours.

The next day, my neighbour Rod helps Eva and me plant the flowers and herbs in some of my better-quality soil that he shifts into the hole in which we've buried Milo's ashes. Eva and I have been hesitant about telling him we've buried Milo there, because we didn't know how he'd react. It's Eva who goes up to him and tells him. He says to her, 'We must put humus there, for the flowers and herbs to grow – I'll help you.' He's incredible, this Rod. Throughout my entire treatment, he's been bringing me many comforting books and cassettes, and, every Saturday, flowers from the Farmer's Market. He's also planted lots of flowers in my garden. He's so very thoughtful.

In the evening, Séverine comes over, and Eva takes photos of the two of us together. We reveal our scars to her lens, because it has her sensitive eye behind it. This session with Séverine is very emotionally intense. When Eva and I tell her what we've done with Milo's ashes, she bursts into tears. She's going to see her psychotherapist tomorrow, and she's happy about it.

Today, dear Yvette gives me a massage with so much love and sensitivity that at one point I start crying. Tears flow without my knowing why or how. My body, having borne such terrible acts of aggression, is suddenly being treated with softness and tenderness: what better remedy? I now feel much better than I've felt all day. Before I had the massage, I had the impression that I was ugly: I'd lost my 'get

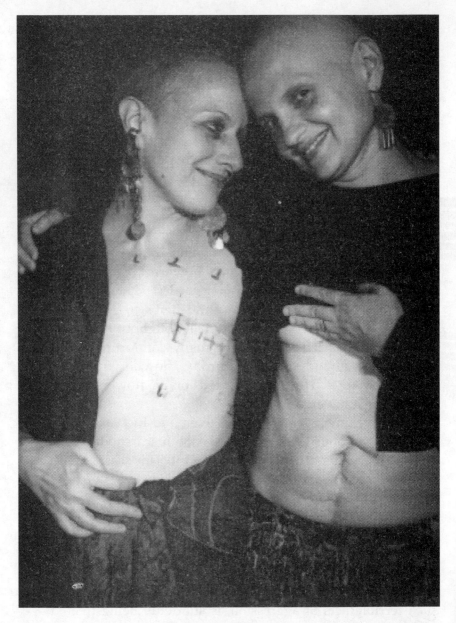

up and go', and I was no longer how I was when I liked myself – before my youth was taken away, and before my body was mistreated. Lately, this word *before* has become a standard one in my vocabulary: I use it to signify 'before I was hit by the disease'!

Should I sue Dr VZ for not being more careful in prescribing those estrogens? I really should give the idea some very serious consideration. I need to get my anger out. I have to find a way to do it, an effective way of telling other people about the dangerous world we're living in. I have to warn people to be more careful with reference to medicine. In this culture, I've been told that the only way to have an impact and make yourself heard is to sue. However, I'm not sure I like that approach, so I'm looking into effective and less damaging ways of dealing with this issue.

Manicha: One must use force – the publicity involved in a court case, and the financial indemnity – to push back the force whereby laboratories and big chemical trusts are using the human body as a terrain for experimentation. Perhaps Dr VZ will start fighting them.

Eva takes some photos of me in a pose that was often struck by Maja, the Spanish painter Goya's model: I'm a postmodern Olympia who has one breast because the other's been mutilated.

Manicha: Is it Muslim culture in which the body is favoured? In Christian culture, it's made a sin!

As is the case with many other religions, in Christianity and Islam, the body is turned into a sinful thing. As a Swedish woman, Eva has a liberated and liberating relationship to the body, and I've always admired her for having it.

8 August 1994

'The essential is always threatened by the insignificant.' I've noted the saying several times in my diary, just as Milo did,

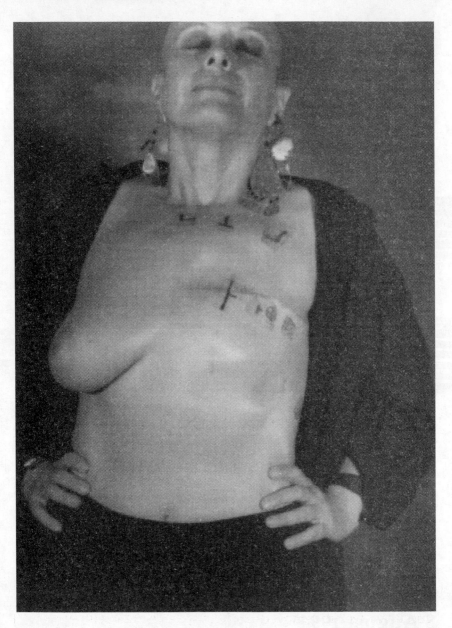

which is why I'm repeating it here. For Milo, it acquired great significance, because when he said it, he put the frustrating events of his day back into perspective.

It's a difficult day today: Eva thinks she might be pregnant, and is nervously excited because she's getting ready to return to Ohio. When she does a home pregnancy test, the 'purple stripe' appears in the test area, whereby pregnancy is supposed to be indicated ... Could I be jealous? I think I'm upset because I remember how much Milo used to want to have a child with Eva, and at that the time she wasn't that rapt in the idea.

Eva: Let me correct that assessment somewhat. I was 29 at the time, and didn't feel quite ready to have a child. This had nothing to do with my love for Milo, if that's what you're implying. I wasn't ready to become a mother at that age, for both medical and psychological reasons. Once I'd become professionally independent, I began to think differently about maternity.

Eva can be self-centred, and she probably thinks I am also. However, I might also be jealous, now I know that Adriamycin might well have had an irreversible effect on my body, by suddenly triggering my passage into menopause almost overnight. I might be envious of someone who might still have the capacity to become pregnant and give birth. I don't like these feelings I have, and want Eva to be happy; however, I think that sometimes she could be more tactful and sensitive in expressing her reactions – which she is most of the time.

Pierrot arrives while Eva's doing her home pregnancy test, before she's to return to Ohio. I find his stories about how he views father and mother to be very tiresome. However, I knew it'd be like this: all that language about 'God this', and 'God that', no matter what subject we're discussing. I feel so removed from my family members when they become dogmatic about things. At the same time, though, there's something very touching about Pierrot. He's come to help me clean the house and to cook for me. He accompanies me to the radiation sessions, and asks the technicians all kinds of questions. He looks very concerned. I know he means well, but I'm not in a good mood. I get depressed very often now I'm having radiation; I'll be so happy when it's over.

And Alban: suffering so much due to his mother's pain and alone-ness, the lack of affection in his family, the fact that his sister is screaming at his mother to shut up because the poor old woman is calling out in the night! Alban, who's become so much closer to his mother over the past few months. Is it because of his relationship with me? His mother is asking him whose son he is – personally, I think she knows it well, but wants to be reassured.

Manicha: Alban is living amid two great tensions: Evelyne's cancer and his reconnection with his dying mother. How's he holding on?

I'm also upset as a result of having a conversation with Dr LE. I go to him with lots of questions, and he tells me I have to continue with the treatment as scheduled, even though I'm feeling the burning sensation and tiredness I'm describing to him. He tells me that if my arm swells up in six months' time, which is possible, it'll result not from the radiation but from the operation. Dr Yoto, my surgeon, has told me the opposite: that the swelling will result from the radiation, but that 'if you're lucky, you won't get it!' Naturally, Dr LE, who believes in technology and radiation very strongly, will never admit to agreeing with this statement!

Manicha: These two Diafoirus characters [a reference to a doctor character in one of Molière's novels] should be placed face to face at some point!

I show Dr LE a passage in the book by Dr Suzanne Képès entitled *Women at Fifty* (Képès: 1987), in which the author states that when a woman takes estrogen, a proliferation of cells, hemorrhages and cysts in the breasts can be brought about. He responds, 'It isn't my area of expertise,' but that he wouldn't have prescribed hormones for me if I didn't have symptoms of menopause anyway. When I bring it to his attention that he surely wouldn't want to have them prescribed for his wife or daughters in the future, he says that his wife and daughters aren't at the age of menopause – he's young: in his late thirties. To that, I stupidly reply, and how I age myself by saying it, 'I mean once they get older!' – as if I myself were old! I'm really depressed as a result of having this conversation, and doubly depressed when Eva tells me her attitude towards menopause: she's completely 'flipping out' about it. Why can't people accept that ageing is a natural bodily process? And the members of the media and advertising industries definitely don't help: they're always glorifying youth, and consider young people to be the only beautiful people!

Madeleine: Beauty? My sweet Evelyne, what does 'old' mean, whether the word is applied to men or women? It doesn't necessarily mean decline and decay! There are such beautiful faces among the elderly that can't be withered because they have wrinkles, because there's something so noble about them, such goodness and concern for other people; one reads such joy in their eyes, which are filled with that wonderful mixture of mischief and intelligence – something that's distinctly lacking in the gaze of beautiful youth. Self-acceptance throughout life is, I believe, part of the secret to having lasting internal beauty. 'Old' and 'young': what do the words really mean, when you get right down to it, Evelyne, my dear?

14 August 1994

I'm fed up with having this radiation. Today, we have to stop because I have blisters under my arm. That whole side of my chest wall hurts, and I 'have it up to here', wondering whether it's really serving a purpose for me to be receiving this treatment; after all, my tumour, even though it was big, hadn't spread.

When I wake up in the morning, I have a headache. David and Sharon come to help me move things from the basement and to get the house ready before I depart. We have a garage sale to get rid of all the things that Fawzi and Jacqueline left here. Diane also comes over to help.

Madeleine: We French readers have trouble understanding this 'garage sale' concept. We aren't used to unloading on to the footpath all the things we'd like to sell off when we move. It springs, first of all, from our basic conservatism, but also, we're much less nomadic in spirit than are Americans.

Today I feel tired, even though I slept well. Yesterday, I show Eva's photos to Keo, Zohreh's friend, who's come with Zohreh, and she finds it hard to look at them. She tells me that instances of breast cancer occurred among her neighbours in India, and that she found the experience daunting. She tells me about a woman called Eve Sedgwick, who works at North Carolina's Duke University, teaches queer theory and has written a book about her own breast cancer. I should try to buy the book, which is entitled *Fat Art / Thin Art* (Sedgwick: 1994).

Manicha: It's incredible how well consensus functions in the US, and in all areas: studies into Afro-Americans, environmentalists, Jews, Latinos, feminists, lesbians and gays, and so on. Everything gets recycled, becomes clean and has 'neat contours and clear structure'. Because academics fear confusion, non-knowledge and complexity – in short, life – everything gets into a discipline!

The painful expression on Sharon's face as she looks at the photos will stay with me. She's hurting. At age 31, she must think that illness is far away, as I thought when Milo got sick. I myself was even younger, and used to think that disease was far, far away – that perhaps it'd never reach me. It's strange, the perspective that young people have. Was I sensitive enough to Milo? I think of David, my sister Adelaide's son, who comes and holds my hand while I'm in the radiation room: he's extremely sensitive and sweet. I appreciated it very much that they've both come to help me. I'm entertained when I see them interacting, teasing each other and playing cheerfully. They seem to have fun together, and I'm happy for them – so much so that I forget my disease for a while!

16 August 1994

I hate the Polaroid photos the radiation technicians have taken of me and put in my records: they look like photos of a concentration-camp victim. I look like a deportee, like a 'number' from a concentration camp – Holocaust analogies keep popping up. I have huge scars that look disproportionate. I'm fed up with my treatment.

Yesterday, Dr LE sees me, and says it's normal and to be expected that I'm getting so red. I ask him whether it's true that my rib bones could become so brittle that they might break. He replies that there's a chance in a hundred it'll happen, and adds, 'I told you that radiation doesn't reach the heart or lungs, but I didn't tell you that about the ribs.' What he won't admit is that I'm the one who always has to ask the questions; otherwise, he wouldn't tell me anything, and even when I ask the questions, they often go unanswered. He almost always seems to be in a rush, but not in so great a rush that he can't ask me whether I like Dr Land. I tell him that what I like about Dr Land is that he answers questions and that I need someone who can communicate. Dr LE asks me whether I've learnt anything new thanks to Dr Land. I reply that Dr Land thinks that if my nodes were positive and were rendered negative through chemo, some traces of the cancer would still be left because the tumour wouldn't have completely disappeared when I had the chemo. When he's asking me these questions, Dr LE takes his time. Why is he so curious about what I think of Dr Land – is it professional rivalry?

Jane: Probably, as well as peer evaluation.

19 August 1994

Now I've had the mastectomy, my surgeon, Dr Yoto, prescribes me a breast prosthesis. *Small consolation!* I think. He tells me I can go to Confidentially Yours or another store that sells prostheses.

Jane: What an ironic name!

Jane's comment is so pertinent: not only is the breast they want to sell me no longer mine; my confidence in my body has been shattered as a result of a mutilation I don't want to hide and keep secret – keep 'confidential'. On the contrary, I want the whole world to know what this civilisation is doing to the women in it!

In the prosthesis store, the saleswomen want to sell me a prosthesis that costs $400, and tell me that my insurance company will reimburse me up to $225! Instead, I opt for the prosthesis the cost of which I'll 'supposedly' be reimbursed 100 per cent. When I go to take the prosthesis, the saleswomen tell me I have to pay $45 as a 'co-payment', and advise me to buy a bra that has a pocket and is on sale for $21! I therefore end up paying $66. The saleswomen are very nice, though. I doubt they make very much money out of their business. What disgusts me is the whole system, in which women's breasts are removed and a business is then made out of the women's misfortune at having lost a breast. Why do these prostheses cost so much?

Jane: Sounds like the food industry, in which people are made obese and are then sold expensive dietary products. Think about the amount that people spend on exercise equipment to work off all that unnecessary, fat-injected food!

I've started receiving the radiation 'boosters', via the last machine in the series: the one that emits flows of electrons. One of the technicians, Sam, is leaving to have a holiday. He's the staff member who retrained to be a radiotherapist after having a stint in the army. I think this is ironic: war connections and connotations with reference to cancer treatments keep popping up! Sam very warmly bids me goodbye, a gesture that's uncharacteristic of someone who's usually very distant and reserved. He seems moved.

Manicha: War is the good fortune of medical researchers!

As for Dr LE, today he comes into the room to give directives about the boosters, then comes back and apologises to me for not saying hello – he's quite sensitive after all.

24 August 1994

I've reached the end of what I can bear: fortunately, tomorrow I'm to have the final treatment. I can't take it any more. I'm finding people to be very strange. I see Suzy, who complains that it's very hot in France this summer and about having to return here; she seems annoyed that she hadn't contacting me sooner. Referring to my cancer, she says,

'You, at least, have a cause to live for!' *The nerve!* I think. Some people are behaving really indecently. I often find Suzy's remarks to be a bit 'off'. As the novelist Albert Camus observed, people are bored with life, and throw themselves into aggressive acts in order to fill the void. Also, there's guilt: some of the people around me are scared of my disease, running away from me and then feeling guilty.

Luckily, I also see Mary Lee Sargent today. She wants to organise a protest based on the conference we've talked about with Miriam Cooke: a march in which women who've suffered from breast cancer link together in order to protest. I love this woman: she inspires me. If it weren't for women such as her, and Cheris and my dear friends Zohreh, Samira and Cindy, I wouldn't feel like coming back to this country at all. I find it to be too materialistic; dehumanising; cold, in all senses of the word; and stressful. Juanita thinks I should bring a lawsuit against Dr VZ and the medical establishment for giving me and other women estrogen as if it were chocolate. Eva also believes I should sue. However, Zohreh is horrified when I tell her I'm contemplating bringing a class action. She tells me about an accident she had, in which a young guy hit her car and that resulted in damage to her teeth and other traumas. Because the young man was at fault, she was told to take the case to court in order to win a big settlement. However, she refused to do so, because she claimed that she could've been the cause of the accident; because when harm isn't intended, you must learn to forget; and because the cost of insurance is skyrocketing as a result of these lawsuits.

I feel torn now. I've suffered too much, and I'm angry. I feel I must find ways to not only express my anger but address the larger issues at stake. At present, the big questions for me are whether my cancer could've been avoided if my doctors had been more vigilance, and if so, why the doctors didn't take these steps. Would filing a lawsuit be an effective way for me to alert the public? Would it be more effective than writing? Who reads? Who follows court cases and lawsuits? What should a person do in this world, in which it seems that a violent voice is the only voice that people listen to? I'm against violence, so what options do I have? Is legal action itself a form of violence?

Manicha: Once more, yes! In the US, it's violence that pays. And the television media are there to publicise court cases.

Jane: But nowadays, doctors are afraid to prescribe anything, so too much caution is also bad.

I agree with you, Jane, but in my case, I feel that caution should've been the order of the day.

Manicha: It isn't doctors as such; it's doctors who become passive instruments of big, competing chemical interests; I'm thinking of the fact that some fast, poorly tested medications are being put on the market. Patients tend to trust their doctors, and when the doctors are being manipulated, the patients' trust is betrayed.

I remember the time I felt I deserved a promotion that I wasn't about to get. It was at a time during which I felt so down that I went to the Share clinic to consult a psychiatrist. The psychiatrist told me to be more assertive and ask for the promotion; her words were 'Wheels that don't squeak don't get oiled.' I pursued my request through my on-campus Affirmative Action committee, which staff and students can appeal to, and through which the interests of minorities or women are protected. I subsequently got my promotion. Was it not a good move to do so? Would I have gotten the promotion if I hadn't asked? I probably would've had to wait one or two more years to get it, whereas I believed I deserved to get it immediately. I would've submitted to this 'injustice' without protesting, and wouldn't have learnt to assert myself the way I did. The issue I'm addressing now is different, but I know I must do something – scream my anger and revolt so other people will hear and be warned. What is the best way to do it? I'll have to ask around for advice.

Mary Lee Sargent tells me she has several women friends who are exhausted as a result of filing a lawsuit, especially with reference to cases against sex discrimination in the workplace. Going to court takes years, your energy is drained, and there are often no results.

Manicha: In France, the exhaustion of battle-fatigued cancer patients would seem to work in favour of the social-security system, which is especially malicious when it comes to giving indemnity to the less skilled members of the working population.

I look at my chest: on the right side, I still have a soft, tender breast, and on the other, my skin is red and burnt. I'm so angry! I shouldn't have taken the EPC my doctor prescribed even though I had no symptoms of menopause. She saw, via a blood test, that my hormone level was low, and because my mother had osteoporosis, prescribed the hormones through which whatever good and bad cells lying dormant in my body were inflamed and activated.

In France, some doctors have told me that the EPC I had is no longer being prescribed in that country because it's too strong. I've also found out that it's being sold 'over the counter' all over the developing world, Lebanon included, at a very low cost, and that you don't have to have a prescription to obtain it!

Manicha: It's good to come back, time and time again – as when a leitmotif is used – to the direct cause of how your disease was brought about and how its development was aided: via prescription of the EPC drug. You have to keep coming back to that, in order to remind your readers that no medical treatment – no drug whatsoever – is entirely harmless. You must make the hormones' effects known to the broadest public possible.

Women take the hormones because their doctors tell them they'll stay young, that they'll remain free of wrinkles or vaginal dryness, and that their chances of suffering heart disease and osteoporosis will be reduced. However, they aren't told that their risk of contracting breast cancer will increase. They find out the side effects, which are many, only if they ask for and read the little paper that comes with the hormones.

In France, some doctors have also told me that doctors should monitor hormone intake very closely, and that the hormone level in a woman of my age – I was 50 when I was hit by cancer – can fluctuate from month to month.

I could've lost my life, and I've now lost confidence in my body. However, what can I learn from the experience? Why must I go through this journey?

Manicha: But the body isn't guilty: it's you, Evelyne, who decided to intervene by having the hormonal treatment!

Why has Claude written me a depressing letter, in which he's aroused so many painful memories about racism in Switzerland, especially the anti-Arab racism my poor father had to suffer at the hands of the thugs in the religious organisation I call Terrorisme Biblique? In that organisation, the members mistrusted father because he was Arab, consider Arabs and Blacks to be inferior, and would never agree to intermarriage.

Jane: They wield their ideology like a weapon!

Why must I suffer so much this year? And why did he, my father, have to die this year?

25 August 1994

Today's my last day of radiotherapy treatment, and I couldn't have stood another moment of it. Dr VZ calls me tonight: she wants to know how I'm doing, before I depart. She's talked with Dr JE, who's given her some news about me. I'm unable to talk to her, first, because Merri has just arrived to see me; second, because I'm too upset as a result of what I've had to go through; and third, because I'm convinced she's responsible for the situation, having provoked my illness by writing that prescription. I tell her I can't talk at present, and ask her to give me a number I can reach her on. She gives me the number, and I hang up. I have a terrible pain in my stomach, and wonder whether it's been provoked as a result of my drinking the gin and lime juice that Zohreh made for me [*later, I find out that any alcoholic beverage would have been difficult for me to drink when I was having the treatment*] or whether I'm feeling angry as a result of the doctor's phone call. I'm still wondering what to do about her.

Diane then phones, and I tell her about VZ. She encourages me to phone the doctor back, because she might have some information for me from Dr JE. I therefore phone her back when Merri has left, and tell her about my depression, my suffering and my hurt. She responds, 'No wonder, after all you've been through. It's normal you should feel this way!' I say, 'But could it have been avoided? Would you prescribe the estrogen to me again?' She replies, 'Yes: you see, when there's an epidemic and we have a vaccine, we'll use it to save people, even if we know that one out of a thousand cases will react badly to it, and might even die from it.' She then tells me a horrible story about her mother, who had breast cancer, and of one of the doctor's aunts. The aunt underwent a double mastectomy and radiation on her chest wall. The radiation was done so poorly that five years later, she developed cancer of the esophagus, which she eventually died from. Despite all this, she refused to participate in a class-action suit proposed to her by other people who'd suffered from receiving similarly poor radiation, because she was thankful to have been cured the first time. This, at least, was VZ's version of the story.

Manicha: VZ is protecting herself: she's probably trying to find out whether there's any lawsuit in the air against her. She's really devious!

Madeleine: My dear Evelyne, VZ doesn't give a damn about your state of health. She knows she made a professional mistake, and she's giving you her spiel to lull you into inaction, by bringing her family story to the rescue, as well as her magnanimity as an added attraction. All this to nip in the bud any whim you might have to mount a court case against her, whereby her reputation would take quite a beating. That's the only reason she's suddenly seeming so concerned. She's a sharp one – nobody's fool!

Jane: This is unfortunately what many doctors have to spend their time worrying about: they also have a career, a family and a reputation to consider. Many of them act in good faith. It's all so complex, isn't it?

Is there a solution to all these questions? I ask myself. Thinking about it now, I realise that VZ's analogy between estrogen and vaccines is unconvincing. The so-called vaccine against osteoporosis she prescribed me isn't really a vaccine, as such. The results of many studies are being published in which the researchers are revealing that the 'vaccine' isn't as effective as it was once thought to be – and why, they're asking, should the patient risk contracting cancer as a result? Among women taking hormones, the risk of contracting cancer is increased by between 30 and 40 per cent, and is far from the 'one in a thousand' stated by VZ. Why give women a cure through which they might be killed at age 50 in order to prevent another disease that they might contract at age 70 or 80? It doesn't make any sense. And why did VZ talk about lawsuits? Had she guessed, or been told, that I was thinking about filing a suit?

Manicha: Sure sounds like it to me!

26 August 1994

Merri says to me, 'What's happening in this country? Everyone we know who is our age is suddenly getting cancer. I'm visiting friends here, and many of them have been hit by the disease in one form or another.'

I'm now convinced we've entered a danger zone: the postmodern era, a time in which the planet and its inhabitants are being destroyed. It's been predicted, and now it's happening. And I'm one of its victims!

Manicha: What you're describing isn't impossible, unfortunately! Everything points to an 'industrialised' society in which the market and science are combined – cloning, 'mad cow' meat, contracting AIDS via contaminated blood, and so on.

Jane: That's it – well put! However, science and the market have always worked hand in hand throughout history, haven't they? It's now a problem of scale, of disproportion, I think.

28 August 1994

Zohreh is against the lawsuit craze; she says, for one thing, that the price of insurance goes up as a consequence. Merri thinks that if you sue because you really need the money in order to right some wrong, it's all right; otherwise, it's a strange way to make yourself heard in this country. I speak with Zohreh about all my questions and worries. She tells me she hoped I'd know how to put all this behind me: that the important thing is to be alive, and that the rest is secondary. She tells me that her doctor thinks that osteoporosis is so horrible that she's prescribing estrogen for all her female patients who've reached the age of 50.

Madeleine: Let's not exaggerate, now! There's no comparison with cancer, especially if one takes care to eat correctly, not American-style!

Zohreh is implying that she understands VZ's reasoning. As for me, I can't agree, if only because osteoporosis comes much later in life – for my mother, it came between when she was between 70 and 80.

Later, when I'm in Paris on sabbatical, I also learn, from a French doctor who's treating one of my friends, that for a woman such as me, who hasn't had children, the risk of suffering from osteoporosis is much lower whereas the risk of contracting cancer is much higher.

Why don't doctors take all these facts into consideration when they're starting to prescribe these critical types of medication? Why are they so careless? I tell Zohreh that one of the problems I've also noticed in my case is that I'll probably never be part of studies through which we might be enlightened about the connection between cancer and estrogen, because my doctors haven't made the link between the two.

Madeleine: Out of intellectual dishonesty: it goes without saying!

When we have an ideology, we're prevented from seeing accurately: blinkers are often put on our ability to make connections. The relationship isn't noted in my record, as such, so how can it be analysed other than through what I'm writing about it now? And how are we to believe in the accuracy of science, or in any scientific meaning or truth, when scientists work in the *milieu* of ideology or fads, such as keeping people young at any cost? In most scientific assessments, predictions or figures, the scientists haven't had all the facts, or all the angles of a given situation or disease.

Jane: I like your treatment of the ethical issue 'To sue or not to sue: that is the question' as it stands in America. In the class actions being mounted against tobacco companies, we have an example of real social action, not simply a means of getting money back. The litigants are trying to prove a point about a large-scale social aberration that's gone on for too long.

Manicha: Sue! Sue! Reaching into people's 'hip pocket' is the only thing that works – such as the big lawsuits through which – so little! – of the course of history has changed: Dreyfus, Nuremberg, the International Tribunal, for crimes against humanity. However, we still must make a noise, get people thinking, and punish the perpetrators when necessary.

Madison, 31 August 1994

I'm at Pierrot's, and I feel down: it's always the same dogmatic discourse, in black and white – shrunk-up visions of life. Pierrot shows me a video of his visit to Lebanon, of father before his death, and of father on his birthday ... Father looks so unhappy, and so much in pain. It hurts to see him like that.

The weather is grey and rainy, and is announcing autumn. Pierrot is still mad at father. He says that father should've put his financial affairs in order before he died, that he shouldn't have left me with the responsibility to meet his wishes, and that his wishes should've been for his family before anyone else! Personally, I believe, and told Pierrot so, that father didn't live exclusively for his family but above all for the Muslim community. It's normal that he should want this community to realise its potential, and I respect father all the more for wanting it. Pierrot says, 'The family comes before anything or anyone else; the family helps in the difficult moments of one's life, in times of crisis.' I tell him that this hasn't necessarily been the case for me, at least not this time: that I've also been helped by some wonderful friends, whose friendship I've been nurturing through the years. Pierrot has to mature. I hope he'll be able to fulfil some of his wishes and, as a consequence, grow up.

Three years later, as I'm completing this book, I'm pleased to note that Pierrot has changed somewhat since the time of writing. He's moved on to have a beautifully different lifestyle. In a way, he's now following in his parents' footsteps. Through father's death, he's been enabled to grow up and outwards. He's no longer putting his family and personal interests first: something he blamed father for not doing! He's regained my respect, and I'm sure that our parents would be proud of him.

I phone some lawyers who operate in Madison, Wisconsin and ask them to advise me about possibly filing a lawsuit as a result of what's happened to me. None of them seems interested in taking on my case. One of them says, 'Breast-cancer cases are messy. In your case, you were given ERT for what's considered to be good medical practice for women, for their welfare. We wouldn't be able to make a case for it, especially because your tumour seems to have come on so suddenly.' Another lawyer says I'd have to show 'real strong medical evidence to back me up'.

Manicha: Lawyers and doctors equal power – and the monetary benefits that go with it. Their respective orders – the bar and the medical association – are associations of racketeering and self-defence, and are as solid as a rock; architects and notaries belong to them too. They're all associations of unquestioned authority figures. All that's missing is a syndicate for politicians!

I'm quite depressed, and I feel a bit better when I re-read the following letters from Amel, which I receive before I leave Urbana.

Bochum, 1 August '94

Evelyne, my friend, what a miracle the telephone is. I was so happy to hear your voice, so clear, so close. After it, I had trouble falling asleep: I felt like staying with you, keeping your voice within me, its intonations. This morning, it's raining, and it's less hot. It's so hard to live far from the Mediterranean: how I understand you, my friend. In Paris, I could ask for the name of a good doctor: tell me if you need advice. I could ask some friends. Maybe you should come a little earlier to Tunisia, starting on the 15th of September. The air is less polluted than in Paris ...

Here, abroad, my fears come back, the ones from which I took so long to calm down ... But I tell myself that I must calm down, and understand my limits in order to keep my distance. I have to take my time. [This sentence is in English in the letter.] However, I remain very impulsive: I rush, but I'll grow up, I'm sure. My friend, I hope I'm making you smile, and that you aren't too sad

for me: there's no need for it. I feel like laughing. How I miss the
sea. We shall go swimming if you want to, in the transparent sea
of Kelibia, if the weather's still fine …

I'm sad not to be present, close to you when you're so tired, my
Evelyne, so courageous. As for the trip to the desert, I hope to be
able to do it, and see how you feel by then about joining us …

I feel like cooking a good fish couscous for you. How's your
mother? I think of her, because the river, edged with trees all green,
resembles Switzerland …

I hope to hear from you soon.

Of all the unexpected consequences of World War II, perhaps
the most ironic is the discovery that a remarkable number of
the new chemicals it ushered in are estrogenic – that is, at low
levels inside the human body, they mimic the female hormone
estrogen. Many of the hyper-masculine weapons of conquest
and progress are, biologically speaking, emasculating.
(Steingraber: 1997: 109)

Certain breast cancers are notorious for growing faster in the
presence of estrogen, which is why prescribing anti-estrogenic
drugs is standard chemo-therapeutic protocol. Many other
cancers – those of the ovary, uterus, testicle, and prostate, for
example – are also known to be, or suspected to be, hormonally mediated. Thus, identifying pollutants that interfere with
hormones is important to public dialogue about human cancers of all kinds. (Steingraber: 1997: 110)

Phtalates, the plasticizers with the nearly impossible name, turn
out to be the most abundant industrial contaminant in the environment. At least two have now been identified as estrogenic,
and traces of both have been found in food. One is used in plastic food wrap, and the other in papers and cardboard designed
for contact with liquid, dry, and fatty foods. Some phtalates are
known to be overtly carcinogenic. (Steingraber: 1997: 112)

A man afflicted with cancer imagined even less that PCBs, toxic residues that seeped into cheap industrially produced hams and packaged meats, stuffed with preservatives, would have estrogenic effects, which is to say feminizing effects, or that they would be harming not only his hypothalamus, a gland in the brain, but also his ever fragile and now exhausted liver, which attempted in vain to obstruct these chemicals.

These strange feminizing effects, due to a combination of environmental contaminants, were to severely perplex American pediatricians and endocrinologists who would attend international toxicology conventions, for these contaminants made little boys grow breasts, experience later and later puberty, they modified behavior, increased males' chances of getting testicular cancer, and women's chances of getting breast cancer, and sterilized to greater or lesser degrees men whose fertility rates were dropping in several countries throughout the world, though no one could actually pinpoint the reason why ... People are still studying and denouncing the link between DDT and breast cancer, which is sharply on the rise. (Séralini: 1997: 164)

Our man will in fact die of the insidious fumes caused by traffic emissions twenty years earlier, having been subjected to the carcinogenic action of all these and other chemicals that accumulated in his body over that period. He will die of liver cancer metastasized to his lungs, not counting the effects on his brain of these alien substances, these pollutants that invade the healthy body. But this same man's best friend, two offices away from his, has been suffering horribly from a malignant lymphoma. He has undergone chemotherapy and radiation, leaving him exhausted and helpless for weeks each time. The treatment helped, but the discomfort was almost worse than the toxic spider web of the disease itself. The number of malignant lymphomas has been on the rise over the past fifteen years, or so say the statistics. The guilty party would once again seem to be chemical and ionizing factors in the environment.

The slightest deviation or excess in this naturally unhealthy life becomes a risk factor, and thus, day after day, the number of malignant tumors keeps on rising. (Séralini: 1997: 165)

8

BREAST CANCER IN FRANCE
WHY SO HUSHED UP?

Cercan, the name of the un-nameable. 'Cercan' is backslang for 'cancer', the title of the book, but also the sign of how impossible it is to come to terms with the name itself. Backslang is the language of those who feel powerless to subvert the order imposed by words. When all their battles have been lost, this facetiousness is all that's left them. A final means of protesting that will change nothing, since the name will ultimately remain the same, but which at the same time expresses a contrary view of the world and underlines our determination not to give up, no matter how great the pressure. (Hyvrard: 1987: 30)

Madison, 1 September 1994

In two days' time, I'll be with my love, and I can hardly wait. The atmosphere of the place I'm in is beginning to weigh on me. An example of why I'm feeling this way is that one day, I overhear the words of a little boy who's playing the role of the moralist with his sister. He tells her she's wrong for showing her Barbie doll undressed to other children on the school bus. He makes such a big deal out of his accusation that I'm sure the little girl will be traumatised as a result. It's ridiculous: he acts as if he's his sister's surrogate parent, and the little girl feels obliged to deny that she undressed the doll in the bus.

Thinking about this situation, I'm reminded of an event that occurred during my own childhood. One day, my Swiss uncle, Jules, found me in his car, lying naked among the fur, silk and velvet of the clothes he sold. I, too, was traumatised, as a result of father's reaction, and thereafter became a rebel. Perhaps the little girl will become a rebel as a result of her experience with her moralistic brother.

I'd like to have another niece like Anaïs: she and that little girl could keep each other company, and Anaïs's fear of losing me would thereby be alleviated. However, Anaïs, don't fear: I have no intention of dying, not yet – I still have too many things to accomplish.

I'm hurt when I see Pierrot's video about father: the poor man seems to be suffering so much in it. I'm hurt when I think I won't be seeing him when I go to Lebanon in the near future. Why must events repeat themselves? Why are human beings seemingly incapable of breaking their chains?

I'm also really annoyed when I read a letter from Bernard, Brigitte's friend. He seems to be suggesting that because of my struggle for women's rights, I became exhausted, and that I should approach the struggle from another angle, by strongly encouraging making men to participate in it. He hasn't read my texts thoroughly enough, because in them I do encourage men to participate: I believe that real change will occur only if women and men work together, hand in hand.

Also, I find the logic behind the words in his letter to be absurd: Mahatma Gandhi wasn't asked to change his direction because he was exhausted as a result of following it – he often carried his dedication to the cause of humanity to the bitter end, often to the detriment of his health. Mother Teresa was also an extremist in this way. Although I don't claim to be a Gandhi or a Mother Teresa – far from it – I respect and admire them, as I respect and admire Jesus, and seek to follow in their footsteps; I know how much Bernard admires

Gandhi. People should look deeper into what motivates them to make statements such as Bernard's: when they say these things, they mean well, and think they're looking after my welfare and health; however, I think their words have more to do with their own fears of making a commitment and getting sick. You can't expect people to be willing to change the course of their life if they don't first understand the importance of the struggle they're about to undertake.

Manicha: A lot can be said about the subject of Mother Teresa, and even more about her ideology. Pain is elevating, she claims; do as Jesus did: suffer on the cross, and you'll get to paradise. And we haven't yet had the last word about the story of embezelled funds, either. [See Christopher Hitchens' *Le mythe de mère Térésa* (Hitchens: 1996).]

I'm thankful to Manicha for opening my eyes to these aspects I was previously unaware of.

On the plane between Chicago and Paris, 2 September 1994

I dream I'm buying money-market shares in a tunnel to be built under Mont Blanc. I'm worried that the tunnel won't work and that the mountain will collapse on it before the tunnel is completed. I analyse the dream with my friend Cindy, as well as with my brother Pierrot. We decide that the tunnel is my journey through cancer. In the dream, I live it as a long tunnel, but it's under a high mountain that's covered with eternal snows: my desire for transcendence, for spirituality and for rising above this illness, through which I'm feeling as if I'm being kept down and oppressed, and living in darkness. I'm afraid I'll be crushed by my desires; however, there's light at the end of the tunnel. My friend Cindy has another interesting interpretation of the dream: that my wanting to buy shares means I want to own my sickness rather than let it own me. I want to appropriate this illness, and be led into the light of day! As for Pierrot, who's a more practical person, he asks me whether I slept well in spite of the dream! There's something endearing about this practical, down-to-earth side of him.

Later, I analyse the dream with Alban, and he detects the tunnels' sexual connotations. A long tunnel can also mean desire to express sexuality. I'm sexually frustrated as a result of this illness: the sexual act is no longer as wonderfully pleasurable as it used to be. This sudden shift into menopause has been provoked as a result of the chemo. My vagina has been shrunk, and penetrative sex is often painful for me; worse still, my self-image has been shattered: ever since I had the mastectomy, I've been looking at nothing but a mutilated body. According to Alban, my dream is about my desire to engage in a sexual act, surrounded with high peaks of eternal snows, which represent my expectation that I'll be taken above my earth-bound miseries.

Madeleine: De-coding dreams is always a subjective matter: it depends on so many imponderables at the very moment we're trying to elucidate them, not to mention all the projections made by the people we confide in about our dreams!

I'm on a plane to Paris now. Lots of young people are on the flight, returning to Paris from a tour to the University of Madison, Wisconsin. I find their freshness a pleasure to behold; they remind me of the young people who live at my brother Théophile's place. Teens from parts of the world other than the States have a different dynamism: they aren't as arrogant as their American counterparts.

Manicha: Have you ever met young Israelis travelling abroad, Evelyne? Generally – like their elders, for that matter – they're horribly arrogant and defiant! The States and Israel: two countries jauntily oppressing others in the name of 'democracy' and 'race'! They're two peoples who've been educated to be forcefully assured and assert their 'superior' ego.

I'm peeling bits of skin off my chest, and I can't believe it might have been a vehicle for cancerous cells to proliferate. I find the whole disease incredible – or Pierrot's favourite word, *invraisemblable!*: 'unbelievable!'. The pieces of skin are hard, like leather.

Yesterday, I speak with Cindy, who tells Pierrot she'd be willing to come and get me from anywhere in the world in order to help me out. I really do have some extraordinary friends: they help me to cope and bear this illness. I feel more fragile during this trip, but at the same time calmer and more focussed than I used to be. I'm remembering Yvette's extraordinary massages.

Paris, 4 September 1994

Last night, I take up some Parisians' invitation to have dinner at their home. The conversation during it is heavy. The guests, especially the men, run through every cliché 'in the book' about the United States. Although I usually don't feel like defending the US, this time I find their remarks so trite I'm obliged to respond. About the subject of sexual harassment, the men remark, 'How can one have a "normal" relationship with women any more?' I tell them that the laws that have been established on American campuses in order to protect students – women in particular – are good because previously there was too much abuse from professors – males in particular, whereby they used their position of power to take advantage of their female students. About the subject of political correctness, the male guests wonder whether you can say anything intelligent any more now you're afraid to even voice an opinion. I don't disagree with this summation, but add that 'PC' has been effective in some domains; for example, at the university I teach at, some fields and subjects, such as Women's Studies and African Studies, have been able to rise to prominence. I'm infuriated when some of the male guests remark that here in France, it's possible to have a wonderful, 'normal' sexual relationship with your secretary! Alban arrives at the dinner late, and the discussion has already ended. I find him to be refined, elegant and intelligent when I see him in the same room as the annoying male guests. I love his vision of life.

I wrote down these dinner-time musings about sexual harassment before former US president Bill Clinton's 'affairs' became public! Now, I understand better that French people could consider the affairs to be 'ridiculous and not worth reporting'. I find it saddening that women who really require protection via sexual-harassment laws get drowned in these politically motivated affairs – which are soaked in money and power – and that women's legitimate requests for help are often ignored by the doyens of the establishment.

Jane: What's irritating isn't the raw facts of PC; it's how the issues are then represented in the media, whereby 'represented' means 'distorted'.

Paris, 6 September 1994

Alban and I go to see Dr EL, my feminist-pioneer friend who's written a book about 'women at 50'. We talk with her about estrogens, and she says there are many valid reasons why women should take them; however, she wouldn't have prescribed them to a woman such as me, who was still getting her periods, and confirms what I've already heard: that the 'EPC' I was prescribed is indeed very, very potent. She seems to regret not having seen me when I came through Paris at Christmas time and was bleeding so much I had called her. It's unfortunate that I was in so great a rush to go and see my parents. I was unable to get in touch with EL's daughter, as she'd advised me to do. When she asks me how my parents are, I almost break down and cry: I'm realising what a toll all this has taken on me.

She tells me she'll contact her daughter – both her daughters are gynecologists: the one who specialises in breast diseases, and that she'll ask her to follow up on my case. She also says I should find a hospital that has all the necessary specialists. Alban informs me that in France, hospitals are also research centres; that hospital treatment costs much less because the hospitals are subsidised by the government; that the hospitals have excellent, knowledgeable specialists; and that it's better to go to a hospital than to a private clinic.

Dr EL tells us about a conference she attended. One of the speakers was a well-known Jungian professor, who stated that women's breasts are among the most sensitive parts of the human body, and are consequently more vulnerable than any other part to all the acts of aggression through which our planet is being destroyed.

Bettina: This is true, in the strictly physical sense: when a patient is in a coma, the doctors often test how sensitive he or she is by pinching a the nipple. It's also true in the psychological sense, because many breast cancers manifest after the woman has had some sort of emotional trauma.

Alban asks the doctor about stress. He says that women of his mother's generation didn't have as much stress as do modern women. EL says that stress definitely has an impact, which is why she's been trying to reduce it in her own life, and why she practises yoga every day. Also, according to a Jungian professor, 'Women's breasts are the receptors of the world's miseries.'

Paris, 8 September 1994

This morning, I phone Dr EL, and she gives me the names of two doctors: an oncologist and a breast specialist, both of whom operate at Hôpital Saint-Louis. She advises me to phone them and make an appointment, and says she'll write me a letter of introduction. I ask her whether she's sent us her article about population – when we visited her, she asked us whether we'd be willing to read it and give her some suggestions. She tells me she's reworking the article, and that she has no confidence in her writing style because she was born in the Rue des Rosiers – one of Paris's Jewish quarters – and that her mother was illiterate. She's opening up to me, telling me about her life, and it's a very moving story.

Later, when I'm more awake, I get the phone book and look up the number of Hôpital Saint-Louis. I dial the number, but there's no answer: the line seems to be busy, but it's hard to tell. I check the number in the phone book again, and find the home number for Dr Esper, one of the doctors that EL has recommended I contact. Alban dials the number for me. A woman answers, and gives Alban another number for the hospital that she thinks Esper might be at. I phone, and the secretary tells me I'll get an appointment quickly only if Dr EL calls Dr Esper herself. I therefore phone Dr EL and ask her to please phone Dr Esper. She tells me she's in the middle of a consultation, that she doesn't have time to either talk to me or phone the doctor, that autumn is always a very busy season, and that she has tons of appointments and things to do. She mumbles something about how hard it is to get in touch with anyone at the hospital. I ask her what I should do, and she tells me she'll call later. Then she hangs up.

I feel embarrassed, sensing I've disturbed – perhaps even irritated – the doctor. But what else could I do? What was I supposed to do? One moment she's ready to tell me about her life; the next, she wants to get rid of me as quickly as possible. Alban concludes that her behaviour is typically Parisian, and that I shouldn't worry: she'll surely call me back to apologise – which she does, in fact, that same evening, to tell me she hasn't been able to reach Esper, that she has five more phone calls to make that evening and that she'll try to call him back tomorrow.

Alban remarks that it doesn't take more time to be nice than to be rude. It occurs to me that he always takes his time with people, and is always kind and patient – and he's probably busier than most people I know! How does he always manage to be kind, sweet and softly spoken while he's very busy? On top of that, he's a Parisian himself – even though he was born in the south of France, he's lived most of his life in Paris. He must be an exception to the rule!

This afternoon, I have a meeting at the Méridien hotel with Mona, Claire Gebeyli and Souad. How I love these women, especially Claire – she's so intense! She tells me that when she learnt about my illness, she was deeply affected and at a loss to know what to write to me. Her best friend, the famous Lebanese poet Nadia Tuéni, had ovarian cancer, for which she received radiation treatment. Seventeen years later, she came down with a cancer that was provoked as a result of the radiation, and this time, she succumbed to the disease. One of her kidneys was burnt – 'roasted from radiation', as Claire describes it.

Mona asks us questions about writing. She's preparing an article about women and writing, for the journal *Bahithat*; yesterday afternoon, when I see her, we talk and talk. She tells me about people who don't grow old well; about her relationship with men; and about her friends, one of whom also had breast cancer and reconstructive surgery. I like her openness and how she deals with her life. I've always admired her.

Claire tells me that Nadia wrote her most beautiful poems when she was ill. Must a person suffer as much as she did in order to discover the sublime? When we're ill, are we able to see relationships, webs and images that we couldn't otherwise? When we succumb to age, become experienced and edge closer to death, do we see life's face rendered more sharply?

Madeleine: Yes, certainly, when one is already in the habit of questioning things.

Manicha: No! For me, what made me discover the 'real' weight of life wasn't my emergency surgery for 'Bowen leucoplasia' *[pre-cancer]* about 25 years ago; it was a passing 'minor depression' I 'contracted' a year before that. I realised that life was a flat wave without either progress or regress, and that it's the artificial projection forward – plans and short-term projects – that gives our existence its salt. I consider that depression is the real human condition: we come from nothing, and go to nothingness! In the meantime, we give ourselves an aim in order to pretend we're 'living' – and it works!

Bettina: I don't like this way of looking at life.

Paris, 20 September 1994

Thanks to Dr EL's phone call, I'm able to get an appointment at Dr Esper's section of Hôpital Saint-Louis. I go with Alban. It's Dr Boi who fills out my medical-history form and asks me some precise questions. She examines me minutely. Then Dr Esper comes in. He's surprised I haven't been given more tests in the States. I remember that I had to insist that Dr JE order the chest X-ray, the bone scan and the tumour markers. I tell the French doctors that the American doctors operate that way in order to save the insurance companies money! I don't know whether they realise I'm being ironic.

At any rate, the doctors order an *ecography*, in which an X-ray machine will be passed over my stomach in order to view any tumour that might be lodged in my liver. I undergo the procedure the next morning. Alban comes with me, and I'm terribly nervous. He keeps telling me he's sure there's nothing there in my liver. I remind him that we were sure it couldn't be cancer when my doctor came to warn us about it, on that cold, rainy Sunday afternoon.

So, while the doctor-technician passes the machine over my abdomen in search of any traces of a liver tumour, I watch her face, trying to detect the slightest trace of suspicion. In the end, when she says there's nothing there, I'm so relieved I could hug her for joy, but I hug Alban instead. How I love to kiss him and wake up in his arms – it's such bliss!

Yesterday, I walk on the Place de l'Opéra: I'm happy to be alive and breathing, and going to Galeries LaFayette, which I thought I might never see again, and I dream of the possibilities of investing in real estate, and of being able to leave my job and devote myself to writing. It all feels like such a miracle!

There's a tiny drizzle. The sky over Paris is grey and slightly rainy, and I enjoy every moment and drink it all in. I stop at a bakery and buy two chocolates, which melt in my mouth. I rarely buy chocolate just for myself, but just for today, I indulge my every whim, and thoroughly enjoy the sweetness of the chocolate and my happiness at being alive in this beautiful city!

I get together with Claudine, a journalist with *L'Evenement du Jeudi*, who I met during a previous sabbatical. We talk about my illness. Her sister had breast cancer when she was 54, and is now 60 and doing very well. She went through everything: a mastectomy, and a year of chemotherapy and radiotherapy. She had a very hard time during her almost unbearable treatment, but didn't want anyone to know she was going through it. She hid her condition by covering her bald head with scarves and wigs, and by covering up her nausea and weakness. Only her family and close friends knew what she was going through.

I first write 'bold head', and Jane quips that it's also in fact a bold–bald head: the boldness would be implied in the baring of the head, if this woman had dared!

Bettina: Right: a bald head, with no attempt at cover-up, is indeed an act of boldness. It's also a reminder of a baby's head, of birth – and of rebirth, in this case.

Manicha: A bald head is a shaven head through which the image of skinhead violence is conjured up, but also the image of the deported, of the patient who's being subjected to violence.

Jane: And of French women who, if they were found to have had sex with German soldiers, had their head shaved as a mark of shame.

Claudine's sister has written philosophy books about the subject of power. I'm reminded of Françoise's friend, a professor of literature, who also went through breast cancer while I was struggling through mine. Françoise tells me that her friend also didn't want anyone to know what she was going through, except for her very close friends and loved ones. Both women didn't want the society around them to know they had cancer, for fear they'd be ostracised and rejected.

Jane: Don't they also fear they'll be pitied? That, for me, would be the worst aspect – and especially so in the case of high-achieving women who have lots of pride!

Bettina: I agree with Jane: it's especially in order to avoid pity that they hide. Pity is worse than the sickness – it's as heavy to bear as guilt.

This illness seems to be even more hushed up here in France than it is in the States. I'm trying to understand the mechanisms for this type of behaviour. Why, for example, does one of my neighbours, Mathilda, speak to me about my illness in so low a voice that she seems to be afraid to talk about it? I think she might know very little about it, until she reveals to me that her mother died from it. And Madame Jardin, another neighbour, who lives in the same building, speaks to me about one of her daughters, who lives in Albi and had breast cancer. The daughter was told she had only two years to live – fortunately, however, she recovered. Madame Jardin is almost in tears when she's remembering the ordeal. She was afraid her daughter wouldn't tell her if she ever had a recurrence because she didn't want to hurt her mother. And other neighbours tell me that their sister or sister-in-law contracted breast cancer after she took estrogen.

The disease has also reached frightening proportions in France, and no one wants to acknowledge it's the case here either. Madame Annick, another neighbour, tells me that France's president, Mitterrand, has prostate cancer that metastisised as a result of grief. The people surrounding him are giving him too hard a time, and that's why he can't get better. Madame Annick tells me that cancer comes upon people because they have sorrow and pain in their life.

Manicha: In Mitterrand's case, I doubt that this cynical lover of power and possession could have been 'touched' by his neighbour's sorrow!

When the Opposition informed him of the events that were occurring at the beginning of the genocide of the Tutsis, and of the massacre of the Hutus by the fascist Rwandan regime of which he was the great protector, he declared, 'In these countries, genocide isn't very important.' *[This comment was reported by the French press in January 1998.]* He was preoccupied with plotting intrigues. In Rwanda's case, the 'Turquoise' operation – a coup d'état in which the French military was involved – was an important initiative!

Bettina: Hold on: we're starting to deviate into politics and to talk nonsense.

Madeleine: Madame Annick's conclusions, drawn from the tabloids, no doubt, don't strike me as being vital in any way, and as a result, Manicha seems to have been provoked into giving a rather questionable reply that's totally off the point.

I read in this week's *Libération*, a French daily newspaper, that every year in France, 25,000 women contract breast cancer and that 10,000 die from it. The proportion of deaths is higher than it is in the States, and the number of deaths equals that of road accidents, as is the case in the States. Why, then, the big cover-up? It should be exactly the opposite: cancer should be the number-one item on everyone's agenda, so that more men and women become aware of their chances of getting it, and do something about it – quickly. I'm revolted by the silence that surrounds this disease, and my anger is exacerbated when I think that women are being complicit in maintaining the silence – especially women who write and are conscious of how important it is to communicate and air issues. Why and how do they justify their silence? Do they feel very threatened? What will they lose if they speak? Are the stakes so high that the women can't speak out?

And why are more women dying from cancer here in

France? Someone tells me it's because they go too late to be treated, or refuse any treatment through which they'll feel robbed of their femininity, which is a more important consideration in French society. It's obvious that women's neglecting to have the necessary tests and seek treatment early is the reason that breast cancer is surrounded by so palpable a silence.

Bettina: Yes: it's very serious.

Jane: I heard Dr Love on NPR *[National Public Radio]* one morning *[9 July 1997]*, and she stated that breast cancer isn't necessarily prevented if it's detected early by way of a mammogram, because one is never sure that those small tumours one finds through early detection would ever have become malignant! I couldn't believe she'd say such a thing. This is all having to do with the debate as to whether the state should be funding mammograms, and at what age a woman should undergo the procedure – 40, 50? It all comes down to money in the end!

However, I'm not surprised to hear Dr Love's reaction, because I've also read her interview with Julie Felner in *Ms* magazine this month (*Ms*: July–August 1997), in which she shows how disillusioned she's become with medicine and with trying to cure breast cancer. She believes that the key is prevention through environmental changes and adopting a different diet. The doctor, who until now has been treating women via the usual 'Cut, poison and burn' treatment, and who's written a major book about breast cancer (Love: 1993), which I read when I was first diagnosed, has decided to cease practising for a while and to devote her time to researching and preventing cancer. She's also becoming increasingly outspoken against hormones. Her recently published book about the subject (Love: 1997) is a must for any woman who's contemplating having ERT. The national debates about early mammograms only serve to reinforce my conviction that very little is known about the disease, and that much more effort and money should be allocated to research and prevention. I couldn't agree more with what Dr Love is now saying!

Manicha: In France also, detection *[mammograms and pap-smear tests]* have recently been reduced in order to 'fill the social-security gaps'!

Madeleine: Where does Manicha get her information? From what I've been able to observe, the situation is exactly the opposite.

Claudine tells me that her sister was treated at Villejuif, a big cancer treatment and research centre located on the outskirts of Paris, and that her sister saw many doctors – among them, the famous Dr Lucien Israël, who treated Resa. Her sister insulted everyone. She didn't want to be viewed as being ill; being rebellious was her way of dominating her disease. When she shouted and cried, and expressed her resentment at the doctors by telling them off, she was able to remain in control of her body. I understand her anger, but shouldn't she, through her rage, have come to an awakening of consciousness, and become committed to her society, and the women in it, in order to facilitate a change of attitudes and values?

Bettina: I have female patients who react in the same way when faced with the disease. I think it's a way of overcoming their fear, and we really can't condemn this kind of reaction. The important thing is to fight according to your own temperament, and not to let yourself slip into despair. You, Evelyne, reacted in accordance with your own personality and generosity, by applying your talent for writing, which is, of course, a more constructive way; however, you have to recognise that there are other ways to combat and overcome the disease.

Manicha: It's easier to take it out on your immediate circle than on 'society' as a whole: revolt isnt revolution!

What else am I going to find out, in this society, in relation to cancer?

I speak with Françoise. She thinks I should carry my analysis further, and talk about my relationship with my body – how I feel as a result of the mastectomy. She thinks that women can be divided between the ones who love their body and the ones who negate it; she thinks I'm somewhere in between. Before, I felt at home in my body, but now I feel mutilated and alienated from it. Sexual problems result when you don't feel good about your body. According to Françoise, I should analyse all this, because I'd thereby help other women understand some things about their body and their relationship with it as a result of having been ill or mutilated; they'd be better able to move forward. Dear Françoise helps me think, and carry my thoughts and analysis many steps further.

Jane: This is where a novel or film could be best put to use!

Madeleine: In my view, there are three categories of women: (1) the ones who like their body, at times excessively; (2) the ones who deny their body and sometimes go so far as to disown it; and (3) the ones who assess their body, gauge it, scrutinise it and know how to get the best out of it. This last category is the rarest, but women like that do exist.

Paris, 28 September 1994

Marvellous get-together today with Andrée Chedid, at La Cour de Rohan, a lovely tea-room in the Latin quarter. It's Souad who organised the meeting with Mona. It's so great to see Andrée after so long. She called me so many times during my illness in order to cheer me up and find out how I was doing. I show her the photos that Eva took, and she finds them very powerful. We talk and talk about important subjects, and compare our ideas about meaningful events, shows and exhibitions that are taking place.

Bettina: I also saw these pictures, and 'powerful' is the word. They said, 'I've been through war and its battles, and here I am, in my dignity and strength, despite the physical and mental after-effects.'

I love Andrée Chedid's vision of life – I'm always uplifted when I've been with her. She's one of those rare individuals whose very presence is a pleasure – like sitting on top of a mountain, breathing fresh, clean air and thinking lofty thoughts: elevated moments you want to keep forever in your memory, and that you want to remember during the dark and difficult days when life is weighing so heavily on you that even breathing is an arduous task.

Amel's letters, such as the following, are also a breath of fresh air for me.

La Marsa, 7 September '94

Evelyne, ma chérie, you're so close, just across from the sea ... Time is bringing us closer: in a few weeks, you'll be here ... In Germany, we visited a couple, both artists from Iran. He's a painter, and his works are very powerful emotionally. The morning of our departure, he had an epileptic seizure in the street. He became epileptic after the torture he received in the Shah's prisons. Now they live in exile – it's hard. That morning, I cried with rage against stupidity, against violence. In Bochum, I decided not to wait any longer for the trip to India. With the money I'd saved, I bought new glasses ['new look' in English in her letter], music and shoes. Once my decision was taken and the waiting ended, I felt as light as a bird ...

I'm expecting Rachida, who's going to spend the day with me. I'm preparing rice and gnaouia [gambos: a green, bean-shaped vegetable that tastes like a cross between spinach, beans and

271

zucchini, and is a bit gluey; you fry it in olive oil and cook it with tomato sauce.] *We talk a lot about you together, my darling friend: how happy I'll be to see you. Knowing you were sick has been so difficult. But I know you're healing now – from your disease, and from what made you sick, my Evelyne. I know how hard it is. I look at the picture you sent me: you're sitting in your garden. Alban is to your right, his hands crossed, yours resting on your knees. You're smiling at Eva, who's looking at you with love, forcing your modesty a bit.*

These last few days, I woke up with anxiety in the throat, so I do my yoga and meditation, and I listen to music and try to write. Writing to you this morning makes me happy ... I'm sometimes so excessive, so cruel. I'm like a sponge: I absorb the unspoken, the hidden pains, the negated fragilities, and it hurts me. How hard it was to experience exile in Germany! Now I'm back in La Marsa, I have more distance; I feel more levelheaded. I've been reading Fragment d'un discours amoureux *by Roland Barthes. It's interesting ... Tell me how you're spending your days; tell me about your desires, your dreams, your worries. I miss you ...*

Several large studies have detected elevated cancer rates around hazardous waste sites. One of them was conducted in New Jersey, a tiny state with an astonishing 112 Superfund sites. Researchers asked whether cancer mortality was associated with environmental factors of various kinds, including the location of toxic waste dumps. Their results showed that communities near toxic waste sites had significantly elevated mortality from stomach and colon cancers. Additionally, in twenty-one different New Jersey counties, breast cancer mortality among white women rose as the distance from residence to dump site shrank. However, many of the clusters of excess cancer occurred in heavily industrialized counties so that air pollution from these sources confounded the results. Thus, a woman with breast cancer in northeastern New Jersey cannot know with certainty whether she is dying because of the air wafting down from the factory stacks or because of the water contaminated by the dump site. (Steingraber: 1997: 71)

Men living in hazardous waste counties suffered significantly higher mortality from cancers of the lung, bladder, esophagus, colon, and stomach than did their contemporaries residing in counties without such sites. Women living in hazardous waste counties suffered significantly higher mortality from lung, breast, bladder, colon, and stomach cancers. Indeed, counties with hazardous waste sites were 6.5 times more likely to have elevated breast cancer rates than counties without such sites. (Steingraber: 1997: 71)

Counties with the highest breast cancer mortality had four times as many facilities that treated and stored toxic waste than the national average. (Steingraber: 1997: 72)

Problems with Premarin: The effects of Premarin on the liver don't appear to be limited to digestion. Even when it's given vaginally, which means that it avoids the digestive system. Premarin has more of an effect on the liver than non-horse estrogens do. There may be something else in the horse urine besides estrogen that causes some of this additional effect. Another problem is that the level of estrogen produced in the blood of women on Premarin consists of three major components. The first is estrone sulfate, which makes up 50 to 60 percent of the preparation. This is a hormone found in both horses and humans. Then there are two horse estrogens that aren't made by humans – equilin sulfate, which is 20 to 30 percent of the preparation; and 17 alpha dihydroequilin sulfate, which is 15 percent. The levels of the equilin estrogens in these pills are many times higher than our bodies' normal levels of estradiol or estrone. What effect does that have? The pharmaceutical companies haven't told us

that. And no one else has studied it. We simply don't know …
To get the urine needed to make Premarin, about 50,000
mares are impregnated each year. For seven months of her
eleven-month pregnancy, each mare is kept in a tiny stall,
barely large enough to hold her. She wears a harness with a
device to collect her urine. In order to make the urine more
concentrated, she is given only minimal water to drink. (Love:
1997: 257)

9

A NO-WIN SITUATION
CELEBRATING FRIENDSHIP IN TUNISIA

As a woman with cancer who grew up in a county with fifteen hazardous waste sites, several carcinogen-emitting industries, and public water wells that, from time to time, show detectable levels of toxic chemicals, I am less concerned about whether the cancer in my community is more directly connected to the dump sites, the air emissions, the occupational exposures, or the drinking water. I am more concerned that the uncertainty over details is being used to call into doubt the fact that profound connections do exist between human health and the environment. I am more concerned that uncertainty is too often parlayed into an excuse to do nothing until more research can be conducted. '"We need more study," is the grandfather of all arguments for taking no action,' says Peter Infante, who, in his daily struggle to set limits on workplace exposure to carcinogens, hears them all. (Steingraber: 1997: 73)

Paris, 1 October 1994

I'm at Orly Airport with Cindy, and she's suffered in the taxi there as a result of the pollution. She's very sensitive, and I love that about her.

Yesterday, we go to Galeries LaFayette. We take the small street located behind Gare St Lazarre, where the prostitutes operate. It's only 11 a.m., but there they are: half-naked and exposing their enormous breasts. Cindy remarks how terrible it would be for a woman in this profession to have breast cancer! She says it in a way that's both funny and sad. I think to myself, *These poor women*, but perhaps they aren't so poor, and are in fact rich and happy. I remember a conversation I had with Françoise Collin, who told me about a conference she organised entitled Sexual Slavery, to which she invited some prostitutes to present a real-life testimonial. The prostitutes said that they didn't envy women who work in the sphere of academia; on the contrary, they felt that they themselves earnt better money and had more fun in the process. *For how long, though?* I thought. *And what about the women oppressed by a pimp?* According to research undertaken by my friend Kathleen Barry, entitled *Female Sexual Slavery* (Barry: 1984), 90 per cent of prostitutes suffer at the hand of a pimp. What do they do when they can no longer sell their body?

Jane: And what about the intellectual prostitution that goes on among academics, vying for tenure, publication, prizes, grants and so on?

Cindy and I wait for our friend Brigitte in front of Galeries LaFayette. Strangely, although we're waiting just a few metres away from Brigitte, we somehow manage not to see her! Later, Brigitte calls us, angry because she thinks we didn't show up on purpose; we, however, had been thinking, *Something unforeseen must've cropped up to prevent her from coming. Poor thing! She must be annoyed, and was probably unable to call us!* Are these cultural or personal differences? French people flare up more quickly, and often regret their action later. I tell Cindy that Brigitte will probably phone to apologise – and sure enough, that's what she does!

It's good to be able to talk about all this with Alban as well as with Cindy, who's one of the most disciplined and straightforward people I know. She tells me she thinks that Brigitte allows herself to talk to me the way she does because she really loves me! I say, 'Wait till she loves you the way she loves me: then we'll see how you like being talked to like that!' We have a good laugh about that one.

Now, on the plane travelling from Paris to Tunis with Cindy, I'm getting very excited about seeing Amel, Azza and our other Tunisian friends. I feel so stimulated, by Cindy's presence as well as at the prospect of getting back to the Arab world again: it's where I really belong, as if it were always calling to me from deep within my soul. Yesterday, my darling Alban says, 'Write! Write! I love it when you win literary awards!' I love this man, who encourages me and is so intellectually alert.

Tunis, 3 October 1994

It's Cindy's birthday, and mine will be in three days' time. We're both Libra: is that why we get along so well? I love and respect her, and feel so fortunate that she's translated my latest novel. What a labour of love; what a gift she showered on me by doing the translation during my treatment! We're sitting on the sidewalk café of the Africa Hotel, which is also called the Méridien hotel. The weather is rainy and grey.

Everything's taking time and effort. Since last summer, the staff at the Clairefontaine bookshop have sold only six copies of my book *Blessures des mots* (Accad: 1993), even though the shop had exclusive rights to sell it. I've forgotten how difficult and time-consuming everything is in this part of the world.

Cindy, Amel and I are spending some intense moments together: talking, discussing, meditating and giving each other massages. How therapeutic, and how good it makes us all feel!

Tunis, 5 October 1994

Cindy and I again sit in the Méridien's sidewalk café. I watch people pass by on Bourguiba Avenue. Flocks of birds sing in the trees. This morning, we swim with Amel in the Mediterranean, the sea that heals. It's beautiful! I feel I'm slowly healing: regaining my strength, and getting rid of all the chemicals my body's had to endure and absorb. It's so wonderful to be with women who are so well in their body and who communicate harmony, peace, love and understanding.

Cindy and I write, and later she gives me what she wrote, as follows.

Evelyne, it's such happiness to be with you once more: we have life to celebrate. I wish you a very beautiful birthday. Your friendship is very precious to me.

> ### Arrival
> *To write as if I could touch it*
> *more deeply:*
> *this street market,*
> *these reddish-whites of afternoon,*
> *this Parisian fog*
> *of walking green-black-blues.*
> *The ongoing outpouring of Saint-Ouen,*
> *Dark cries of 'Papa!' mixed with*
> *whiffs of a golden, warm baguette.*
> *Facing me,*
> *this woman flying a smile –*
> *birds in her eyes –*
> *who draws me into her world,*
> *touching East and West,*
> *her hand freeing itself*
> *to take mine.*

On the plane between Tunis and Beirut, 7 October 1994

I'm about to land at Beirut Airport, and there's nervous anticipation in the air. Last night, I dream that mother is being transported on a stretcher that looks more like a casket. Alive and radiantly smiling at me, she's coming up to me, and going to meet father: images of life and death, of meeting and departing, of leaving and arriving.

What a beautiful birthday the women give me at Amel's home yesterday evening. I'm deeply moved, and when they – especially Amel – start reading *Blessures des mots* (Accad: 1993), my novel about their feminist movement, I cry. They'd like to produce a stage version of it, and it'll be great if they follow through. I feel so close to this dear friend Amel. With Cindy I also have some fantastic, intense moments. Yesterday, we swim in a raging sea. I find these swims incredibly soothing, even when the waves are high. I've always loved the sea, and now I find it even more meaningful and intense – as if I were going through a rebirth. The salt numbs the pain on my chest wall, and the sea and wind caress and revitalise my skin. I feel I'm healing not only physically but spiritually.

Yarzé, 11 October 1994

I've been in Lebanon for a few days now. Claire Gebeyli remembers I'm arriving on the 7th, and phones to arrange to see me. It's sad not seeing father, but at the same time, mother is marvellous and serene. It's Adelaide who's worrying me. She tells me that if she had breast cancer, she'd refuse to be treated: she'd prefer to die. I don't believe she would, but I'm saddened to hear her talk like that. It's so evident that she isn't happy. Her lifestyle is a mismatch with who she could be: she's a vibrant and passionate woman, waiting to fly!

Mother is often making me laugh, in spite of her illness – she's extraordinary.

The phone rings at my friend Mona's place, in which I'm staying at present. No one picks it up, and I wonder why. Mona's friend Néna comes tonight and shows me her reconstructed breasts. She tells me that if she could help other women by doing so, she'd be willing to show her breasts and talk about what happened to her when she got breast cancer, during the middle of the war. She thinks she contracted the cancer as a result of being stressed. In both the States and Lebanon, I've heard many statements and read many books in which breast cancer is linked to stress – and there certainly was plenty of it around during the war in Lebanon. Néna tells me that there's too much ignorance about the subject of cancer, and that there are too many taboos surrounding it.

However, I'm noticing here, as I've noticed in other places, that people need to talk about cancer. Mona Kouloub has opened up to me and told me about the surgery, chemotherapy and radiation she underwent. The dean of Beirut University College, a woman I've often had the chance to interact with and who I deeply admire, cries as she tells me that her son had to go to the States to have a bone-marrow transplant in order to treat him for a very aggressive lymphoma. He's only 18! Also, some members of The Women's Institute would like me to address a special meeting about my experiences as a cancer patient.

Tonight at Mona's, Néna, says that a woman never completely overcomes the traumatism of going through breast cancer: she can never again be at ease with her body. However, I think that Néna's reconstructed breasts look rather good – they have the shape of a young woman's breasts; I understand her feelings very well, though. I'm touched that she's confided in me, and I admire her for being frank and open.

At first, I used the word *trauma* rather than *traumatism*.

Madeleine: After breast reconstruction, it's better to speak of 'traumatism', because Néna is referring to the whole set of physical and psychological disturbances that are triggered within the organism as a result of cancer; in fact, there exists a relatively strong psychological traumatism due to the violent emotional shock that the patient has had to deal with on his or her way to being cured.

I miss Alban.

I find it isn't easy to live in Lebanon these days: it's very hot at present, even though we're already in the middle of October, and the traffic is unbearable. During meetings I attend with the Bahithats ('Researchers': Bahithats is both a women's organisation and the name of the organisation's journal), it's obvious that unbreachable divisions with reference to power and control exist among the women researchers, as is the case in Tunis; this is despite the fact that the Lebanese women have received a substantial, five-year grant from the Ford Foundation: an advantage that my Tunisian friends would no doubt envy.

Jane: I'm surprised you say 'despite': I believe that money often becomes an aggravating factor, because the people involved have to fight for their share by discrediting their competitors' work.

Unfortunately, this is to a great extent true; however, I could've hoped that if the material conditions had been better, some of the practical aspects of the research could have been improved and some problems alleviated, so that the working atmosphere could've been more harmonious.

Madeleine: Not all women are like you, Evelyne, blithe spirit. What do you make of pride, jealousy and selfishness?

Beirut, 12 October 1994

If it weren't for mother's presence, I wouldn't be staying here, in the family home: there's too much dissension, and I can't stand it when Adelaide says she'd rather die than have the kind of treatment I was subjected to. I can't absorb her suffering the way I used to, I can't continue to absorb other people's suffering, and I'm tired of hearing people say that we Lebanese have to be patient because the country is coming out of a war. Many people and countries emerge from a similarly major trial stronger, more beautiful, more serene and more 'together'. Here at home and in society in general, I believe it's too easy for everyone to complain and remain complacent because they've been hurt. I no longer have the patience I had before I came so close to death.

Cindy: That's a good thing. Your need to protect yourself might be hard for other people to understand, but you have to look after yourself.

I'm saddened that Rose can't bear to look at the photos of my wound, scar and mastectomy. I tell her she might find them interesting in the context of her art – I'm thinking of my photographer friend Eva and the artistic statement she was making. And I'm hurt that some people are telling me they couldn't sleep after seeing the photos, and that I shouldn't show them because they're disturbing. Why this hiding from life's painful realities? Was I like that before I became ill? Did I avoid looking at suffering? I don't think so; however, looking at suffering has taken on a different meaning for me.

Two years after I've written these words, I think about them more. I remember that 12 years ago in Paris, when Resa was recuperating in hospital after having her breasts reconstructed, she offered to show them to me but I actually refused to look at them. It's strange how we can change with time and as a result of life's experiences, and how we can forget our reactions. For this reason, it's useful for me to be keeping a journal and writing down, as much as possible, what's happening every day.

Cindy: I wonder why we're so afraid to see evidence of another person's pain.

Jane: We find these photos disturbing because when we're being raised, we see photos of sexy women who have perfect breasts and a perfect body, or we see artists' paintings and sculptures of an ideal body; we therefore feel uneasy when we look at a photo of an 'ugly' but perfectly healthy body, let alone a photo of an unhealthy or mutilated one. Our society has a low tolerance level for any representation of imperfection. *[My own mother had her teeth 'fixed' not because there was anything wrong with them but because they didn't look good in our family photos!]* This is why Diane Arbus's photos are so startling. She often photographs so-called freaks of nature, and insane people and people who are very marginalised in society.

Why don't people express more love for each other? Last week, I can't bear to listen to a conversation between my friends Myrna and Farid: it's unbearably empty. Nor am I able, any longer, to participate in vacuous dinner conversations: I have neither the time nor the patience to be routinely polite. Life's too short, and I still have so many things that'll take time for me to accomplish properly.

In future, I don't want to come back to Lebanon unless I have my own place to live in. Depending on other people is too difficult: I'm used to doing things on my own, and getting about here is a real headache. One of my acquaintances, Julia, is living in a milieu in which the people she's interacting with are quite spoilt, despite the reversals they suffered during the war; I wonder whether she's aware of this situation I've observed.

Beirut, 21 October 1994

I'm at the airport, about to head back to Tunis. Lebanon is nothing but a big construction site – there are buildings going up everywhere! The country's artistic activities and cultural life in general are picking up at an extraordinary pace. It's the victory of life over death. However, materialism is becoming entrenched. I'm told there's a lot of theft, and I see 'oceans of misery surrounding islands of wealth': an expression that Alban often uses to describe cities.

Although I find mother to be very serene, she's suffering intensely from both losing father and enduring her many illnesses. She tells me that father suffered a lot at the end of his life, not only from his disease but from being treated as if he were a child. I hurt when I think about both reasons for his pain.

Here at the airport, I see a young bride, all dressed in white. She's leaving to get married in another country. What will life bring her? She seems so carefree. She takes the plane to Frankfurt: a young Lebanese bride going to a German groom?

This time here in Lebanon, I go through another big health scare: Dr ES, who our family doctor recommended to me, tells me I should have another four to six months of chemotherapy in order to make sure all the cancerous cells have been eliminated. Why didn't the other doctors I've seen make this recommendation? I'm in a no-win situation: if I go through the extra chemo, I'll have to be tortured all over again – nausea, hair loss and so on – whereas if I don't go through it and the cancer comes back, I'll regret my decision. I ask Alban to make me an appointment with Dr Esper, and I send Dr ES's report to Dr JE and ask her to advise me.

I'll have to make a decision soon, because if I undergo another four to six months of chemo, I'll have to start right away.

Manicha: It's unbearable to think that the patient must make up her own mind – make that agonising decision – about what to do for her treatment! How come there's such divergence of opinion and such obvious inconsistency among doctors?

It's why I decided to write this book, Manicha: to reveal, to scream out, these inconsistencies and the difficulties that cancer patients face, not only in choosing options but – most of all – in lacking options.

I'm on a Middle East Airline plane, returning from Beirut to Tunis. I remember the days when I worked as a cabin-crew member on the same airline in order to pay for my fare to the States, to study. Things have never come easily to me: I've had to earn them the hard way. However, being a flight steward for a little while was rather fun, although tiring. I was able to travel to many countries, and learnt many things I'd been shielded from in my protected life.

Adelaide has tears in her eyes as she says goodbye – she's so sensitive. Fortunately, she's very sweet and mild mannered with mother, who's also very sweet and softly spoken – personality traits through which harmony is generated around her.

Yesterday, I visit some friends. We speak about illness, especially cancer. We discuss the sad story of Nadia Tuéni, one of the greatest Francophone (French North African, Middle Eastern, Swiss, Belgian, Vietnamese and so on) poets the Arab world has known. Nadia watched her seven-year-old daughter die of kidney cancer – which today is a treatable type of cancer. After she went through that horrible ordeal, she became pregnant again. She went to the doctor, and he asked her whether she was taking any medication. When she told him what she was taking, he suggested he give her an abortion because there was a risk that the child would be born deformed. It was tremendously painful – physically, mentally and emotionally – for Nadia to have the abortion. Later, she became pregnant again and gave birth to her second son. Seven months later, she found herself pregnant again, and was surprised at how close the two pregnancies were. However, it wasn't another pregnancy; it was a cyst on her ovary, which turned out to be not only malignant but the worst kind of malignant cyst. She went to Paris to be treated at the Institut Curie, at which she was given radiotherapy. Seventeen years later, she developed what's called a 'therapeutic cancer', on one of her kidneys; the kidney had been burnt as a result of the radiation she received during the earlier treatment. In 1983, Nadia Tuéni died from that 'therapeutic cancer'. I think, *She absorbed her daughter's kidney cancer; she died as a result of suffering and grief.*

Also, I notice how frequently the number seven, the number that symbolises perfection and wholeness, recurred throughout Nadia's life: she was a great writer, and I feel that the number could be a marker for the perfection that was evident in all that she did. I think about this remarkable woman's pain, but I'm also drawn to thinking about her beauty and the poetry she wrote. For this reason, I can't resist quoting from one of her poems, which she herself translated for the 15 July 1982 issue of the *Chicago Tribune*, about a year before she died. I've taken the poem from *July of My Remembrance* (Tuéni: 1991: 31), a collection of poems that Nadia compiled as (Tuéni: 1991: 4) 'a souvenir album, Nadia's gift to her "house of the zodiac": born Cancer, she offered, for reasons not unknown, her last poem to July.'

A body whole, unscathed,
is beauty to behold.
Beyond the final gasp
my life goes on, resisting
like a sun many times dead.
So open wide the window;
let in the sounds of night.
They shall be my bier,
they shall be my shroud.
On Lebanon draw down the shade.
Let just the memory remain
which, mingling with the air,
brings back my short-lived prime.
Let the mountain on me spread
its gravel, wind and thyme.
A name I shall become, imprinted on the shore,
and for you, sometimes, that butterfly of night
whose soared wings crackle from the scorch of light.

Tunis, 23 October 1994

I'm at the Club Tahar Haddad, for a singing rehearsal with
dear Amel. I'm filled with all kinds of emotions in this place,
in which I experienced so many intense and wonderful
moments. The weather is very cold, grey and rainy. The sea
has been unleashed, and I'm sleepy.

Amel has made an appointment for me with her doctor,
Hassen, to see what he has to say about the Beirut doctor's
diagnosis that I should have another four to six months of
chemotherapy – an idea I find terrorising but that I have to
live with for the moment. As my sweet Alban says, 'With
this disease, everything's so approximate.' At this time,
Alban tries to reach Dr Esper, but is told that although the
doctor doesn't give appointments before January, he'll take
my call if I have a specific question to ask. Alban also calls

Dr TU, who operates at the big centre called Villejuif, on the outskirts of Paris – the Beirut doctor, Dr ES, has recommended him – and makes an appointment for the 8th of November.

Here I am, making all kinds of plans to present my books and address conferences; however, I'm not doing it with a light heart, because I'm wondering whether I'll be able to fulfil all my commitments if I have to undergo another round of chemo. I've lost the joy of recovering that I had before I visited the Beirut doctor, who really gave me the blues. I'm worried by his advice, because no matter what option I choose, risks are involved.

Khadija, the director of the Club Tahar Haddad, tells me that Amel didn't tell her I had breast cancer, only that I was a bit sick. Even my friends are afraid to name this disease, the *marad illi ma btitssama*: 'the disease that can't be named'. People such as my poor Amel are frightened to call the disease by its name: she's seen close friends and relatives, including her own father, die from it. She thinks I'm healed now, and that I shouldn't have another round of chemo; instead, she's made an appointment for me to see her doctor, who she really trusts and who has a lot of experience in the area of breast cancer.

Paris, 27 October 1994

I'm back in Paris now. Yesterday on the plane, I want to write, but I have a bad stomach ache, having caught a bug in Tunis that a lot of people had come down with. There are so many things I want to write about, such as what happened in Tunis, and my visit to Amel's doctor.

Yesterday in Tunis, I make a vegetable broth for lunch. When Amel returns to the house, she brings some fish she's bought at La Goulette, an area located on the outskirts of Tunis, close to where she teaches. Was it eating the fish that made me sick? Had the fish been gutted and washed carefully enough? Alban tells me that fish eat anything, even the most rotten and disgusting waste matter.

Amel accompanies me to visit her doctor, Dr Hassen, who operates in the city's Saint Augustine clinic, which is run by nuns. We sit in the waiting room, in which there are a lot of other people: people who look sad and anguished; people with cancer. A woman comes and sits near us, and asks us to make her laugh; Amel and I have been talking and laughing, as we're often doing. We talk about cancer with the woman, and she tells us her story. There's no history of breast cancer in her family – her two grandmothers lived till they were 90! She doesn't understand how or why she contracted the disease when she reached 50 – *Just like me*, I think, and tell her. She had a mastectomy. She had radiation therapy on all the nodes of her chest wall and under her arm – the nodes weren't removed during the operation – as well as on her ovaries, and after that, chemotherapy. She tired a lot as a result of the radiation. She was horrified that the door of the radiation room bore a sign, in French, the warning on which was *Bombes cobalt!*: 'Cobalt bombs!' – the containers of radioactive cobalt used medically. She asked herself, *Why do they use such terrifying names, and why do I have to go through this? Why me, and what produced it – was it the government-subsidised cooking oil?* Amel tells me that Tunisians are suspicious of the cheap cooking oil they use, because it's a mixture of various kinds of vegetable oils.

Jane: Especially after the oil scandal in Spain! Everyone's sure that adulterated oil is now the root of all evil!

Amel tells us that when she cooks, she uses only pure olive oil; however, the woman says her family doesn't like it. Both Amel and I ask her a lot of questions. She tells us she experienced her cancer as a castration. It is indeed a castration, and on top of everything, when you've had chemotherapy, you gain weight, and that does nothing for your self-image. The woman tells us that because her financial situation was tight, she had to forgo two expensive medical check-ups. Now she's worried because she has a pain on her right side and a funny taste in her mouth.

I tell the woman my story. When we discuss hair, and I describe the shaving session I had with Samira and Zohra, Amel starts crying. This sweet friend of mine is surrounding me with so much care and affection, yet she's almost too sensitive. I hate giving her this amount of pain.

We go in to see Dr Hassen. He asks me lots of questions, and is astonished that I was given estrogen under minimal surveillance and that the tumour grew so quickly. He tells me that although the prognosis for lobular carcinoma is better than it is for most other types of cancer, the patient's other breast has to be watched very carefully, because the cancer often *bi-laterises*, that is, spreads to the other breast. He asks me whether I had a biopsy of the other breast, and I tell him I didn't have it. He says he would have done it, just to be on the safe side. He draws a diagram of the breasts to show me which place lobular carcinoma is usually located in: exactly the place that mine was located in and developed. I'm very impressed by him, because he's knowledgeable and precise. He tells me he's sure my tumour was provoked as a result of the estrogen I took, and adds that scientists have given laboratory mice high doses of estrogen and the mice have consequently developed mammary cancer.

He then examines me while a nurse – a nun – takes my blood pressure. He asks me whether I'm planning to have reconstruction. I reply that I haven't decided yet, and that I'm mainly thinking about healing. He says I should think about having it, because I'm still young. He then asks me how much a mastectomy costs in the States. I reply that although

I'm not entirely sure, I believe that the operation itself – what the surgeon charges without hospital, anesthesia and other fees – costs only $2500, but that the whole treatment, including chemo and radiation, can run up to $50,000. He goes to wash his hands, while I get dressed and return to the other room, where Amel is waiting.

We ask him whether he thinks I should have another round of chemotherapy, as the Lebanese doctor has suggested. He says he doesn't think I should, and that the chemo I've already had is very potent and toxic for the heart. For the type of cancer I had, the signs for recovery are favourable: the nodes were negative, despite the size of the tumour, so the cancer had a non-aggressive quality. I would've suffered much more damage if I'd had an aggressive cancer of that size. Whether the malignancy is bad isn't always determined by its size: some very small tumours can behave much worse.

Dr Hassen says he wouldn't do anything more to treat me. He says that although I mustn't live in a constant state of fear, I must remain vigilant. He gives me the name of another doctor, TU, who's a friend of his who operates in Paris.

⧗

I read some of the letters that await me in Paris, and include extracts from them as follows. I feel courageous and energetic when I read them.

Nathalie: *What can I learn from this ordeal? Indeed, what can you learn? Nothing – everything ... to learn to go back to the root of things ... Isn't life about awareness, the knowledge and understanding of the self and then other people, the world? ... Nature always sends us signs ... always puts us in situations, in order to help us rise ... if we run away, it will follow us and we'll never experience a state of ignorant bliss. I know you'll travel through the tunnel and that once you've reached the other end, you'll be even more beautiful than before ... Evelyne, nothing is coincidence, even our friendship ...*

Gilles: *What matters is that you give me the impression you aren't doing too badly. If the process* [of cancer] *had been once again unleashed, it would show. And French medicine is excellent. That said, one can never know for sure, with this bitch of a disease.*

Jane: The French would say ' a whore of a disease': notice they're all feminine epithets!

Enough is known, in your case, to heal you. But you must remain vigilant, and you're so right to want to understand: today, medical attitudes having evolved, the patient knows what's happening step by step, as much as the doctor. And you aren't wrong to practise relaxation: morale plays a big part in cancer, and anguish plays a big part in morale ... As for here, nothing's new; fortunately, nothing's all I can ask: nothing in everything ...

Paula: *It was so brave of you to confront your illness and subsequent operation as you have, and your determination to grow from this dreadful experience is very admirable. By giving voice to your difficult journey, you've given heart and courage to so many women. The way the medical profession behaved with the hormone therapy is shocking; it made a great impression on me, because I'm on hormone-replacement therapy and weighing the risks associated with it. Until the medical establishment finally pays attention to the health concerns of women – and that attention is still slow in coming – many more women will be the victims of drug treatment that can cause cancer.*

The best news is that you're recovering. Although it might feel slow to you, there's definite progress being made, thank God. Both Lisa and I are so happy you're feeling much better. And I personally can attest that a person can be free of the disease. One of my best friends had lung cancer diagnosed 10 years ago. After having her lung removed, followed by chemotherapy, she is and has been free of the disease. The only reason her cancer was discovered was that when a concerned physician learnt that both the woman's parents had died of the disease, he insisted she have a thorough examination.

With my very best wishes and love

The most basic lie in this matter consists of having people believe that the effects of treatment are well known and under control. Specialists euphemize, employing the term 'side effects', i.e. harmful undesirable effects, to signify something therapeutic ... In the case of chemotherapy, what good does it do to warn of the disappearance of white cells that can't even be seen, and then to hush up problems having to do with menstruation? Particularly when it's a question of breast or uterine cancers, whereby one needn't be a cancer specialist to understand that these are entirely female cancers. Not to mention the early onset of menopause and sterility, triggered by these treatments. Could we not at least call for a bit of consistency in attitudes with reference to the side effects of these treatments? ... A choice has to be made: either not to inform at all, so as not to suggest the kind of problems that only might occur, or to inform, as best possible, to enable the patient to make an enlightened decision – at the very least, not to leave patients in a state of anxiety and abandon as they face the problems that are bound to arise, with no knowledge of what has caused them, how long they are going to last or how to relieve them ... Imagine the terror of a sufferer who gradually discovers he can no longer lean over, sit, walk, stand – in short, who realizes he has aged forty years in the space of one, without any kind of warning. Imagine, too, how he feels when, no longer able to move, his muscles begin to atrophy, and a corpse-like stiffness sets in. When compared with this, nausea and vomiting seem reassuring, because as horrible as they are, at least they have been indexed. The list of troubles that accompany chemotherapy has yet to be drawn up in full. (As a side note, the hideous sensation of poison entering the veins would provide enough material to fill several pages, and still would not fully render the shock of chemical therapy.) An easy way to sum it up would be the following: you have the feeling that you are dying of a continuous poisoning. (Hyvrard: 1987: 170–2)

Our biosphere has reached the endpoint of its potential to safely shelter us beneath the world's sky. The crucial lack of fresh, bio-available drinking water will inevitably make itself felt across all continents, even though some privileged places still wear the blinkers of apparent or provisional abundance. We must learn as soon as possible how to desalinate the oceans on a large scale, and especially how to develop other, less wasteful consumer habits. Drought is likely to spread even further, with the impending greenhouse effect. Even if sporadic flooding as a result of atmospheric warming trends is frequent, ... even if these floods occur with increasing frequency, and with increasingly disastrous consequences, because we are not equipped to receive water at so great a rate, this liquid of life, once on the ground, is useless for the purposes of human consumption. (Séralini: 1997: 111)

10

PARIS BREAST BLUES
THE FEAR OF RECURRENCE

The worst suffering is the one that cannot be shared. And cancer patients, more often than not, feel this suffering twice as much: twice because, once sick, they cannot share with those around them the anxiety they are experiencing; also, however because beneath this suffering lies another, much older, dating back to childhood, which has never been shared either, never seen by anyone. Yet I believe that if I can share with you my suffering, I am already halfway towards healing … even though I am going to die. I am healed psychologically, which is already an enormous gain. (Lambrichs: 1995: 98)

Paris, 3 November 1994

I've written a letter to my doctor here, Dr Esper, asking him to advise me, and enclosing a copy of the letter from the Beirut doctor, Dr ES. Today, Dr Esper phones to tell me he doesn't think it's necessary for me to have more chemotherapy, because my lymph nodes were negative; if I were ever to have more chemo, I should've had it when I was being treated – not now, five months having already elapsed since I had my last chemo session. He remarks that treating breast cancer is an uncertain endeavour, because there are always pros and cons, no matter what choice the patient makes. I like him because he's frank, and appreciate the fact that he's called me.

As for Dr JE, my doctor in the States, I've sent her a similar letter, but I haven't heard back from her yet. I've asked some friends in the States to contact her and let her know I'm waiting for her to respond, and I intend to write to her again.

These past few days, I've been feeling anxious. I have pains in various parts of my body, and imagine I have lumps here and there. I'll be able to relax and know I'm free of any recurrence only when I've had the first check-ups and the doctors have concluded there are no problems. However, even if I do get a 'clean bill of health', how can I ever relax now I've had this disease? I feel as if I have the sword of Damocles hanging over my head.

It's worse than being shelled during a war, because unlike when you're having shells raining down on you, you don't know how to protect yourself. And it's worse than hiding in a bomb shelter with a lot of other scared people, because you feel very alone, and believe that no one can really share your anxiety. I realise that when I was in the States, I felt better when I was able to speak with other cancer patients in the support groups I'd joined. I now think I should find some support groups here as well.

I tell Alban that in a way, cancer is worse than AIDS, because in the case of AIDS, nowadays everyone knows the do's and don'ts, although many victims continue to be claimed as a result of poorly screened blood transfusions and mother-to-child contamination. I contrast, cancers, apart from the types that are related to specific lifestyle choices, such as smoking, arrive in people's sphere of reality without warning, whereby the victims don't know 'where', 'how' or 'why', or what to do in order to avoid the disease. When I'm with Martine and I make this comparison, she remarks that AIDS is terrible because it's hitting young people who are in their prime, and no relief is in sight. I comment that cancer is hitting younger and younger people, and that the death tolls are now very high. However, why bother to compare the levels of evil of these two horrible, twentieth-century plagues?

Deirdre: Suffering is a very individual experience that can't really be measured.

Here in Paris, I feel too isolated with my disease: I should seek out other cancer patients, support groups and people who are willing to share my anxiety.

Tonight, one of Alban's daughters, Patsy, phones me and gives me the address of her acupuncturist. She says she's been helped as a result of going to him for acupuncture sessions, because her energy is made to circulate. She finds the procedure calming and soothing, and is pleased that her immune system is reinforced as a result of the treatment.

Paris, 5 November 1994

I must learn to live with my anxiety: the fear that I'll have a recurrence and my uneasiness about my mutilated body. I must work on myself to feel less anguished, and to be more relaxed and joyful. I'm noticing that Alban hurts when I talk about illness, and my state of anxiety and nervousness.

However, I find it very difficult when I wake up with a vague headache – I no longer have terrible migraines, which were probably caused by the hormones my body produced – as well as pains in my mutilated chest wall and the lower part of my leg, on the side I was operated on. I'm scared: 'What if the cancer has come back in these places?' Perhaps, though, because I had pain in the same spot in my leg – the spot that mother had a phlebitis in – before I became ill, I shouldn't be so anxious.

I'm finding it difficult to live with my mutilated body. When I wear the breast prosthesis, I feel pain because the device is heavy, and rubs on and scratches my skin; however, when I don't wear it, all my clothes shift on that side. My body is completely out of balance. I think about how it was before I got sick, and remember that I used to like the way it looked. I had two breasts for more than 35 years, but now, one side of my chest is breast-less, as I was when I was a child – and nipple-less as well. Learning to live with so drastic a change is extremely difficult. Even when I tell myself that worse things could happen, I can't adjust to the changes that have been inflicted on my poor body. I think I'll feel better when I start writing again.

I learn that Séverine has lost 10 kilos – more than 20 pounds – and that she's had to be operated on for intestinal fibrosis; fortunately, the fibroids weren't cancerous, and she's getting better. When I hear from her, I feel sad, wish I could be near her. Why does she have to suffer so much?

We also learn that the author and our friend Noureddine Aba is back in hospital. Although he's had cardiac therapy, his heartbeat has started to increase excessively, and as a result his lung has been seriously bruised again. We're all alarmed to hear of his state. Alban still has an infection in his reproductive system, and will have to have a biopsy. As for me, I feel I'm not 'out of the woods' yet, and am anguished. I must learn, and try to view things differently.

Paris, 8 November 1994

I see Dr TU at the Institut Gustave Roussy, located in Villejuif, one of France's – and probably Europe's – biggest cancer-research centres. He agrees with what his friend, Dr ES, the Beirut doctor, has said, and that I should have another four to six months of supplementary chemo. I wish I could've avoided showing him ES's letter, so he wouldn't be influenced by what ES said, but I couldn't avoid doing so. Hearing what he has to say, I become frightened. He says it's possible that the analyses of my lymph nodes, hormone receptors and DNA weren't precise; in other words, he says that everything could've been misread and inaccurately analysed.

Jane: I can't believe he put you through this, and cast doubt on all the positive prognoses: I would've punched him!

Bettina: Me too!

Madeleine: In the case of good specialists, all tests and analyses that aren't undertaken according to their specific method and under their supervision are deemed suspicious and liable to be erroneous. In France, this is the prevailing mentality among all the country's head physicians. And they're even more wary of their American counterparts, who they judge to be too cavalier or hasty in making their conclusions.

Dr TU says the reports contain too many contradictions, and that because the tumour grew so fast, it might've been an inflammatory one – very virulent and therefore very dangerous. He doesn't share my conviction that it was caused by the estrogens. However, in the pathological report, the fact that it was a multi-focal lobular carcinoma is clearly stated; surely the reporting doctor couldn't be that wrong. I don't know what to do any more. Dr TU wants me to resume having the chemo right away, and also wants to have a catheter opened on my chest. When I hear his words, I'm terribly scared, and when he examines me, he's very rough and he hurts me – a characteristic I haven't experienced with other doctors.

I decide I'd rather continue my follow-up with Dr Esper: he's much closer to where I live and more 'human', plus he's a breast specialist. I feel I can trust him. Although the two doctors who want me to have more chemo are very competent in their field, they aren't breast specialists – they're cancer generalists.

Manicha: At a time when cancer is so widespread, how can we still have doctors, like him, who are so brutal and have so little 'psychology'? They seem to be totally lacking in solidarity with cancer patients, if not totally lacking in compassion! Unfortunately, his kind is still quite common. They should be denounced by their patients, boycotted and banned. These doctors must change!

Paris, 9 November 1994

I wake up when I hear a noise in the kitchen. I've been dreaming. I can't remember the dream very clearly, but say to myself, 'Something's wrong in the house.' Is the dripping water that's been annoying me no longer dripping? The cause of my worrying is my visit to Villejuif and the talk about restarting chemotherapy: I don't want that poison coursing through my veins any more. Water dripping, drop by drop, like chemo being injected in an IV drip, drop by drop; a hole being opened in my chest, to let the chemicals in. I'm disgusted and revolted by the idea.

What should I do?

Alban tells me it's a gamble, like tossing a coin to decide what to do. There's no certainty. If I have the chemo, I'll mess up my body, which is already weakened, in order to eliminate malignant cells that mightn't be there, whereas if I don't have it, I might later find that the cancer has metastasised. However, it seems less likely that the latter scenario will occur, given that my lymph nodes were negative – a finding that Dr TU doubts – and that the cancer came suddenly, caused by the estrogen: a fact that very few members of the medical establishment want to admit, because it's considered to be good medical practice to administer ERT.

Bettina: But not enough time has elapsed. I'm all the more sceptical because past generations of women for whom this substitution treatment wasn't available were no worse off for not having it.

Alban notices that there are no windows in Dr TU's office. However, the doctor seems very proud to be part of the Villejuif establishment, and when I remark that's located too far from where I live, and ask whether I can be treated somewhere closer, he seems surprised that I don't want to make the effort to go to so prestigious a place, which, in his assessment, has the most knowledgeable specialists – how could I even consider going elsewhere?

To me, though, Villejuif seems like a big, soul-less factory. Every year, 100,000 cancer patients are treated there. It's incredible how this disease is spreading and no real cure has yet been found, except in the case of some leukemias and lymphomas. Why is the amount of discussion about cancer so minimal? Nowadays, one out of three Americans is hit with the disease; from what I'm reading, the number is as high here in Europe as it is in the States.

Jane: From my own lay perspective, it seems it is discussed, but always in terms of big headlines about medical breakthroughs, which are often thinly disguised 'info-mercials' that are paid for by big laboratories and drug companies. Other headlines are simply 'sound bites' about the latest food or children's product that's been found to be carcinogenic. The longer, in-depth articles published in the *JAMA* [*Journal of the American Medical Association*], *The New England Journal*, *Nature* and so on are probably not read by the general public.

Madeleine: Here, Evelyne, I think you're overdoing it a bit: there isn't only one type of cancer – the disease takes many forms, and has a multifarious nature when it comes to cause, localisation and the necessarily specific terrain it develops in. Therefore, there can be only general axes along which treatment must be individualised. There's no miracle cure – but I do understand your anguish and need to revolt.

Madeleine, please allow me to respond by quoting a scientist, Sandra Steingraber (Steingraber: 1997: 40–2), who also revolts, and has statistics in hand:

> In recent years, breast cancer mortality among white women has begun to slow down, declining 6.8 percent from 1989 to 1993. However, the death rate is still higher than it was when Rachel Carson died of the disease in 1964, and is still rising for black women. Moreover, breast cancer incidence rates are still rising for localized disease even as they are falling for more advanced-stage diagnoses (a shift probably indicating that breast cancer is being detected and treated earlier); the proportion of women developing the disease at all remains at the highest level ever recorded.

Paris, 14 November 1994

Andrée Chedid is phoning me a lot, and warms my heart: what a marvellous person she is, and what a friend she's turned out to be. She advises me to phone Danielle Evian, a distant friend, to discuss my medical options with her, because Danielle has gone through a similar experience; also, Andrée promises to speak with her husband, Louis, about the options. I've been very troubled, not knowing what to do: I haven't received any response from Dr JE, my doctor in the States, and I'm wondering whether my decision to stick with the Hôpital Saint-Louis is a sound one.

When I phone Danielle, she's extremely kind and helpful, and we talk at great length about illness. Time takes on a different meaning when you discover you have cancer. Before Danielle became ill, she always believed that every possible horrible thing would happen to her; as a consequence, she wasn't surprised and didn't rebel when she was told she had cancer. Unlike I, who asked, *Why me?*, she said to herself, *It will be. It had to be me. If it's going to hit someone, I'll be the one.*

She tells me it's very important to choose the right doctor, to feel I can discuss things with him or her, and eventually to even change protocol in the middle of treatment. Four years ago, she already suspected that something was present in her colon, and had tests done. Her doctor told her everything was all right, and even patted her on the shoulder to reassure her. Three years later, she was losing a lot of weight, had become anemic and was feeling unwell. One of her friends, realising how unwell Danielle really was, got her to hospital in a hurry. Danielle had an already advanced tumour in her colon. Back home, she checked the results of the tests she'd had done three years earlier. She discovered that the area that was photographed had been cut off, at the exact spot at which her tumour must've already commenced growing. I think about how important it is to listen to our body.

Bettina: That's where prevention begins.

Danielle makes a deep impression on me by sharing her story and pain: she expresses herself profoundly and precisely, and analyses her situation in a very interesting way. Two days later, she calls me to tell me that after making some inquiries, she's found out that the Hôpital Saint-Louis is one of the best centres for cancer treatment and research; that Dr Esper has a great reputation as a breast-cancer specialist; and that although Dr TU, at Villejuif, is also a good doctor, he perhaps isn't the most tactful practitioner and isn't a breast-cancer specialist. Consequently, I'm truly reassured that I've made the right decision: to trust Esper and follow his advice.

Today, I go back to Villejuif, accompanied by Alban. We have to wait two solid hours to see Dr Lass, the friend of Dr Hassen, of Tunis. Dr Lass doesn't agree with Dr TU's assessment, even though both doctors operate at Villejuif. He says that if I'd had an inflammatory cancer, at least 10 of my 11 lymph nodes would've been infected, and that 11 is a sufficient number of lymph nodes to have in order to determine whether or not the nodes are infected; at the time, Dr TU, however, insisted that the number of nodes checked was insufficient for determining whether or not the disease had spread. And Lass adds, 'Of course, the estrogens you took inflamed the cancer cells you might've had – definitely so!' He advises me to watch very carefully to detect any local or remote recurrence, but tells me I'd be ill-advised to have chemo again at this point. At the end of the consultation, I feel it's worth it for me to have wasted the whole morning, having taken the metro and then the suburban commuter train in order to get to Villejuif, and then having waited to see Dr Lass: I've been reassured, and Alban has been so sweet in accompanying me.

Manicha: If love is unable to triumph over fear, or over weariness in the face of disease, what good is it? On the other hand, though, friendship is able to!

Madeleine: Does Manicha know what real love is, and what it's able to bear? Love and friendship are two very strong feelings, but they're very different.

Paris, 15 November 1994

Do the doctors who want me to have extra chemo realise how much pain and suffering are involved in the treatment: the torture a person endures through having this poison? They talk about it as if it were some common medication, like taking aspirin. These past few days, I've been thinking, *If I don't take it, and the cancer comes back, I'll tell myself I should've accepted having more chemo, because if I don't have it I'll have a faster death.* It's death I'm thinking about when I come upon some biblical verses, including the following one, from the Book of Wisdom (4:7).

The premature death of the righteous: The just, even if he dies before his time, in his youth, will find rest. Honorable old age is not given through long days; it is not measured through the number of years ...

Reading this verse, I'm consoled, because I can't help still thinking in terms of the way I was raised: I believe I might've brought this misfortune on myself by behaving badly – by not 'sticking to the straight and narrow'. According to this verse, though, the opposite is true: it's often the 'righteous' who are taken early to glorify His name; however, most people can't understand the mystery.

Later, Misu, my Japanese neighbour, brings me an issue of the Jehovah's Witness journal *Watch Tower: Wake Up!*, which is devoted to the subject of breast cancer (*Watch Tower: Wake Up!*: April 1994: 2–25). It includes an article entitled 'Breast Cancer: The Obsessive Fear of All Women', which contains a lot of interesting research about the subject.

I read Misu the biblical verses I've just been reading, and she tells me that the Book of Wisdom isn't in the regular Bible: it's an Apocryphal book, which is a book that's not considered to be divinely inspired, and therefore doesn't belong to the 'revealed' texts. I'm reassured when I hear this, because it's as if by coming upon the verses as I have, I can expect to die young. It's strange and amazing how torn I can be as a result of how I was raised – will I always feel so torn over these issues?

Cindy: When a person reads biblical verses and has expectations, the message of the verses is often confirmed.

I agree with you, Cindy.

⌛

I try to obtain my medical records from Villejuif, but the registry staff member tells me they're sent to doctors only. When I insist on obtaining a copy of them, I'm told it simply isn't done, and that I can have access to only parts of the records. Alban tells me that under French law, everyone has the right to obtain his or her medical records. I decide I'll phone the registry in order to obtain the records. I'm finding all these formalities tiring, though: why can't I see the records without having to pretend they're for a doctor to see? And why isn't my doctor in the States answering my letters?

Bettina: It doesn't make sense that we have to beg for our own medical records. By definition, they're more important for the sufferer herself, because it's only by knowing and understanding the disease that she'll ever be in a position to effectively combat it, win it over and get it under control. There's no way you can fight if you don't have knowledge.

Madeleine: Because not everyone is able to understand medical jargon without having some kind of explanation beforehand, the medical records made available to patients are often simplified

summaries, in which all the technical terms have been left out –
and this is fortunate, because some fragile sufferers would be too
sensitive to deal with the whole story: go back to your own passage in which you write about the effect that the French words
Bombes cobalt! *[Cobalt bombs!]* had on that patient in Tunis – and
yet this is the right technical term for the treatment.

Manicha: The patient: always considered to be a 'minor'! What
she's first and foremost concerned about – her body, her being –
are sealed away from her! In order to obtain her own records, she
must obtain yet another 'authorisation', by the good graces of the
members of the medical establishment.

Madeleine: Let's make sure we aren't just doodling around here:
the legal right of access to medical records comes with all kinds of
precaution – which are admittedly a double-edged sword. The
doctor has to evaluate the intelligence and sensitivity of his
patients before he reveals to them, at their request, the full extent
of their disease or ailment. Some seriously ill patients ask to be
told nothing about their illness, out of sheer fear.

Paris, 17 November 1994

Yesterday, I see Andrée Chedid, a woman who always gives
me hope, courage and energy. She offers me a beautiful
green-jade necklace, and I'm wearing it as a lucky charm
because she wore it. I'm uplifted and I feel so good when
I'm with her. She's considerate and attentive, a role-model
and an inspiration.

Alban is also helping me tremendously. These days, he's
worried because of the circumstances surrounding his living situation. He occupies a room in his son's apartment,
which used to be his until he was forced into retirement and
could no longer afford to keep it on. His son now wants to
buy a house outside Paris, and is threatening to leave the

apartment. At present, Alban's daughter, Patsy, has a lot of problems, and nothing is going right for her: not her women's circus troupe, and not her relationship with either her lovers or the fathers of her children. I think Alban is also preoccupied with my health concerns, and wish I could avoid causing him any more anxiety. I hope I'll feel well again soon.

Paris, 18 November 1994

I must buy another notebook. It's grey over Paris today. My mutilated chest wall often hurts, and the arm from under which the lymph nodes were removed is also sore: the cause of the pain must be the humidity in the air.

This year, I'm noticing the drug addicts in my district. One summer, when my niece and nephews were staying here – sometimes with me and sometimes at some friends' place in the district – in order to work with the addicts, they told me that the area is a 'hot spot' for drug addicts; before, however, I didn't notice the unfortunate souls as much. Today, I see a beautiful but ravaged blonde woman sitting on the sidewalk at Place Clichy, urinating. She's accompanied by a black man, and the other day I also see them together, near La Fourche.

Two days ago, again near La Fourche, I see a young man sitting on the toilet inside one of the green street urinals that are an initiative of Jacques Chirac, when he was mayor. The toilet door is wide open, and the young man is preparing himself a fix. His pants are down, and on the floor are a packet of cigarettes and – for reasons unknown – a half-broken egg. He's completely unaware of the picture of desolation he's presenting to passers-by.

Bettina: The egg: maybe it meant a half-broken life.

Danielle Evian sends me some of the psychiatrist Carl Jung's thoughts about illness, which I translate from the French (Jung: 1964) as follows. Danielle writes,

This page, an extract from Jung's book *My Life*, still has a lot of resonance for me. I thought you might also find some help in it:

My disease also had other repercussions: they consisted, might I say, of an acceptance of being, of an unconditional 'yes' to what is, without subjective objection, an acceptance of the conditions of existence, as I see them, as I understand them, an acceptance of my being, simply as it is ... It is only after my illness that I understood how important it was to accept one's destiny. Because this is how the self does not waiver when the incomprehensible arises. A self that holds on, that bears truth and is commensurate with the world and with destiny. And this is how defeat can also be victory. Nothing is upset inside or outside, because one's own continuity has resisted the river of life and time. But it can happen only if our pretension does not prevent destiny from manifesting its intentions.

Paris, 20 November 1994

I'm experiencing pain in my chest wall as well as in my arm. I'm doing some exercises. I'm afraid I'll get a 'fat arm': a common problem for women such as me, who've had lymph nodes removed, plus radiation. Alban is giving me massages, and is so sweet and good at giving them – I'm having a lot of relief as result. It's three months now since the treatment finished, and I have a blood test as a precautionary check-up. I'm nervous, though, and anxious because of a pain I have in my lower left leg. With each pain I experience, the fear of cancer is awakened in me. Will I have to live the rest of my life accompanied by the fears and anxieties that are with me today? I can try to silence my anguish – but isn't it better to listen to it in order to be more vigilant? Or is it better to not listen to it in order to quell my nervousness? Which is the better way to overcome my worries? It's an insoluble dilemma – just like this insoluble disease.

Bettina: That's the whole problem – right there.

Cindy: What a tough choice!

I find the notes that Alban took when we went to see several doctors over these past few days. Dr TU, who operates in Villejuif's Institut Gustave Roussy, makes the following assessment.

(1) The number of lymph nodes removed and checked, eleven, were not sufficient for a good evaluation.

(2) Possibility of dissemination substantial.

(3) Chemotherapy was done for possible metastasis, but a mere four cycles would seem inadequate.

(4) Cancerous cells in the breast are detected only when they have reached a high level.

(5) The conservative treatment I received [chemo before surgery in order to try and save my breast] *was useless.*

(6) Reasons to undergo another set of chemotherapy: (a) large size of the tumour; (b) rapid growth of the tumour;(c) negativity of the receptors; (d) small number of lymph-nodes dissections.

(7) His recommendations: (a) six cycles of CMF [Cytoxan, Methotrexate, 5-FU]; *(b) get back the biopsy slides and the*

results for another evaluation. No mention of the estrogen taken at the beginning, which I told him seemed to have provoked the whole process.

However, Dr Lass – same institute (Villejuif), same place, the following week – gives us quite a different assessment:

(1) No lymph-nodes involvement; no reason for another chemo.

(2) TU thinks it's a very rapidly evolving tumour. This could be true, but there's no reason to start another chemo now; better watch it closely.

(3) Recurrence could happen locally or at a distance (bones, lungs, liver).

(4) Control tests should include blood tests and tumour markers.

(5) Lobular cancer isn't always fast.

(6) Novaldex could be given as a palliative measure.

And Dr Joyer, who's been advised by Dr Hin, the Chinese doctor who gave me an acupuncture treatment when Patsy took me to see him, has the following things to say.

(1) Take mistletoe (Viscum Album) as adjuvant therapy.

(2) The importance of the meridians. There's a method of relaxation of the meridians, TchiKong, which involves regularly making sounds and gestures.

(3) Allopathy and the patient's anxiety must be taken into account.

(4) About estrogen: menopause isn't a disease: why treat it as such?

Bettina: I couldn't agree more.

(5) A second chemotherapy would be ill-advised: chemotherapy involves risks, for example leukemia; it attacks vital organs: heart, liver, spleen and so on.

(6) I must be followed very closely and undergo traditional control tests.

(7) A patient must be in control and take charge of herself or himself; self-discipline is very important.

For me, Dr Joyer prescribes a Chinese topical cream – Crème de Perle – that I'm finding to be very effective when I apply it to my mutilated, radiated chest wall, as well as mistletoe (*Viscum Album*), which I've started taking.

Jane: Emphasise this aspect of your quest for cures: it's one of the most important parts of the book so far, and should be expanded on. Your search for alternatives, while you're keeping 'one ear open' to traditional, mainstream medicine, is fascinating; also, philosophically speaking, it can be applied to all aspects of life.

Cindy: The information given here is vital and important!

Paris, 24 November 1994

Yesterday, Alban and I go to see a gynecologist, Dr Mici, who's the daughter of my friend Dr EL. She lives in the 16ème, near the Lebanese restaurant owned by Narsay and Nayla. Because there's a transport strike – as well as other types of strike – I'm afraid I'll get there late, so I leave early in order to get to the doctor's office, which is located in an 'uptown' quarter, near the Champs-Elysées and the Arc de Triomphe. When I arrive in the district, I see lots of 'bums' about the place, and one of them is even urinating for all to see and speaking very loudly. Alban tells me that bums like to go to rich districts because the begging is lucrative there.

Dr Mici reassures me: I feel secure when she's hearing my questions and asking her own, as well as when she's establishing my medical record and examining me. She tells me that with reference to my tumour, the only thing I have to worry about is its size. Feeling somehow intimated, and not daring to ask her about my main concern, I tell myself, *The reason the tumour was so big was that it was multi-focal, and I took estrogen.* The doctor reads the grading of the tissues removed during the biopsy, and tells me that the adjective used is 'mild', and that this is a very good sign. I ask myself, *Why didn't Dr JE explain these things to me, and why didn't she answer my letters?* I find Dr JE's attitude upsetting, to say the least, and Dr Mici's very reassuring. She prescribes me a topical cream for the pain I'm having in my veins and arm; a medicine for me to drink in order to reinforce my veins; and a non-hormonal internal cream to re-hydrate my vagina. She knows how to speak, listen and reassure, and I like her manner. I'm so pleasantly surprised – even astonished – that I leave in a euphoric mood, which Alban immediately notices; he urges me to write about the visit so I'll remember the details later.

Today, I have dinner at Catherine's place, with Monique. Catherine prepares a delicious meal: flaky dough filled with smoked salmon; a salad of prawns, avocado and corn; various cheeses; and a delicious chocolate cake, all served with an excellent Bourgogne wine. However, it's too much for me: I can no longer eat meals that have this many courses; Monique is the same. I tell Catherine I appreciate her concern and that I feel surrounded with love.

Monique is afraid to return home on the metro: she tells me it's become dangerous. It's true you see more misery, drug addiction and homelessness on the metro, but I love it: it has an incredible variety of people, and I'm always happy to watch them. And when I'm with Alban, who notices everything and describes people's life as he imagines it from the way they act, I see the richness of life even more – I'm stimulated and no longer scared. Even when I'm alone and filled with Alban's vision, I'm not afraid.

Monique and I decide to take the metro together. When we part to go to our separate platforms, I get on my train and find a seat. I notice a man and woman, both dressed in dark-coloured clothing and a bit 'high', holding each other, gazing at each other and kissing. A man sitting next to them is doing a word crossword puzzle. The woman leans over to help him, and the man, sitting opposite him, manages to find the right word for him to write. It's a very warm atmosphere, there in the carriage.

Alban tells me that if many Parisians start avoiding the metro because they reason as Monique does, the system will definitely become dangerous. The way to keep it safe is for 'normal' people to use it.

Madeleine: I'll go along with you on that one.

Manicha: The Paris metro isn't all that 'friendly'! If you get verbally – or even physically – attacked, your co-passengers will turn their heads or get off as soon as possible! This lack of solidarity is due, I believe, to selfishness that's typical of both the new generation and the 'yuppies': 'Me first!' In that way, the metro is dangerous: you're alone.

Madeleine: You feel alone when you feel afraid: that's all.

Paris, 25 November 1994

Since I've become ill, people have been talking to me about cancer. People in my building are even stopping me to ask me how I'm feeling and to tell me their story. For example, Mathilda, one of my neighbours I used to talk to a lot, stops me to talk and tell me about her mother, who died of breast cancer when she was 58. Mathilda tells me that her mother's very insensitive doctor said to her mother, 'You've come to us very late, dear madam.' The tumour had already metastasised to the mother's lungs, and the doctors had to excise a big chunk of her chest and arm muscles. When Mathilda describes the experience, I shiver. She tells me that for a long time, she herself lived in fear, and frequently had check-up tests done. However, she adds that with time, fear diminishes. I remember, though, that she did say to me once, 'You do ask, *Why me?* When my husband died, I too asked why it had to happen to me, although it isn't the same thing as being hit in your own body, is it? And why all these cancers? Do you remember the concierge we had before? She died very quickly from an incurable case of breast cancer. She left a family behind.'

I reply, 'It's all the pollution; the pesticides; the things we eat. Look at Paris: why isn't leaded gas forbidden? And why aren't cars restricted to specific areas, or banned altogether when the level of pollution reaches a dangerously high level?'

'Yes,' continues Mathilda. 'My daughter, who works in Vienna, tells me they reduce car use on the days when there's heavy atmospheric pollution.'

She then tells me about a soup she used to make, in which she used pumpkin and leeks. Now, it doesn't taste the same: vegetables are treated in such a way that they no longer have the taste they once had. I tell her it's worse in the States. I realise that Mathilda wouldn't have talked to me like this before I had cancer.

Manicha: Nowadays, many people – even ordinary folks – are making the connection between health and the environment. However, to ask that radical changes be made is another story.

I'm reading the article about breast cancer in the issue of the Jehovah's Witness journal that my neighbour Misu has given me (*Watch Tower: Wake-Up!*: April 1994: 4). The article contains several useful references, which I include as follows.

(1) 'According to some estimations, by the year 2000, approximately one million new cases will be diagnosed every year.' [And this is stated just like that – matter-of-factly!]

(2) In the journal Science, *the writer, Devra Lee Davis, states that according to the evidence, there's a clear, although hard to define, link between breast cancer and environmental factors. Because the breast is the most* radio-sensitive *part of the body, that is, the part that's most exposed to ionising radiation, the risk that a woman will contract cancer in it is higher. This is also the case for both men and women who have contact with toxic-chemical products.*

(3) Three out of four breast-cancer victims are incapable of designating a precise factor as having contributed to the manifestation of the disease.

(4) 'Body fat produces estrogen, a female hormone which can have harmful effects on breast tissue and provoke cancer.' On page 4 of a 1992 issue of the British Medical Bulletin, *the writer estimates that 'non-contraceptive estrogen raises the risk of breast cancer by 30 to 50% when used over a prolonged period of time.'*

I've also been reading an issue of a Canadian journal entitled *Les Cahiers de la Femme* (*Canadian Women Studies*: Summer 1994: volume 14: number 3), which is devoted to the theme of women and health. It contains several two articles about breast cancer: 'Breast Cancer and the Environment', by Megan Williams (pages 7–11), and 'Women with Cancer and the Meaning of Body Talk', by Cynthia Mathieson (pages 52–7), as well as many articles in which important points about health are included.

In Megan Williams's article, the writer notes that Devra Lee Davis, who's an epidemiologist and a senior advisor to the United States' Office of the Assistant Secretary for Health, is one of the few researchers who've begun to explore the link between the factors commonly noted in research into breast cancer and pollution. According to Davis, the key is estrogen-producing toxins. She writes (*Canadian Women Studies*: Summer 1994: volume 14: number 3: page 8), 'All risks have one thing in common: they are all tied to total lifetime exposure to estrogen. The more estrogen a woman is exposed to during her lifetime, the greater her risk of getting cancer.' Here, the link with estrogen is made very clearly – why don't doctors want to acknowledge it?

I'm reading a beautiful letter from Amel; it's always uplifting to hear from her. I quote from her letter as follows.

Evelyne, ma chérie, I'm at La Goulette train station. It's half past noon, and I'm going to Tunis to see films. I hope to see many of them and to meet people: Jocelyne Saab, Assia Djebar, Farida Belyazid ... As you see, I'm in the middle of a festival, living through other people's images, imagination ...

I saw Chahine's L'Emigré *[The Immigrant]. I found it tender, a bit crazy, like Chahine: a rare Arab man who has an unleashed imagination, an outlook in which he's in love with men, women and life. And he filmed the desert I'm just returning from. I spent all of last week resting, sleeping; the desert experience was very powerful. The first few days, I didn't feel like going out: I wanted to keep in me the vision of immense space limited only by the horizon, where only sand prevails. It helped me get centred on myself, or rather to locate myself in space, in life. And at night, a round and immense sky would envelope us, erasing everything else – a luminous sky of stars, so close. Oh, the discomfort of the desert: no faucets, no toilets, and above all, voracious flies, pursuing us relentlessly through all openings, all holes, with an unceasing noise; at night, they were replaced with mosquitoes. The next day of the first evening, we woke up with bites on all parts of our body that had been exposed. And at night we were itchy. Then we learnt to better protect ourselves, then to get used to it, to no longer pay attention to flies or mosquitoes. Two miles from the camp, there was water: a spring in the desert, cool in the morning and warm at noon – a real miracle, in the middle of the desert ...*

One morning, we got up very early – at six, or even earlier – and miracle: a blessed moment without flies or mosquitoes, and a sky with fabulous colours: mauve, green, yellow and red. After the desert, my house seems luxurious, even if the toilet flush still isn't working and the cooking gas is barely coming out ...

The film festival's over now. There's a beautiful sun-sky, the air's slightly cool, and I miss you. I did my yoga this morning. I feel full of energy; I have so much to do. Moufida's film [Les silences du palais – Moufida is a childhood friend of Amel] *won the Tanit d'or* [first prize]. *I saw Farida* [a Moroccan film-maker friend of Amel], *who's more mature and surer of herself after all the trials she's through. She's writing scenarios, but hasn't yet found the money to produce a second film ...*

I saw a short film by Dina El Joundi: Beyni wa beinak, Beyrouth [*Between Me and You, Beirut*]. *I thought of you. Wounds get healed with time, and with the desire to dwell among the living. I have so many other things to tell you ...*

Paris, 28 November 1994

Yesterday, Alban and I go to Nogent to visit Agnès and Paul Sanders. Catherine Mokh is also there, visiting. She and Agnès are showing slides of their work in Lebanese women's prisons as well as in the Beirut camp of Sabra, where mostly Palestinian but also some Lebanese people are living. Agnès tells us the terrible story of a Romanian woman who'd come to Lebanon to try and earn some money by working in a bar, without turning to prostitution, in order to be able to send some help to her very poor family living in Romania. The woman was swindled by a drug-trafficking Lebanese man, who gave her a double-bottomed suitcase that was filled with presents but that also contained hidden heroin. She was caught at the airport and thrown into gaol, whereby, if it hadn't been for Agnès and Catherine's visit, no one would've known what had happened to her, and she would've had to wait an eternity before she was able to do anything.

I find the photos of the Sabra camp very disturbing: run-down houses, misery, poverty, and filth that's causing all kinds of infection and disease. It's terrible, all this suffering – the conditions these human beings are living in are worse than animals'.

I'm reading another letter from Amel, to cheer me up, and I include extracts from it as follows.

... I'm so glad you're doing well. I went to a kinesiology workshop [the relationship between the body organs, the brain and the meridians]. *I'm so glad you're doing lymphatic drainage – it's important for you ... It'd be so wonderful if you and Alban could live right across from me; I'm trying to arrange it ...*

Rachida came and slept here with Randa, an Algerian friend who was in Lebanon. She liked it a lot, but was shocked to see the class differences, to do with the standards of living. She went to Tyr and Sidon. She showed us pictures. It's beautiful – we shall go together, Evelyne.

In the garden, there's a dove that's quietly walking. The weather's still beautiful: no rain; almost hot; the sea calm; the sky luminous. It seems that in Beirut, it was cold. I hope you can have a serene time in search of yourself. It's also painful; however, my darling friend, you mustn't get sick any more, and I'm sure this is possible. Avoid negative energy, and relax ...

Thank you, Evelyne, for being here, full of energy. I need to hear your voice and your laughter ...

Paris, 29 November 1994

Yesterday, Alban and I make love. However, for me, making love isn't as it was 'before'. It has nothing to do with Alban – on the contrary, I probably love him more than I loved him before; our love is always growing and deepening – something I feel very strongly. No, it has to do with my body: the relationship I now have with my body, which is no longer as it was before. First, as a result of chemo, I was plunged into menopause, which is why my reproductive system is 'getting atrophied' – the exact words used in my pap-test results) and my mucous membranes are drying out. I no longer have as much desire and pleasure as I used to, whereas before, I was almost always excited about the prospect of making love. The image I have of my body, and the image my body projects, is that it's a mutilated body, incomplete, and no longer feminine. Even when I tell myself that all these perceptions must be 'in my head', I recognise that the canons of beauty and femininity are culturally based, and are formed by way of the education system and the media, through hard-to-resist ideas that are constantly transmitted to us.

I view my body as if it were masculine on one side, because I'm lacking a breast there – but it isn't even masculine, because there's no nipple, and a scar has taken the place of my breast; on the other side, I see my breast, and am reminded of the one I'm missing –is it an androgynous body? There's also the issue of my hair: it's growing back frizzy and woolly. I don't like the head I have now – perhaps

I should've brought the wigs with me that I wore last year in order to create another 'look', one I could live with better.

Madeleine: Your hair? All that is so subjective. I assure you, Evelyne, that you look lovely with your hair all in curls. This flattering style sets off the oval shape of your face.

But why is the image we have of ourselves so important when we're making love – shouldn't it be the image of the other person that's important? I believe that both images are important. However, as I'm now discovering, a lot of narcissism is involved in the act of love.

When I consider, the question of narcissism, I'm taken back to a discussion I had with Marie Claire. She told me that for her master, Jacques Lacan, the famous psychoanalyst after Freud, love was a narcissistic act, a summation I was angered at hearing. I used to refuse to acknowledge this notion of narcissism. Is the importance of my own image during the act of love, an image I'm discovering today, a reflection of narcissism? At first, I thought it was; now, though, I'm no longer sure. If the other person were non-existent during the act of love, why would my image be so important?

Am I in love with myself. Why? Because I am so taken with you, because it is you that I love and you alone and everything that in truth is yours. And it is thus that I love myself, because my self belongs to you. (Kierkegaard: 1943: 315)

Isn't love an exchange? In this act of exchange, the image of yourself undoubtedly holds an essential place, and this image cannot be only narcissistic, because the value of my image in the act of exchange can't come from me only; to a great extent it's a social construction: the image I'm able to construct is confronted with the image constructed by the other, by other people; it composes itself with another image, and with other images. In the act of love, there's negotiation; there's exchange – equal or unequal – of images, and the adjustment of images. What is essential, in my existing situation, is the relationship of exchange negotiated at a given time, which is brutally broken as a result of my mutilation. The re-evaluation of the conditions of exchange is therefore a condition *sine qua non* of the perpetuation of the act of love. Because of the 'excision', the mutilation, inflicted on me, the image I used to have of myself in my relationship to other people and with Alban has been blurred. Will I be able to overcome this moment? Will I be able to create a different image of myself – one with which I'll be better pleased me and through which I'll feel at ease when I'm making love, perhaps not as much as I felt at ease before, but through which I'll feel more pleasure than I feel now? Will Alban and I be able to reconstruct the incredible fusion of our two bodies that we attained through love, through our desire, and through the relationship of our two bodies and of the images we had of them?

Jane: The most interesting aspect of this chapter is the balancing act you perform – like Alban's daughter's circus! – in the midst of all the conflicting opinions, which are in turn rooted in various medical interests, be they academic, professional or even routine. In addition to absorbing these official diagnoses, you managed to seek out gentler alternatives, by navigating what are essentially unchartered waters! This is getting to the heart of the matter.

What we are questioning is not the ignorance of the species or its powerlessness in the face of disease; we feel no bitterness in that regard. It is rather the fact that we were subjected by a corps of physicians to a barbaric treatment that has left us weakened, without informing us of these effects or asking our opinion. This attitude is unacceptable. What we are questioning is that we were not warned; we were not offered choices (though it is likely that we would have opted for the treatment). (Hyvrard: 1987: 174)

We also criticize the fact that the corps of physicians overall refuses to listen to our living testimony. In this ridiculous face-off where what is at stake is Truth and the possible progress of a kind of medicine that will rely on the real effects of treatment, the white coats win every time. The playing field is uneven, for the patient risks his life but the doctor risks nothing. Cancer specialists are untouchable, so intense is the fear, and so dense is the mystery. This is true to such an extent that cancer patients are no longer people with normal rights. Anything can be done to a cancer patient, and no complaint will be addressed, because death is the norm. Even if he is left to die of the cold, this will be considered normal because, in any case, his destiny is death, by cancer or by something else; it does not matter. The true motto of this cancer world is surely 'Abandon all hope, ye who enter here.' (Hyvrard: 1987: 175)

Dumping began to take place out in the high seas; tall smoke stacks spewed emissions into the upper air, with little filtering or purification, for there was no immediate consciousness that the world is a closed system. Refuse in all forms was being dumped: solids (less serious, because they are at least visible and therefore removable) or chemicals, and all this in areas very, very near to where we live, millions and millions of times more than we ever had before, a function of the frightening multiplication of people on the earth, itself a product of all this progress. In the space of one century, everything has been contaminated: air, water, food … many epidemiological studies have clearly shown the link between peak pollution and increased mortality due to serious respiratory ailments. In addition, cancers, immune deficiencies, and neuro-toxic ailments occur at a much deeper level, with much longer-term effects. The ways in which pollutants act on our hormonal system are as countless as soldiers in some perverse army, as witnessed by way of the number of mentions in basic- and applied-toxicology journals ... soon, life expectancy will be reduced, despite medical progress: in peace time, of course. The worsening public health crisis in Russia is already attracting attention, whereby the life-expectancy rate is in free fall: from 64.9 to 57.5 for men, for example, between 1987 and 1994. In addition to an inadequate health system as compared with Western Europe's, radio-ecological pollution in Russia has become a disaster, in a country in which nuclear-power stations are in ruins. (Séralini: 1997: 142–3)

11

BEIRUT, WAR AND CANCER
KAHABRA *BRINGS* KAHABRA

In order to make myself cross the threshold of that big metal door that leads to the other side of life, I told myself the legend once again: an SS officer stands with a skull atop his cap, a *Totenkopf verbanden*, one of those old friends of the Birkenau camp, the lordly estate of Auschwitz, Oswiecim-Upon-Vistule, where I visited only in my dreams. Then, taking a deep breath, I murmured to myself in Yiddish (that scary language, as Kafka used to say, the only one that makes you confident enough to stand your ground when faced with that fear), and I said to myself: 'Lolkele, my little lamb, don't *krekhtxes* (moan ridiculously, croak). As long as we're not at the door of the gas chamber, there's still hope.' (Francos: 1983: 47)

Me, like a madwoman, I ran into the room, slamming the door, held my head with both hands and began to bang it against the wall — as she used to do so often as a child. And I said to myself: 'I am a civil war.' (Francos: 1983: 47)

Paris, 4 December 1994

The disposal unit that connects my Japanese neighbour Misu's small studio with our building's main drainage has

many problems. When I think about plumbing, I'm reminded of the human body, especially how some diseases are
treated by way of cutting and burning, and reconnecting
bits and pieces here and there.

Today, Adelaide phones, to tell me that Eloïse,
Théophile's wife, has to have an operation to remove a
small tumour in her breast. I'm terribly depressed when I
hear the news, and each time I try to phone Beirut, I fail to
get through. Will Théophile now go on his trip as scheduled
or postpone it to be with Eloïse?

I realise how much Alban, as well as my friends in the
States, have stood by me during my trial. Here, though, it
isn't the same: people seem to think more about themselves,
and no one has the time to give to other people.

Salwa phones, and tells me that Séverine has started
walking again, but that she still has a tube attached to her to
feed herself, because as yet she can't quite do it herself. I
worry a lot aboutmy little sister, and am distressed when
Salwa reminds me of her condition. It's so unfair that she
has to go through so much pain and suffering. All illnesses
and diseases are unfair, but this one is especially cruel. It's
just too horrible and unbearable to think that someone her
age, who's already suffered through her own mother's
death from the same disease when Séverine was exactly the
same age as her own daughter, Laura, now is, should have
to re-live the scenario and have her daughter witness her
suffering.

Paris, 8 December 1994

Today, Alban and I spend the day running around in order
for me to have my hand, arm and scar massaged; have
Alban undergo 'urinary re-education'; and visit my apartment's insurance centre, in order to discuss my building's
plumbing and security. According to Alban, all insurers are

crooks. At the insurance centre, after we're made to wait for quite some time, we're greeted by a nice receptionist, who explains we have three options for the insurance, all of which are very expensive. I'm weary of having to address these minor problems: they seem so petty juxtaposed with a life-threatening disease.

At Alban's doctor's office, while we're waiting to see the doctor, I read an article in a French-language issue of *marie claire* (*marie claire*: October 1994: 134–42), written by Ewa Evler and Jackie Séguin and entitled 'Cancer du sein: Parlons-en'. The article contains the testimony of four women who've been hit with breast cancer. The women talk about their struggle against the disease, and declare – and how I agree with them! – that in France the problem is much too trivialised. I think, *And it's much more trivialised than it is in the States.* When I read some of the women's stories, I shiver in recognition of the plight of some cancer patients. The women state that doctors don't explain anything to their patients. I include a few self-translated extracts from the stories (from pages 134, 134–6, 136–8 and 138, respectively) as follows, in order to illustrate how prevalent this lack of communication between patient and doctor has become. It's a real problem, and must be made known and resolved.

F. B., 38, diagnosed at age 35

Today, I'm no longer the same. I feel that my time is limited. It makes me live everything more intensively ... What revolts me is that breast cancer is so trivialised. People say it's nothing, no big deal – but it isn't their health that's at stake! It isn't 'nothing'; it's dramatic when you have to go through it. And though it's hard for me to admit it, I was ashamed, at times, for having breast cancer, for being so vulnerable, lost, alone. I hadn't been told it would be long, difficult, painful. No one ever talks about it. This silence must be broken. Breast cancer isn't a shameful disease.

A. S., 47, diagnosed at age 33

I've changed in my head. Fewer things touch me. People who complain about small things get on my nerves. All the things that annoy me I drop now ... You can't constantly live in fear, so I get rid of all the negative things, and I struggle. I struggle for my life.

M.-L. J., 35, diagnosed at age 29

It took me three years to feel I'd overcome it. Now I've crossed the five-year hump, I'm considered healed. However, I believe that cancer is still in my head, for life. Because my cancer was hormonal, I must receive an injection every month, which has triggered early menopause. It's a hard thing to experience at my age. I no longer have my periods; I can no longer have children. I've had hot flashes for five years. During a yearly check-up, I heard my doctor say, 'She's castrated.' Castrated? What a horrible word! What does it mean: that I'm no longer a woman? But I'm not old! Today, I'm fed up with the medical establishment ... And the frustration I felt about the lack of information I was given is still there. I still don't know what kind of cancer I had, or at which stage it was. I must admit I'm upset with my doctors. They didn't understand that I wanted answers to my questions.

M.L., 46, diagnosed at age 33

I'd like to pass on two messages. The first one: 'Think about prevention!' It's a guarantee for healing. The second one: 'Don't close yourself off into the world of disease: continue to work at any cost.

I consider myself healed. I didn't have reconstruction. I'm sure it'd be fabulous, but I don't want to undergo another operation. What annoys me most is that I still have a swollen arm, which is noticeably bigger than my other arm. Most doctors think that the problem of lymphedema ('fat arm') is secondary. I don't agree: it's very important, and very crippling. I'd like women to know that this problem exists, that it's important not to let it get settled in, but to find a good physical therapist who'll practise real manual lymphatic drainages. It's important to be informed, and above all to watch the problem constantly.

The day before yesterday, we visit Dr Esper at the Hôpital Saint-Louis. Apparently, all the results were negative – what good news! Esper seems to be very knowledgeable in his field. Unfortunately, though, Dr JE, my doctor in the States, has sent neither my *block-slides* nor my examination results, both of which should've been in my file here.

I'm unsettled by these acts of negligence. Esper says that if my chest wall is still sore, it's because the muscles are growing back, and the area is restructuring, or re-forming, itself as a result of the various aggressive procedures I've been subjected to. He explains that it takes between a year and 18 months for 'things' to become normal again – *Minus the breast*, I think to myself. For my left arm, he prescribes sessions of manual lymphatic drainage massages so the swelling won't settle in. He says the problem will stay with me for the rest of my life. I tell him I'm afraid for my other breast: that I'm worried I'll have to be subjected to another mutilation and therefore the same handicap in my other arm – that both my arms will thereby be crippled. I ask him whether it wouldn't be better to prevent myself from being doubly afflicted in this way by doing what the doctor in Milwaukee has suggested: having another mastectomy. He says that the risks of having a car accident are greater than the risks of having a recurrence in the other breast, and that he's against ordering preventive mastectomies.

Jane: Good on him! When was the last time you heard that a male doctor had ordered a man to have his balls removed preventively?

329

Paris, 9 December 1994

Dr JE still hasn't responded to my letters; nor has she sent my block-slides and examination results to Dr Esper. I find this negligence totally unacceptable: it seems she doesn't care a bit about my case. When I had the operation, she charged $60 to see me – and why did she come at that time? It wasn't really necessary; also, she charged $160 for my first consultation with her, and $75 for the 5- to 10-minute consultations I had with her after that one. I deduce that to answer a patient's letter for zero money would equal the fact that she had zero time to do it and that I'd consequently get zero response. The other doctors I've consulted here in France take only $30, and take their time to answer their patients' questions. Alban tells me that the prices are so low because the research hospitals are subsidised by the government: health is socialised. Although the system's fairness appeals to me, I wonder how long it can last. The French government is in deep debt, and is probably unable to keep paying the bills indefinitely. The system has to be reformed, but I hope its reformers don't end up imitating the system that's in place in the United States, the government of which the French tend to follow in too many ways.

Madeleine: In France, all hospitals are considered to be public-service centres, not just the big university hospitals. Many private clinics also have arrangements with the department of social security, so they receive state subsidies.

This afternoon, Théophile phones because Eloïse, his wife, is on the operating table. The doctors haven't yet detected whether her micro-calcification is cancerous. If it does turn out to be cancerous, they're saying they'll have to take out a quarter of her breast. Théophile is very depressed, and phones me many times, during which the phone line is

constantly cut off. He says, 'Eloïse and I now better understand what you went through – I'd much prefer to be on
the operating table myself.' I tell him that Alban said the
same thing when I was in hospital about to be operated
on. I try to reassure him by pointing out that the tissue
taken in most similar biopsies turns out to be benign. I
also try to phone him but have the line constantly cut off.
I'm frustrated because I can feel that my brother is very
anxious, and regret that I'm a long way away and unable
to comfort him.

Tonight, Adelaide phones to let me know that Eloïse's
biopsied tissue wasn't cancerous. I'm so happy for Eloïse
and Théophile, but I can't help thinking, *Why didn't it turn
out the same for me? Why was mine in the 25 per cent of biopsies
that turn out to be positive for cancer?* Is this how my friend
Elizabeth would've felt if my biopsied tissue had also
turned out to be benign? I think she probably wouldn't
have, because her attitude about the 'Why me?' reaction
was to ask, 'Why not me?'

I'm feeling pain in my arm at the point at which blood was
drawn from me yesterday at a private lab, so I'm upset again.
Why aren't the nurses more careful when they're drawing
blood? I find that when hospital nurses are doing this procedure, they're much more careful than private-laboratory
nurses are. I've noticed that many Parisian-hospital nurses
are immigrants – usually from North Africa, an African country or the Caribbean – and that they're usually nicer, more
cheerful and more careful.

Jane: Your comment is interesting, considering what a horrendous reputation nurses have in the Maghreb *[North Africa: 'the
country of the setting sun']*: they're reputed to be negligent, cruel
and disdainful, and to be always looking for tips, stealing materi-
als and so on.

Alban: It might have to do with the way Arabo-Islamic people view the body; blood, in particular, is considered to be dirty and something to be avoided.

It's true that most of the Parisian-hospital nurses who drew my blood were of Caribbean or African origin rather than North African. The fact that they work under better material conditions could also be the reason why there's a difference in attitude between nurses working in Paris and nurses working in their own country.

Madeleine: People from the Maghreb who are working in hospitals here are mostly of Algerian or Moroccan origin. However, they're rarely in a nursing position. On the other hand, there are many excellent doctors from the Maghreb, and at the other end of the spectrum, workers from the Maghreb often have a service position as a janitor or kitchen hand. However, some young people of Maghreb origin but who were born in France are now attending a nursing school.

Paris, 13 December 1994

Again and again, I can't help but ask myself why Séverine is having to suffer so much – and to think I wouldn't be as conscious of her pain if I hadn't gone through so much pain myself. My poor, dear Séverine. I'm revolted by the unfairness of it all: how could all this be happening to one person?

I can't bear to listen to the complaints of people who are suffering through 'little' ordeals. One example is Brigitte, who's experiencing problems with her teeth and back: I tell myself I should be more compassionate, that things are relative, and that for Brigitte, her problems are a 'big thing'. I know I should be as sympathetic as I used to be, but I'm finding it very difficult to be that way now. I'm even finding it difficult to sympathise with Alban's daughter Patsy, who has huge money problems. I tell myself, 'She'll overcome it; she's young; things'll get better for her – after all, it's only money!

Recently, after Alban spends two weeks with me, Patsy makes some rather curious remarks to me. She tells me the story of Lacan, the well-known psychoanalyst and the biggest name in the field, after Freud, and his daughter, who I'll call Aurore. Apparently, Aurore is now revealing to newspaper journalists all kinds of unpleasant facts about her father, and her accounts reflect how bitter she feels towards him because he was always absent and pretended he was in places he wasn't in at all. She says that when she came forward to talk to him, he had one of his mistresses psychoanalyse her! Patsy has concluded that Lacan, who wrote publicly about truth, privately never stopped lying. I tell her it isn't true that he wrote about truth, and ask her whether she's read his writings. She replies that she hasn't.

However, what she's really insinuating is that on the grounds mentioned in the newspaper articles, Lacan and Alban, her father, are similar. I tell her that Alban isn't at all like Lacan, and that the latter is unlikeable, at least from things I've read both about him and by him. He didn't aim to be truthful, and thought that woman was the *manque* – lack – of man and not an entity in herself. In Luce Irigaray's book *This Sex Which Is Not One* (*Ce sexe qui n'en est pas un*) (Irigaray: 1985), Irigaray criticises him for espousing this philosophy, and states that he kicked her out of a seminar he was conducting because she dared to take a stand against his views.

Originally, instead of writing the word seminar, I mistakenly wrote the word *seminary*, which is a place that men go to study in order to be a priest.

Jane: In the case of Lacan, the word is perhaps appropriate, because he was the 'high priest' of psychoanalysis.

I believe that Patsy needs her father to give her attention, and that she might be a bit jealous of me and of my relationship with him. I remind her that she once told me that Alban was very present during her childhood and adolescence. He spent a lot of time with his children, and even took them to Iran when he was conducting some of his research into anthropology there. The trips have been the basis of some of Patsy's *imaginaire* as well as of her ideas for some of the scenes in her women's circus.

Jane: I hope you're wearing your *yed Fatima* ['Fatima's hand': a small piece of jewellery in the shape of a hand and often in silver, which is considered to protect its wearer] to ward off all the evil eyes, the jealous eyes that the marvellous relationship you have with Alban is no doubt attracting to you!

From Monique, I learn that she wants to stop taking the hormones her doctor has prescribed her. However, her dentist is concerned that her teeth might thereby become demineralised, and has told her it wouldn't be a good idea. She's feeling tormented and anxious about what to do. I feel that her reactions might have something to do with the effects that hormones have had on me: most of my friends have been affected by what's happened to me, and as a result, some of them have interrupted their hormone 'treatment'.

On the plane between Paris and Beirut, 20 December 1994

I wonder why I have to live minus a breast, and most of all, why I have to endure this fear of a recurrence. Even when I'm telling myself I shouldn't think about it, that it's very unlikely to happen – as likely as having a bad car accident, to use Esper's analogy – I'm frightened by each little ache, each pain, and my life is put back into question.

I'm in the same plane I was in last year during the same period, when my cancer had probably already started, and when I was taking the hormones, which were like fertilisers for the mad cells that were happily proliferating in my body, thanks to this 'great food' I didn't know I was providing the cells with, and that nobody had warned me about. This time last year, I was tired and sad to be heading home to see my sick parents. Today, father's no longer here, mother is still very sick and her condition is getting worse.

As for me, I've had this cancer I wasn't expecting at all and didn't know would hit me. Why? Why is life so threatened by death, and in so personal yet random a way, so that you ask, 'Why was I singled out? Why now? Will I overcome whereas other people haven't? Will my body triumph over the crazily dividing cells: and why, why, are they dividing so furiously? Is it really the body that does it: did my body do this to me? No, it's all the waste that's being emitted into the environment – I'm sure of it, even if no serious studies have yet been conducted into this cause of the problem. Even during the most intensive shelling during the war in Lebanon, I didn't experience fear in quite this way.

Although I tell myself it was the hormones that were the cause – that it was Dr VZ's fault for prescribing them: how I curse her every day – sometimes I question this summation also. Was it really those hormones, even though the evidence is right there for all to acknowledge: my breasts swollen in less than a month when I started taking the hormones, and the bleeding, the bleeding, the unending bleeding?

Alban: Hormones, atmospheric emissions and so on belong in the same category. It's like violence done to nature; aggression perpetrated on nature; the will to brutally transform nature without taking into account its own rules; the will to transform some discrete segments of nature without knowing, asking about or taking into consideration its whole – in other words, it's progress gone mad, de-natured.

I'm concerned about my dear friend Amel, and yesterday try to call her before I leave. Her aunt – the one I know from Bizerte – has died suddenly, when Amel tells me, she sounds really upset. I don't have many details about what happened; I only know that the death was apparently unexpected. Life is so fragile.

I'm feeling old. How can the relationship you have with your body change so much in less than a year? When hormones are involved, things progress neither slowly nor subtly.

I cry over lost time, even though I've already achieved quite a bit in my life. Why am I so traumatised? Why do I miss father so much, even though he traumatised me when I was a child and an adolescent? Towards the end, though, we were able to be reconciled, to clear up our misunderstandings and to become friends.

I'm watching a fashion show on the in-flight TV. I decide I'd very much like to see the catwalks filled with models wearing ultra-chic clothes but bearing only one breast, in an act of defiance against accepted 'normal' fashion, and against this civilisation that's given me this horrible disease! I'm sure it's given it to me! I've always been a rebel, and I recognise the people who are the same. I believe in rebellion: I think it's healthy. When you're a rebel, you're better able to grow, mature and create, and to not follow blindly, like a sheep.

Was my breast acting out environmental disturbance when it contracted the cancer? Will the other breast act out the disturbance too? Why do breasts react to the environment as my breast reacted to it? Is it that extra-sensitive space that's stirred by pollution? Why, then, don't all breasts react to pollution? Why so only one in seven breasts react to it? Is it like everything else in human nature: that some living things are more sensitive than others? Is it good to be so sensitive when sensitivity can lead to death? Can you be sensitive and creative yet not be threatened with madness and death?

Bettina: I often ask myself the same questions, but have never come up with an answer.

Jane: I'm not quite sure what you mean by 'act out'. Psychotherapists say, for example, that children playing games are 'acting out' their fears. I rather like the idea of a traumatised breast acting out the trauma in the same way a child acts out her trauma in playing her games or doing her artwork, and this is often the case with young war victims. I wonder whether your breast is expressing the environmental aggression it received?

I can't live as before; in fact, I shouldn't live as before. My body's saturated and tired. A 'crab' tried to devour it. I overcame the experience. My body has triumphed: I know it; I feel it. But it's tired, and it hurts. It's crying from all its wounds. And I'm crying too.

Beirut is approaching, and soon the plane will land. Night is falling over the city. Beirut: the magic city. Beirut: the sensitive city, so many times the victim of folly and close to death. Beirut: eaten up by a cancer, a devouring war, which it triumphed over. Beirut: city of my childhood and adolescence. I miss father, father who won't be there to greet me, with that broad smile of his. Father, who tormented me during my childhood and adolescence, only to apologise later and tell me I was an overly sensitive child. He shouldn't have been as strict with me as he was. I cry over having lost him, and over having lost my youth.

337

Beirut, 22 December 1994

I'm in Beirut. The hairdresser who came to do mother's hair tells me he's used to seeing hair that turns out like mine as a result of cancer treatments. It's radiation that especially makes it curly in this strange, electric way. In Arabic, he tells me, '*Kahraba* (electricity) brings *kahraba*.' Before, I didn't believe people when they told me that hair reacts different-ly to these treatments: that hair that used to be curly becomes straight and that straight hair turns curly – I thought the stories were just 'old wives' tales'. And I can tell that people think I'm making it up when I tell them that my hair wasn't curly like this before; in fact, I'm having a hard time accepting my head at present, because my hair is in an in between state that I don't really like, and I'm disturbed when I see and feel its woolly texture.

Jane and other people loved my hair this way, especially in the summer of '95, when we were in Tunis – Jane says I looked angel-ic! However, I had a hard time with it. Why is how you yourself feel about your look more important than what other people say about it?

The Beirut hairdresser tells me there are two types of cancer: the feminine and the masculine. The feminine is much more virulent than the masculine: it's very aggressive; a real killer. I ponder over his remark, which is about gender dif-ferences as applied to illness. I've always been interested in gender differences; it's the subject of one of my books, *Sexuality and War: Literary Masks of the Middle East* (Accad: 1990). In that book, I analyse how gender differences are closely linked to war, and examine how sexuality and war are interconnected. I consider that the popular image of can-cer as a battle is reinforced in my analysis, in which I show that the fear men have of women is manifested even in their portrayal of disease. The female brand of a disease – is there any such thing scientifically? – is much more dangerous than the male one; it kills faster. Where did this idea come from?

Alban: The question is also 'How did the idea come: how was it born?'

Is it because of the rapid, mad division of cells? Why would that be more female than male?

Alban: It probably has more to do with the rapid growth of a tumour in the body, whereby it reached the size of a fetus: the analogy between pregnancy and a tumour.

Jane: And don't men commonly think of women as excessive creatures whose sexuality is boundless? Whereas men are relatively limited by the sex act itself, women are thought to be insatiable – or at least that's the myth that's been handed down.

At any rate, it's an interesting popular notion of cancer. I wonder whether I'll find other notions like that one – popular sayings, proverbs, folk tales – and what I'll learn from them about the disease.

Aïn Saadé, 13 January 1995

My stay in Lebanon is coming to an end, and I must say I'm not sorry. I'm saturated with the setting – the pollution; the family; too many people. I feel I've accomplished my mission: I've finished correcting father's book, which is to be sent to its editors, and I've taken care of mother. It's enough to have completed those two tasks. I'm now anxious to leave and be back with Alban.

339

At Beirut Airport, 16 January 1995

How quickly you adjust to anguish. How quickly you adjust to departures and arrivals! How quickly life goes away filled with these anxieties, these departures and arrivals, these joys and pains. I've had a wonderful stay at Théophile's; his wife Eloïse is extraordinary, and her devotion is unsurpassed.

Jane and Cindy: What's noticeable in your writing now is how, along with your healing, there seems to be an equal hardening, or toughening, going on. This isn't to say you're becoming callous or indifferent to other people's suffering – on the contrary; however, at this point you're less vulnerable and more defiant – even proud of your triumph.

The citizens of Cape Cod and Long Island have struggled mightily to bring scientific attention to the link between cancers and environmental contamination in their communities. Still, the resources they command are starkly different from those among Normandale's residents. My meetings with the breast cancer activists of Long Island have taken place on college campuses and convention hotels. I have spoken with the cancer activists of Cape Cod in a beachfront conference center. When I met with a community leader in my own hometown, we held our discussion in the back room of an auto repair shop and towing company.

Said a man from Normandale who lost his wife to ovarian cancer, 'I think the state has a way of putting things to the side or overlooking what's the real truth.' (Steingraber: 1997: 86)

Taped above my desk are graphs showing the U.S. annual production of synthetic chemicals. I keep them here to make visible a phenomenon I was born in the midst of but am too young to recall first hand. The first consists of several lines, each representing the manufacture of a single substance. One line is benzene, the human carcinogen known to cause leukemia and suspected of playing a role in multiple myeloma and non-Hodgkin's lymphoma. Another is perchloroethylene, the probable human carcinogen used to dry-clean clothes. A third represents production of vinyl chloride, a known cause of angiosarcoma and a possible breast carcinogen. They all look like ski slopes. After 1940, the lines begin to rise significantly and then shoot upward after 1960. (Steingraber: 1997: 89)

And yet we're not protecting plant life on a global level. Instead, we are behaving more like parasites, like their predators. What's more, given that everything is constantly being exchanged and that very little actually degrades (otherwise it would not be considered as polluting), whenever we contaminate a field with insecticides or herbicides in order to enhance production, we are also polluting the cattle that graze there, and polluted cattle means contaminated hamburgers and steaks, which we then consume. What we are carrying out here is essentially a low-burn collective suicide, because our body is in constant development ... The world's resources are not infinite. This fact was not absolutely essential in the 20th century, but it has become so at present ... We must attempt to foresee how the things we manufacture now are going to affect life cycles in the future. Children must be taught to understand the laws of nature as they relate to the environment, to health and to our consumer habits. Because, once again, it is a matter of our society's survival into the 21st century. (Séralini: 1997: 211–13)

12

SEARCHING FOR ALTERNATIVES
INCOMPREHENSIBLE PAINS

You know, Medicine operates according to one-size-fits-all protocols that are then adapted to each individual, but at the same time, they have very little latitude. We, on the other hand, function on a tailor-made basis. We count on the special competence of the individual, and try to call it forth. (Lambrichs: 1995: 52)

Everything that happens seems to be premised upon meaning as the first condition for survival. The absence of meaning could lead only to suicide or madness. In order not to die or to sink into dementia, the sick person who wishes to survive spontaneously seeks a meaning to his illness. Confronted with the news of a fatal disease, he will rebuild his entire history on the basis of this new event, which becomes its logical consequence, one might say. Could the quest for meaning of illness not then be considered as the expression of the will to survive? (Lambrichs: 1995: 83)

Paris, 12 February 1995

I'm back in Paris, but I'm not writing: I'm simply too tired, it's too cold, and I'm too anxious. I even go to Dr Mici, my gynecologist, to have her examine my breast. She reassures me, tells me she can't feel any lumps, and gives me an order for a mammogram in case I'll be more reassured in having one. My arm hurts. Luckily, I can have it massaged by some wonderful physical therapists I've discovered in my neighborhood. One of them, Pierre, gives extremely good massages, but he's just gone off on holidays with his woman friend.

The most helpful therapist is Bettina, the first therapist I meet when I return; I ask a pharmacist in my street to give me the name of a good one. Bettina can't take me at first, because she's over-booked. Later, I tell her how much I wished she were available that first time, and she admits she felt the same way about seeing me. We connect immediately. For my most recent massage, she replaces Pierre, and I like her technique and presence, and very much enjoy talking with her. Her father is Egypto-Armenian, and her mother is German; she herself was born here in France. She's very beautiful and sensitive.

She tells me the story of a friend of hers who had breast cancer. The woman was only 35, and had a child. She had a premonition she'd contract the disease, and insisted of her doctors that they order a mammogram – and that's most probably what saved her life. Her arm swells up, especially when she's travelling; I remember that Mona's friend Néna told me that her arm swelled up whenever she went on a long flight. I've found out that as a result of cabin pressure, the lymphatic liquid travels to the arm and thereby makes it swell up.

Bettina's massage is very soothing. She drains the lymphatic liquid effectively by applying soft pressure with her fingers, and tells me about her father's family members, some of whom live in Cairo's popular Shubra district, and others of whom live in Héliopolis, one of the city's more middle-class suburbs. She remembers that her grandmother used to lower a basket on a rope from her balcony in order

343

to get her groceries – mainly fruits and vegetables. Listening to Bettina's story, I'm reminded of my mother, who used the same shopping method in Beirut: she bargained in Arabic, and lowered the money in a basket, which the greengrocer then filled with fruits and vegetables.

When mother and father were engaged and she was waiting in Switzerland for him, my father designed a whole correspondence course in order to teach her Arabic. He entitled the course *L'Arabe sans larmes*: Arabic without Tears. However, someone stole the package when we lost our Ras-Beirut apartment to Muhajareen – displaced people who lived in houses or apartments that people left during the summer or at other times during the war in Lebanon. We were never able to recover the manuscript of the course, even when we got the apartment back; by then, father was too weak to try and salvage it. Through visualising Bettina's story, I remember my sweet mother, who was so alive and present, and who made us so happy when we were children by singing her songs, and by always being soft and kind.

Bettina is very attentive. She reminds me of my Swedish friend Elizabeth, who also has long hair, a sensitive gaze and a passionate outlook; we have a real affinity. I give her a copy of my article about breast cancer, which she reads in one stretch and appreciates. She also thinks that French people must become more outspoken and talk about the problem more. I feel so lucky that our paths have crossed, and that her office is located on my street, Avenue de Saint-Ouen.

I'm so happy to have Alban here at present: I'm better able to overcome my anxiety, forget about my swelling arm, and accept the grey, unending February rain that this year is causing France's rivers to overflow.

To cheer myself up, I'm reading some of the letters that keep pouring in. I include extracts from three of them as follows.

Mary Lee Sargent: *I devoured your journey journal as soon as it arrived today. It was inspiring, brave and intelligent, and contained valuable information. I wish every woman could read it, truly. You've been in my thoughts so often during the past few months. It wasn't until I spoke with you about breast cancer and your experience of it at the Women's Studies year-end party that I finally began to keep a file on the subject ...*

Our system gives us an abundance of things most of us don't want, and deprives us of basic necessities – education that everyone has access to, decent transportation, un-poisoned food, health care, and affordable housing. We get tons of junky material goods and cancer in the US. Are we not fortunate? I think the thing that upset me the most in your journal is that you were given [the EPC] *simply because your family had a history of osteoporosis. Is there any form of hormone-replacement therapy that's safe or safer, I wonder? I heard a wonderful program on NPR* [National Public Radio] *about a book called* The Menopause Industry, *by a woman from New Zealand, whose name escapes me at the moment. She is, in part, reporting on a massive study of the effects of estrogen therapies that was undertaken by the New Zealand government. Her message was that estrogen should never be taken for more than five years, and that in some cases, for some women, it should never be prescribed ...*

I've also gotten obsessed with making videos using the fancy, new equipment that's now available to the faculty at Parkland. I've made a video of a male friend of mine (a father of four) doing housework and talking about doing housework ... If you're at all interested, I'd like to make a video of you – and possibly other women – talking about your experience having had breast cancer. Thank the universe, spirit, that your tests are negative, which is positive. We'll all keep reminding the spirit to keep up the good work in our own ways ...

Amel: *Evelyne, ma chérie, since yesterday, you've been in Paris. Yesterday morning, the sun came out after several grey days (there's even been some snow), and I thought of you, flying from Beirut to Paris. My very dear, your voice from Lebanon on the phone was so happy. In it, I felt the love of your people, your mother and Théophile in particular, and the warmth of Lebanon. Your voice was filled with the sun and the vibrations of the air you were breathing on your balcony in the mountains. And it made me feel so good, this friendly voice calling me from so far away, from the other side of the Mediterranean.*

I've suffered a lot lately. Chemna – the aunt from Bizerte you met – died on the 16th of December, unexpectedly, from pulmonary embolism. She'd come to spend the night at my sister Zbeida's, and Zbeida had called to ask me to stop by. She seemed to be in good health, and spoke with Zbeida the whole afternoon. I was taking a nap, being exhausted after work. When I got there, at 5.30 p.m., she was having a terrible attack, and a few minutes later she was dead. We were around her: her son, my brother-in-law (a doctor) and me. It all happened so quickly. I just couldn't get over the suddenness of this passage.

The same night, we went to Bizerte: my sister; Héla, my aunt's daughter, who's pregnant, and me. The next day, I took part in the funeral. At 2 p.m., she was taken by the men to the cemetery. I loved her as if she were my mother, who she resembled: she had the same good humour, generosity and simplicity. She was a friend, a big sister to me – only seven years older than I. Forgive me, Evelyne, for talking to you about these sad things, but they're the stuff that life is made of.

The nodes in my throat became swollen, and for the first time, I went to see a homeopath. Despite the fact that my brother-in-law, brother and sister were applying pressure on me to take antibiotics, I didn't want to take them, and I'm feeling better ...

My darling friend, I'm so happy your mother's doing better; I'd so much like to know her. You know that my vision of death and life is changing. I understand that we can't prevent someone from dying – it's like birth: it can't be stopped. I spoke with a friend, Irène, who I did the kinesiology workshop with. She's going to

loan me Patrick Drouot's book about death, which he treats as a
passage. I feel more serene ...
　So, I'm slowly emerging from my grief. I'm tired of my job at
present. I don't have much energy. At the end of this month, I'll
have four days of kinesiology ... Last time, I wanted to work on
my desire to change jobs, but what came out was torture [20
years earlier, Amel had been gaoled and tortured for political reasons]; *it was very painful ... This session helped me; it*
was completely unexpected, and very powerful..
　My darling friend, I see you laughing, and I'm smiling. You
must be saying, 'What's Amel talking about: what are these sto-
ries about kinesiology and meditation?' ...
　How are you, ma chérie? How's your lovely frizzy hair? I read
the interview you had with Rachida – I love it when you're angry.
It hurt me to feel the hurt and nausea you've had from this bar-
baric therapy. How hard it must have been for you: this pain in
your own flesh, of which no one can partake, which belongs to you
only – but you're so much loved, because you give without meas-
ure. I miss you, Evelyne, and I'm so happy to know you'll soon be
here with Alban ... I wish you a happy New Year.

Diane: *I'm thinking of you. I feel you close to me, in my heart ...*
All my life I've been seeking to learn, to look for guides, to have
this rare exchange through which I'm inspired by knowledge to go
beyond myself. In your presence, I've learnt to have confidence, to
become someone worthy of confidence and conscience. I'm learn-
ing to give form to dreams, to share ... More importantly still, I'm
remembering that one mustn't make excuses for failing to express
consciousness, compassion and love. Thank you, dear friend, for
all you bring to this world, and for all that you awaken in me ...

Paris, 14 February 1995

It's Valentine's Day. Tomorrow, I'm going to Hôpital Saint-
Louis to have a total check-up: mammograms; ecographies;

347

X-rays; blood tests; the whole bit. Luckily, Alban's coming with me. I'm worried most about the blood tests, because when the nurse draws the blood in a rough way, as the nurse drew it last time, at that private lab in Paris's 16th district, my arm hurts for weeks afterwards; however, when capable and gentle people do the job, the experience can be very smooth and painless.

Today, Patsy goes to the Paris suburb of St Quentin-en-Yvelines in order to meet local officials to discuss starting up a circus centre and school. I hope very much that the meeting is a success, and she's given the opportunities she so much needs if she's to get her women's circus off the ground. Once, I accompanied her to the Emile Snyder Award ceremony, at which she met the district mayor and other public figures, all of whom were charmed by her wit, looks and vivacious intelligence and were interested in having her start up a circus centre and school in St Quentin-en-Yvelines. When Patsy is joking around and acting, she's a charmer. Some of her shows are hilarious and well performed. However, it costs a lot to pay the female-only actors, and to pay for the costumes and sets. Patsy has been staging the shows courageously, all on her own and with very little outside help. I admire her for doing so, and hope she can get moving with the project.

Mother isn't doing well these days. She must be recognising that March is coming up: father was born the 6th and died on the 24th – a tragically odd coincidence.

Paris, 19 February 1995

When I wake up this morning, my chest wall is sore. When I touch it, I feel it's my ribcage that's hurting, and that the pain's in all the places that have been touched by the radiation. However, I'm also worried it might be the cancer that's returned there – metastasised – and am unnerved to think so. This disease is so frightening: we live in fear, always anxious that the disease might've returned, and that this time there won't be any way to heal it. We can at least accept living with pain in the arm, just as we're used to coping with migraines or other everyday aches and pains; however, the prospect of having to live with mad cells that might be gobbling up healthy ones in our body is frightening, even when we know that some people have been able to overcome the recurrence.

Jane: When I read this, I got a flash of the image of the stalker: the man who scares women out of their mind by always following them everywhere. You always have the feeling he's there, somewhere, even when you can't see him, and even when people tell you there's nothing to worry about. I was thinking about one of our graduate students in the French department, who left because she was worried about a man like this!

This morning, luckily, I'm able to cuddle up to my sweet Alban, and I feel reassured.

I wonder whether I'll ever be able to come out of this state of fear. Will I always be questioning my whole life as a result of having all these aches and pains?

When I read some of Nadia Tuéni's last poems, I feel she was convinced that cancer was leading her towards death, especially after the disease recurred. I include one of her prose-poems, from *La terre arrêtée* (Tuéni: 1984: 19), translated, as follows.

I and Time

From easy utopia, to death's grand inventory, there is my life, incapable of reproducing itself, suffering from incomprehensible pains. Condemned by birth to the uneasiness of existence in time, all at once unhappy to be subjected to the state of being, and panicking at what

> *alone could put an end to it, meaning death, I am going*
> *away, rolling like a pebble, from adaptations to discov-*
> *eries, from struggles to sleep, until that unknown*
> *beach, where tossed by the wave I come to land. My time*
> *has come to an end.*

How poignant and sublime Nadia Tuéni's writing strikes me as being! It resonates in me as music does. I feel I've crossed the Valley of the Shadow of Death and have emerged from it, saved. Why, then, am I feeling so anxious at night when I wake up, or when I'm in pain? All the demons wake up then too, and all the horror I've lived resurfaces.

I must write about the visit that Patsy and I pay to the acupuncturist. Patsy insists I go with her to see him, at the beginning of my stay in Paris, when I tell her I've had breast cancer. I phone her one day when I'm newly arrived in the city and feeling depressed. She tells me she wondered why her father, Alban, was so nervous over the summer period. We talk at great length over the phone, as she likes to do. As always, she's understanding, sweet and comforting, and she tells me to meet her at the Belleville metro stop tomorrow.

The acupuncturist, Dr Hin, is an old Chinese man. He instructs us to go into separate treatment rooms, which look more like sanctuaries: filled with all kinds of objects, spiritual images and the smell of incense. He asks both of us to remove all our clothing except our panties and to stretch out on a bed. He massages us, and presses on specific body points that connect the meridians that are part of the body's immune system. He then plants special acupuncture needles in the points. Apparently, the treatment is soothing and is undertaken to reinforce the body's immune system. For Patsy's treatment, the Dr Hin plants the needles on one side of her face. We laugh a lot when he calls her *monsieur* because the needles have formed a pattern in the shape of a beard. She falls asleep, and later tells me she always falls asleep when she comes for treatment because she's so relaxed during it.

After our treatment, we talk with Dr Hin. He tells us he's read, in an issue of the British medical journal *The Lancet* that was published several years ago, that estrogen has indeed been proven to cause cancerous cells to proliferate. He prescribes me some Chinese herbs, which I'm to buy from a store located close to where he lives, and gives me the name of a woman doctor whose office is located close to where Monique lives. The doctor, Dr Joyer, practises traditional as well as alternative medicine. He tells me she'll be able to prescribe me mistletoe (*Viscum Album*) and relaxation sessions, which my insurance company will refund the costs of. I don't know how much better I'll be as a result of this treatment, but find that my anxiety has been somewhat relieved. And at least I no longer feel I'm just wallowing in my fears: I'm dealing with them by doing something and seeking alternatives.

Paris, 21 February 1995

I'm re-reading my sweet Séverine's letter of the 5th of January, as follows, which I find when I get back from Lebanon. I shiver when I think she has to suffer so much.

My dear Evelyne, no: I haven't forgotten you, but I've been so sick I couldn't write a word! However, I've regularly had news about you from Alain and Samira, and I received your letter of the 1st of December. You'd sent me word, through Alain, to speak to my oncologist about your problem, but I wasn't able to do so: I was in the hospital, and above all, my oncologist, who'd been so great, 'disappeared' approximately two weeks before my hospitalisation, and hasn't yet reappeared. No one at the Nicolle clinic in Urbana wanted to tell me what had happened, but I finally came to understand he had all kinds of problems, the poor guy! His replacement is a former colleague who'd retired, a horrible person I didn't get along with at all.

The 6th of January: I'm continuing to write while listening to your singing: it gives me the impression I'm with you. The horrible story of my oncologist is as follows.

He hospitalised me because he was convinced I was full of tumours – ovarian. I knew it wasn't that: my symptoms would have been different. In short, when he didn't find any cancer, he wasn't interested in me any more. He started by telling me I'd never had breast cancer (interesting!), and went on to say that the intense nausea I felt was all in my head. He didn't listen to me once, and after I'd spent a month in the hospital, he sent me back home, sick as a dog. When I phoned him to ask him for an anti-nausea drug, he responded – through his nurse – that I didn't need it, that I was overly anxious, and that I'd do well to see a psychiatrist! I'm not exaggerating. His nurse sounded very uncomfortable to have to give me this message, and advised me to call the doctor on duty the next day.

I've spent a month in the hospital, a month that's been a real nightmare, at the mercy of this fool and of a surgeon who shouted at me because I wasn't getting well quickly enough. Luckily, there was a gastro-enterologist – a woman, of course – who listened to what I was saying, and who persuaded them to operate on me because as a result of all the symptoms I'd been complaining about since July, a partial intestinal obstruction was suggested, even if the medical tests didn't show it, and the first (minor) operation had revealed only adherences due to the preceding operations.

She was right, and they had to remove part of my intestines. During the operation, they also had to put an enormous tube in my stomach. It went all the way to my intestines in order to feed me during my convalescence. The presence of the tube itself gave me unbearable nausea. I felt seasick all the time, and for about two months could neither read nor watch TV. When I went home, I had to be fed for almost another month through this tube in my stomach and a catheter in my chest. It was the gastro-enterologist who decided to remove the tube just before Christmas and to replace it with a small tube that was much less invasive. It was a real miracle: the next day, I started feeling better and eating.

Now, I'm eating completely normally and I feel much, much better. What upsets me is that my nightmare could have been shortened if these guys had listened to me rather than treated me like a fool or a hysterical woman.

I'm now seeing Dr PJ; for two months, I wasn't able to do chemo, of course. I might have to start again on Monday – another three cycles. Here you have the whole story of my medical misadventures. To amuse Alban, I'll tell you that the hospital bill for the month was $61,500, and this doesn't include either the operations or the doctors' daily visits! No comment.

I'm glad you've found a doctor you can trust. I believe there comes a time when one has to stop asking for other opinions, because each time, the doctors are going to tell you something different, and it can drive you crazy! I can ask JE for your biopsy slides, but I'm not sure she can send them like that ...

I wonder how your stay in Lebanon is going at present. You must be enjoying your mother, in spite of her illness; I know you would have liked to be there for your father ...

I see Alain from time to time. He's always so kind: he brought me caramel custard to give me an appetite, and a Kuglof – this delicious Alsatian cake ...

Zohreh phoned me many times. She wanted to come and see me, but is very busy; I'm going to phone her to tell her I feel better. She's so devoted.

Samira is still here – what a miracle! I'd finally accepted the fact she was going to leave ... I believe I was one of the first to know she'd finally decided to stay. She's been so great, as usual – she often came to see me at the hospital, and phoned me regularly. I'm lucky.

I'll have to stop writing now. Charles is in Chicago for a conference, and I have to fix something to eat for Laura. We'd

planned on going somewhere, but it snowed too much today and
I can't take the car out.
  How's Alban? Kiss him for me. I kiss you affectionately. Happy
New Year, and Good Health. – Séverine

I re-read this letter, and realise how much my poor Séverine
has suffered and is continuing to suffer. It's all so unfair, and
when I read her description of some of her doctors, I get
really mad. There's simply no excuse for them not to listen:
isn't listening their most basic duty in treating her as a
human being? And doctors' fees and hospital bills: they're
'going through the ceiling' – it defies belief! Where in the
world does all this money go?

And yet, in the midst of her misery, Séverine finds time
to think of other people, to ask about me and to be concerned. I find her thoughtfulness so touching, given her
circumstances.

I'm reading Judith Brouste's book *L'Etat d'alerte* (Brouste:
1994), which was reviewed in the issue of *marie claire* that
contained all the testimonials about breast cancer. The
reviewer stated that it was a good book about the subject,
and advised readers to read it along with another book,
Elizabeth Gille's *Le crabe sur la banquette arrière* (Gille: 1994).
So far, I've found only the former book, and I'm disappointed I haven't found the latter.

Brouste's book isn't about breast cancer; it's about the
narrator's philosophical searching for 'something else' in
her otherwise empty, deadly boring life. Personally, I can
identify with only the beginning of the story, when she's
writing about her chemo sessions and her relationship with
her body, her disease and the threat of death, but also about
the idea, which I find that everyone who's gone through the
experience has, that you'll never be the same; in fact, perhaps she's narrating about how she 'touched bottom': the
possibility that her body, as well as her sexuality, would die.

When she finished her treatment, she then had a sexual relationship with her doctor. Theirs is a sado-masochistic arrangement: he ties her up to make her reach orgasm. He chains her up to dominate her, and she lets herself be subjugated to go all the way to the end of what she can bear, to the end of her suffering, in order to be reborn to life, to love. The 'S&M' process is a metaphor for what she had to go through when she had chemotherapy: having to experience suffering, and the death of good and bad cells, in order to be reborn to a life free of cancer.

Madeleine: That should teach you not to always trust these so-called women's mags: it's a category in which, in France at least, the aim is to have a pretty low common denominator. The books promoted in these magazines tend to be a bit sordid, or corny, happy-ending novels; whatever the case, I'd stay away from them if I were you.

Nevertheless, it was in magazines such as these that I found the very moving breast-cancer testimonials I've quoted in Chapter 11, and that I sometimes find interesting articles in. And Judith Brouste's book, *L'Etat d'alerte*, is published by Le Seuil, which to my knowledge is a respectable publishing house.

I analyse this novel with Alban. In reality, it's an illustration of my thesis that chemotherapy is barbaric – the torture of the twentieth century. While the doctor is caring for his breast-cancer patient, in the midst of her nausea and suffering, he takes the liberty of telling her all about his divorces and his numerous adventures with many mistresses. When his patient is 'healed', she throws herself into his arms, and as their – almost purely sexual – relationship is evolving, he uses chains and leather, ties her down, treats her as a sexual object, and tortures her as he'd tortured her before with chemo. Finally, she runs away from the relationship; she comes out of it 'healed', knowing she wants a 'true' love. Nevertheless, the whole situation is disgusting: I find it revolting that a doctor could behave in this way, and that a patient-narrator could disguise the problem of breast cancer by superimposing a sordid 'love' story on it – even if the story is a symbolic illustration of my subject.

Jane: This is what sells books! And what gets her invited to go on *Pivot [a French TV program that writers dream of being invited to go on because they get a lot of publicity that way]*, on which she'll be asked invasive questions such as 'Is this a true story?' and 'What's it like to be chained up?'

Paris, 22 February 1995

Alban and I go to see his doctor, Dr Hues, the endocrinologist at the Avicenne hospital, near St Denis-Basilique. The doctor studies the X-rays of Alban's hypophysis gland and his level of prolactine, both of which haven't changed much since last time the doctor studied them. When he asks Alban whether he's taking the medicine, which I'll call PLD, as well as the testosterone – male hormone – he prescribed him, I'm quite surprised to hear Alban's answer, in a shaky voice, 'I've been too upset this year to think about that!' As a result, we talk about my breast cancer, as well as about hormones. Dr Hues says, 'Of course, all the experiments show that estrogens make cancerous cells proliferate; however, in medicine, you have to know how to "measure out": strike a balance between avoiding decalcification by achieving an adequate level of hormone without bringing about a cancer.'

'But why,' Alban exclaims, 'were we never told that in this way?'

The doctor again tells us that in France, the EPC I had isn't being prescribed any more. He asks me what kind of estrogen I was given and whether it was combined with progesterone. When I ask him why the EPC is no longer prescribed in France, he replies that nowadays, more natural and less potent kinds of hormone product are available.

Tonight, I watch a TV show that features Claude Roy, a guest who had cancer and wrote a book about it, entitled *Permis de Séjour, 1977–1982* (Roy: 1983). The title could be translated as being 'residence permit', which would be a play on words: the idea of getting a licence to remain, or stay, in the sense of having the right to exist.

Jane: Who has the right to exist, to reside on this earth, and who doesn't? And who decides? Is it, as poets say, just a throw of the die, or what? Do we need a licence to be?

The book is about humans' capacity or incapacity to look truth in the face. According to Roy, 'The human animal liar has received the grace or the curse to be able to lie to himself.' When Roy contracted lung cancer, he felt compelled to ask many questions that I find interesting. I translate some of his words (Roy: 1983: 12–13) as follows.

I seek the picture in the tapestry, the hidden connectedness among things that seem remote. Confronted with cancer, with The People's Republic of China, which I found seriously ailing in 1979, with the surgical operation I underwent in 1982 and the police operation that Poland was subjected to as a result of the military *coup d'etat* in 1981, the same problem interests me: how to know the truth? Is it good to know the truth? In public as in personal life, the same phenomenon always fascinates me: the art Man applies in order not to see what would hurt or upset him, to believe the unbelievable, whatever he can live with … the patient who closes his eyes in order not to confront his situation directly, or in order to have the strength to bear the unbearable …

Paris, 23 February 1995

This morning, I'm saddened to hear on the radio that Emmanuel Roblès has died. I remember when Emmanuel came to my university to give some talks. Afterwards, I invited him to my place for a Lebanese meal with some friends. We subsequently became friends, and every summer I spent in Paris, I met him for meals at the George V Restaurant, on the Champs Elysées – one of his favourite restaurants. I enjoyed talking with him and listening to him tell his many stories: he had great gift for storytelling. I learnt a lot from him about various subjects, such as writing, and writers, from Camus to Mouloud Feraoun, both of whom he knew, but Feraoun on a more personal level. His private and public talks were always fascinating and well organised. He had a way of making the most dull topic come alive and of injecting passionate into it. When I hear the news that he's died, I feel strange, because only the night before, when I was watching the TV show that featured Claude Roy, I was thinking about him and wondering whether there'd be a similar show about him.

When Claude Roy on TV is talking about cancer, he becomes extremely emotional. I feel it hurts him to talk about it, especially when he mentions the fact that one of his friends died from the disease whereas he himself has come out of it healed. In his book, he states (Roy: 1983: 343–4),

> The theories about what causes diseases reflect, successively, the cultural conceptions of a given historical period: disease as divine punishment in societies dominated by the sacred. In religion, disease as malediction, curse, result of 'the evil eye'. In archaic societies under the spell of the shaman, or the sorcerer, disease as sociological mistake, bacterial contamination through neglect and absence of care … I am a contemporary of the theories inspired by Freud …

disease is the result of an internal conflict that has been neither elucidated nor overcome. It is this theory that Susan
Sontag violently attacked when she herself was hit with cancer: to add to the weight of disease the guilt of the patient
seems to her absurd ... However, not everything is explained
by referring to the organic or mechanical causes: I was hit
with lung cancer because I smoked too much during a great
part of my life. This is true. But why did I smoke too much?
Why was I inhabited by a nervousness through which I found
relief only by ingesting toxic smoke? Also, I have lived and
still live a conflict, literally historical, a struggle, a tearing
apart that besieged me, obsessed me, sapped me, wore me
out until cancer.

I'm similarly struck by Alban's expression of emotion yesterday, when we went to see his doctor. He's been so shaken
by my disease that he's no longer thinking about his own
health, to the point he's forgetting to take his medicine.
Ironically, this neglect might turn out to have been a blessing
in disguise, because, at least with reference to testosterone,
it's thought that these hormones stimulate cancer cells: a
process that later in this book is proven to occur, in Alban's
case as well.

Paris, 28 February 1995

I have a day of suffering and fear. I think I must be going
through some hormonal change in my body and all kinds of
effects are being produced that I recognise as 'before', when I
was supposed to have my periods. The sensation is the same
– except that now I'm afraid. I'm imagining the worst: that
hormones are arousing within me all the cancer demons, and
that these monsters are invading and devouring me.

Today, I drag myself around, feeling listless and lethargic,
as if I have the flu; I'm running a temperature – if only it were

the flu; I have a vague headache; and I ache all over. A few days ago, I make the mistake of reading a small book about cancer 'follow-up', which cancer all patients are given when they've been treated. According to the book's author, you must be very careful during the five years after you've been treated, because 60 per cent of all breast-cancer recurrences arise within the first three years after the first treatment, 20 per cent within the next two years, and 20 per cent in subsequent years. You're advised to watch for pains – in the shoulder, lower back or kidney area – as well as for changes on the scar or breast, for fatigue, for headaches, for blurred vision, for dizziness, and so on. It seems I only have to read this stuff to have the fear-driven symptoms come on.

Alban and I go to hear Vénus Khoury-Ghata read her poetry. It's a nice change, and we have a very uplifting evening. Vénus talks about her 'unceasing need to talk about death' as a result of her experiences during the war in Lebanon and the death of some of her loved ones in Paris, in which she's been living for more than 30 years. Her poetry is characterised by brilliant, unusual images, and I've always admired it. I translate some of the lines from her book *Mon anthologie* (Khoury-Ghata: 1993: 8, 180) as follows.

> *Nail your shadow;*
> *nurse your amputated gestures;*
> *cross this nocturnal sun;*
> *calm your objects caught in anxiety;*
> *dry the sweat from your heart and your books;*
> *tighten the stitches of your blood ...*
>
> *Do not fear*
> *when obscurity pours its ink on your walls:*
> *it is only the night's writing,*
> *the hybrid flight of darkness,*

skimming the roofs of tombs to upset their sullen
dwellers.

By design, petroleum-derived pesticides have the power to kill because they chemically interfere with one or another of nerve impulses. The weed killer atrazine hinders the process of photosynthesis. The phenoxy herbicides bring about death by mimicking the effect of plant growth hormones. (Steingraber: 1997: 91)

Throughout all of these routes, we find ourselves facing a rising tide of biologically active, synthetic organic chemicals. Some interfere with our hormones, some attach themselves to our chromosomes, some cripple the immune system, and some overstimulate the activity of certain enzymes. If we could metabolize these chemicals into completely benign breakdown products and excrete them, they would pose less of a hazard. Instead, a good many of them accumulate. In essence, synthetic organic chemicals confront us with the worst of both worlds. They are similar enough to naturally occurring chemicals to react with us but different enough to not go away easily. (Steingraber: 1997: 92)

Everything accumulates. The diversity and toxicity of fumes emitted by car engines or other mass combustion go far beyond anything that nature could be emitting on its own. In France, lung cancer is the worst among males, and has been increasing unabated since 1950. Cancer will soon become the disease that every family will have to cope with, and will likely be the most frequent cause of death before the age of 65 if the incidence of cancer cases keeps progressing at current rates. Of course, 85% of all lung cancers are ascribed to tobacco use, which is also the cause of half the deaths resulting from cancer of the bladder and a quarter of the ones due to pancreatic and kidney cancers, and a factor in many others. We should wonder, nevertheless, about the nearly 600% net increase in deaths among males due to tobacco, if we take only the period 1950–1985. That does not include other pulmonary ailments. According to many sources, the concomitant rise in atmospheric pollution cannot be considered a mere innocent additive here! And again, cancer is but one of the diseases taken as an example, among the many harmful consequences. Young people are being affected at ever increasing rates. By stifling ourselves like this, we are in the process of losing the improved quality of life and the increased life expectancy that modern medicine made possible, and that our mothers and fathers worked hard to achieve throughout this century. (Séralini: 1997: 51–2)

13

TRAGIC IRONY
ONE HEALED; THE OTHER HIT

Cadmium intake by humans is mostly from direct consumption of contaminated plants, especially fruits and vegetables. Cadmium is classified as a probable human carcinogen. In animals, it is associated with sarcoma, lung cancer, and prostate cancer. High rates of lung, prostate, and testicular cancers have also been reported in workers who inhale cadmium on the job – but the question of incineration, cadmium ingestion, and cancer risk remains unexplored. Somewhere between 50 to 75 percent of the cadmium in the waste stream – about thirteen hundred tons – comes from discarded batteries. Dead batteries, if incinerated, do pose a cancer risk, reasoned one epidemiologist after analyzing the numbers. (Steingraber: 1997: 222)

Paris, 1 March 1995

I'm reading Lynn Payer's very interesting book *Medicine and Culture* (Payer: 1988), in which the author reveals to what extent treatments for various health problems can vary from country to country. For example, she compares French people, who are always talking about their liver, with German people, who blame their heart for their fatigue, even when there's nothing wrong with them; she also compares the medical systems of Britain and the States, and concludes that surgery is performed much more frequently in the latter country. Payer, an American, writes about European medical issues for various journals, and is therefore in a good position to explore the differences she's uncovered. She's come to realise that many of the practices she once took for granted didn't result as much from scientific progress as from American cultural biases, whereby in some cases the effect was harm rather than help.

One of the issues she develops that's related to my area of inquiry has to do with how aggressive American medicine is. I quote from her book (Payer: 1988: 124) as follows.

> … even as Europeans were developing the simple mastectomy and the lumpectomy as less mutilating ways to treat breast cancer, American doctors were advocating the superradical mastectomy and prophylactic removal of both breasts to prevent breast cancer.

Compared with French, West German and English doctors, American doctors conduct a greater number of diagnostic tests; they use higher doses of drugs and more-aggressive drugs; and the surgery, which they perform more often, is likely to be more aggressive. Compared with her French, West German and English counterparts, an American woman is two to three times more likely to have a hysterectomy. In the United States, more than 60 per cent of hysterectomies are performed for women who are younger than 44. Many American doctors consider hysterectomy to be the best treatment for many pre-cancerous conditions that their European counterparts treat less radically. Compared with their European counterparts, American doctors perform prostate surgery more often. In the States, both doctors and people in general view the patient who 'beats' cancer as being superior to the patient who fights the disease but succumbs to it, and in turn view the latter patient as being superior to the patient who refuses to fight: American doctors aren't very good at treating chronic diseases, because their strategy is to do something and do it very fast. Because of this tendency to go for the 'quick fix', American doctors don't look too kindly on surgical procedures that might have to be repeated; for example, they often prefer to perform a hysterectomy rather than a *myomectomy*, which is the operation to remove fibroids but conserve the uterus, but which might have to be repeated and which, compared with a hysterectomy, often takes longer to perform.

I again quote from Lynn Payer's book (Payer: 1988: 146–7), as follows.

> Once a substance is branded as 'bad,' all complexities about whether it might be good for some people, or good in small quantities, vanish. Pregnant women, and even women trying to become pregnant, are told to avoid all alcohol, even though most studies have shown that drinking up to two glasses of wine a day throughout pregnancy does not increase the risk of harm to the fetus. New York City has legislated that all restaurants and bars post signs warning pregnant women that alcohol can cause birth defects, giving the impression that alcohol is some kind of nutritional thalidomide that can harm the fetus no matter how small the dose.

Bettina: That sounds like nonsense: when alcohol is taken in moderation, there are no such risks.

Jane: Plus it's hypocritical! Once that super-protected fetus becomes a person, and enters that same New York bar, he or she is encouraged, through the advertising machine, to smoke, drink, buy guns and eat junk! Are any warnings posted then?

Payer concludes that choice of diagnoses and treatment isn't a science, and that the benefits that ensue and the risks taken will always be on a cultural scale. Unfortunately, most doctors continue to hide behind the screen of 'scientific' medicine, which is somehow given precedence over patients' 'unscientific' desires.

Manicha: North Americans are full of *nouveaux riche* arrogance: nothing is big enough for them, from the Hollywood star who has the biggest breasts to the guy who drives the biggest car, and on and on.

I feel better today because my anxieties are flying away; it's amazing the difference it makes when you feel better. I must've been going through a hormonal change to have felt so bad. Dark thoughts assail me when I feel weak, and I imagine the worst.

Dol, 4 March 1995

I'm staying at Souad and Pierre's place in Brittany, and I'm remembering the days I spent with Alban in St Malo, almost seven years ago. It was an exquisite time, when illness was something we didn't even think about, let alone imagine it'd ever affect us.

At the time, Alban had been invited to give some talks about Islam to a group of religious people. The talks were organised by monks, or something of the kind. We – I especially – delighted in shocking the monks by displaying our 'forbidden love'. There we were, in the garden of the château, walking and hugging, and ready to make love at every turn. For a bit of mischief, I sang the *muezzin*, the chant to Allah that's sung in the minarets of the mosques in order to call the faithful to prayer! I fondly remember our walks along Brittany's beach, when Alban embraced me as if each embrace were our last! I also remember the times I took the TGV to Neuchâtel to visit my parents. How quickly life changes, and how quickly our ability to live crazily and with excitement is transformed.

I remember that it was on the 2nd of March, 1994 – a year ago – that I was diagnosed as having cancer. The horrible memories of that time are now becoming dimmer. Luckily, time has a way of dulling them, but unfortunately the good ones are also dimmed, although not in the same way. Françoise tells me that my face looks healthier than it did last October, when I'd just arrived.

Souad and Pierre are making us feel very welcome. It's incredible here: the food; the warmth; the walks; the beauty of the landscape, and of dear friends; and rediscovering Brittany, which is laden with so many unforgettable memories.

I feel I'm slowly healing and regaining my strength.

Paris, 7 March 1995

Yesterday, I phone mother: it's the 6th of March, father's birthday. Mother isn't feeling well, and must be close to the end of her life. Will I see her again?

Today, in the metro, I see a beautiful woman of my age who has very short hair – 'salt and pepper', like my hair was when I came out of the treatment. She asks me what time it is. I feel we're somehow on the same wavelength. I look at her from the corner of my eye, and wonder whether she's also been mutilated by having her breast cut off – I think it might be so. If all women who've been subjected to the operation 'came out of the cancer closet' by revealing their mutilation in public, or by wearing some visible sign, we'd create a chain of solidarity through mutual recognition.

This is what Audre Lorde also writes about in her breast-cancer journal (Lorde: 1980). She wishes that all the women who've had a mastectomy would stop concealing it. She's against breast reconstruction and prostheses. I'm not sure how I feel about those remedial options, but I think that if, in taking them, women can better overcome their fear and despair about seeing their body mutilated, and if their self-image is thereby improved and their health not endangered, they should consider them. I believe it's up to each individual women to choose, even if the choice has huge political implications. I know I have problems with my self-image at present. Even though my sweet Alban keeps complimenting me, I can't help but feel that my femininity has been diminished, and that feeling this way isn't good for my morale.

Bettina: I agree with your line of reasoning.

Paris, 9 March 1995

Today, Alban and I visit Dr Esper to have my check-up and find out my lab results, which I do every three months. The doctor tells me everything's all right, except that I have a high cholesterol level and a few micro-calcifications in my other breast, which we'll have to watch. He has a good attitude, and I feel secure when I'm talking with him. He reminds me of Alban: calm; poised; careful to weigh every word he says; sure of what he does, but very humble.

As he did during our previous visit Dr Esper, Alban fantasises about what the doctor is doing while he's making us wait. The first time we came to see Esper, Alban imagined the doctor was having lunch somewhere), but this time, he decided he was making love in in his office! When Alban makes these funny remarks, he's being typically French. Actually, however, the explanation for Esper's unavailability today is he has a whole class of young female interns in his office, and is teaching them. When we go in and I feel the young women's gaze on me, I feel a bit edgy. One of them, though, gives me a very sympathetic look, and another shows expertise when she examines me. Consequently, my anxiety fades away.

I phone Kathleen and spoke with her friend Emilie, who three years ago also had breast cancer and is now being refused a loan from a Paris bank in order to purchase an apartment. Alban wonders whether it's legal for the bank manager to refuse her the loan on health grounds; however, the manager seems to be refusing the loan with impunity. I must speak out about all this discrimination: it should be stopped.

Bettina: This problem has to be brought out into the open: it's pathetic to have to lie about your health in order to apply for a loan!

This young woman, Emilie, is scared because she's going to a United States university for a year in order to do research, and she'll have to have medical insurance. She's been informed that in the States, no insurer will insure someone who has a pre-existing condition, and this summation is correct. I wonder what she'll do; perhaps the university she's going to can get her a policy – I hope so.

Paris, 12 March 1995

Today, I have lunch at home with Tom, Carole, Ruth and Kathleen: the first time, since I've had the disease, that I've invited so many people to eat together. Ruth brings me an article she's written about my work, entitled 'The Poetics of Pain' – what an appropriate title! I'm always surprised to see women such as Ruth and Cindy writing about my work and helping me discover aspects of it that I wasn't aware of.

Today, when we talk about cancer, Carole tells us about all kinds of strange diseases, along with cancer, that are occurring in Urbana, and that even children are being hit with them. She knows a woman who lives in a northern United States city who, surprised at seeing many of her neighbourhood's children dying of leukemia, led an investigation and asked a lawyer to become involved. She and the investigators discovered that many big companies and industries had serious leaks and weren't cleaning up their toxic waste. The lawyer was daring in investing big sums of money in the case, knowing his clients would win and that he'd get the money back; however, if the government swings to the Right, and big-business interests prevail, even mounting a case will no longer be an option.

Carole also tells me about a lump she had on her neck and that she was worried about having removed: thyroid cancer runs in her family. Many years ago, just before she left to go to Africa to do research, she had a similar lump removed that turned out to be cancerous, and had her lymph nodes removed without being told they would be.

Cindy: Unbelievable!

She wasn't warned, and, like most people, didn't know, that lymph nodes are vital to the immune system!

Paris, 15 March 1995

Yesterday, I invite Uncle Marc and Claire, a young woman I find very likeable, to lunch, not knowing they're going to announce to me that they're getting married next week! Uncle Marc is almost 75, Claire barely 45. I admire their courage in overcoming the age difference and rising beyond it as a consideration. He's my mother's brother, and when mother heard he was remarrying – his wife died a few years ago – my mother, with her usual humour, exclaimed, 'Expect the unexpected from this brother!'

What bothers me about this uncle is that he doesn't

realise he makes racist comments, and I can understand why father suffered so much because of him. I remember some misunderstandings through which mother was torn apart. For example, I conveyed to Uncle Marc what some people from Terrorisme Biblique – the name I give to the religious group they belonged to – had said about the possibility that a young man from the group would marry me. The young man's family's response was 'Never to an Arab!' Uncle Marc reacted by saying I didn't really 'look Arab', and that I looked even less so when I was younger! My Aunt Mireille reported to me and my middle brother Augustus that my mother's family found Augustus to be the best looking of all the family's brothers and sisters because he was the least distinctively 'Arab looking'! I wonder whether they realised what they were saying, and the racist implications of their statements.

I also remember all the difficult steps and endless procedures that father had to go through in order to obtain Swiss nationality, and how my mother's family members made fun of him rather than help him. Father finally obtained Swiss nationality only one year before he returned to Lebanon, two years before he died. I always tried to figure out why it was so important for him to have Swiss nationality. Similar to most immigrants, he feared he'd be ostracised, and subjected to racism and repression in his host country, especially because he came from an Arab country and culture. Once, when he was complaining to me about the lack of help he was receiving from my mother's family – Uncle Marc especially – I asked him why he was going through so much trouble to obtain his Swiss nationality. He replied, 'What if your mother dies before me, and they kick me out of here?' At the time, mother and father were living in the Swiss city of Neuchâtel because the war was still raging in Lebanon and we'd lost all the houses they could've lived in.

Father had a lofty notion of love. I remember how upset he was with Uncle Marc when Marc put his wife, Aunt Julie, into a nursing home. My uncle had taken care of her during her 10-year illness, and resorted to putting her in a nursing home only when it became unbearable for him to continue caring for her. Aunt Julie died a few weeks after she entered the nursing home. Father couldn't understand how Marc could've been so cruel as to put her in the home when she'd always said how much she didn't want to go to one. He had no sympathy for Uncle Marc, who'd reached the limits of what he could bear.

My father would definitely never have left my mother in a place such as that. Of the two – mother and him – he was the more romantic. He was madly in love with her, and died mostly because it made him sick to see her so ill. He wanted to die. Hadn't he, one day, whispered in my ear their most cherished secret: that they were praying to God to take them together? Why did he have to die before she died? Why didn't God listen to their request? Mother is still here, incredibly serene and retaining her great sense of humour! It's hard for her to be the one left behind, but it's less hard for her than it would've been for my father now if he'd been the one left alone. Perhaps, then, God knows what He's doing after all!

Is my illness also the result of hidden pains: buried sufferings I don't want to acknowledge? Should I bring them to the surface, analyse them in order to exorcise them and not repeat them? I know I was very disturbed as a result of my divorce from Jay, my subsequent relationship with Gilles and my situation with Alban – especially at the beginning of that relationship. Then mother and father got sick, and I watched father being struck down and losing all his strength and vital energy in the midst of an implacable storm: the twentieth-century disease that, along with AIDS, is so unforgiving. And I was stressed out professionally.

Fortunately, I have Alban. It's incredible how beautifully my relationship with him has evolved, and how secure I now feel. Because of our relationship, I have strength, confidence and happiness; therefore, in that way at least, I've moved on to something else: blissful confidence. It's on the professional level that I should learn to say no: to bureaucracy, and to the aspects of academia that take time. Rather than take on empty duties, I should accept only the meaningful tasks, assert myself more, and set my priorities high and stick to them.

Jane *[encouraging me]*: *Hak badna yaki, ya Evelyne!*

Thank you, my dear Jane – I need this reinforcement!

Paris, 16 March 1995

Today, I go with Ruth to a seminar conducted by Françoise Collin. Orlan presents a video-taped show, and tells us about the *auto-transformation* – she doesn't want us to call it mutilation – of her body; the title of her conference is I Gave My Body to Art. Monique comes to the conference for only five minutes, and then has to leave: she can't bear to watch a face being cut with knives and scissors, and blood being wiped away. I also find the video difficult to watch. However, I feel that Orlan's analysis – a discourse that accompanies the cutting and fixing of various parts of her body, by the doctors who agreed to operate on her – has a distancing effect and that the participants are thereby able to reflect about identity and the body. The experience is a bit like how I felt when I had my mastectomy, and I'm able to express my thoughts during the discussion. We also discussed traditional norms of the bodily beauty; what art is, or should be, or has now become; and our capacity to transform and thereby sublimate our body.

Jane *[asking me to make this point clearer]*: Was it plastic surgery?

Orlan is a woman who's made a name for herself by asking willing doctors to perform operations on her that aren't necessarily esthetically pleasing, such as adding little lumps to her forehead, above the eyebrows – funny, isn't it, Jane: thinking about you, who were made, through social pressure, to get rid of the lump on your forehead!. She asks for the least possible anesthesia in order to stay alert during the operation; she's had several operations – transformations of her body, especially her face. She has people film the whole ordeal, during which she talks to herself. She then comments on the whole performance: why she does it; why and how she gave her body to art; how she's thereby enabled to express another form of art!

Cindy: Unbelievably strange!

Madeleine: Strange? That's putting it mildly. I don't see the slightest connection with art: it looks like sado-masochism to me.

⧖

Tonight, I'm a bit disturbed, because I've just talked to Alban, and he's told me his doctor has found the marker of his PSA – what measures the likelihood he'll get prostate cancer – to be too high. I'm now worried Alban has contracted cancer, and we're barely out of my traumatic experience, as well as my father's. I can't imagine it'll be repeated in my sweet Alban – I don't even want to think about it.

Paris, 18 March 1995

I have dinner with Marie Claire, in her stunning apartment located on l'Ile St Louis, the beautiful island on the Seine. Marie Claire gives me a warm reception, and tells me that

Maurice, the man she loved passionately, died of cancer at the age of 59! When he was 57, he had pains in his stomach, but didn't pay too much attention to them. Two years later, when the doctors opened him up to operate, it was already too late: the cancer had metastasised. The doctor took Marie Claire to one side to tell her there was no hope for Maurice. For the last four months of his life, he stayed with her in this apartment. He suffered terribly.

I tell myself, *Another one!* Is it me noticing it more, or is cancer increasing? Years ago, Marie Claire told me about the then love of her life, who'd died of cancer; I wasn't receptive back then, and didn't ask her many questions. Now, however, because I've suffered, I can better understand her plight: I have more compassion for people who have these major problems, and I'm able to ask meaningful, precise questions. Unlike that first time, Marie Claire and I are now speaking the same language.

Marie Claire tells me she didn't like Orlan's show: she found it gratuitously exhibitionistic. In her view, Orlan was forcing brutal images 'down our throats', being violent with us and getting pleasure out of it – it was her own personal 'trip' through which she hoped – to immortalise herself and 'go down in history'.

Cindy: I agree: the performance sounds highly sadistic!

This evening with Marie Claire is indeed intense, and these kinds of relationship – warm and enriching – now count so much in my life. Things aren't the same any more: I flee shallowness and superficiality. I've changed: as a result of my illness, I'm transformed – for the better, I feel – and I'm communicating better with people who, like me, have 'crossed the high seas', who have another dimension in their life and who want to communicate on a different level. It's a beautiful experience, crossing the Pont Marie to meet

Marie Claire in her beautiful apartment that overlooks the Seine.

Rodez, 20 March 1995

I'm staying with my married friends Sylvie and Dédé, in Rodez. It's tense, because the weather is lousy and the couple are fighting about insignificant things. I'm reflecting on how trivial it is to get angry about life's little miseries, which to these two probably seem huge. Yesterday evening, I notice that Dédé's bad mood has come about because he's telling me the story of his mistress, Amélie, who died of breast cancer. When I ask him precise questions, he gives me rather vague answers, such as that Amélie was probably poorly treated by a doctor in her district, who must've prescribed her hormones – she was 50 when it happened – *The critical, fatal age*, I think to myself. She'd delayed having her breast removed – having a mastectomy – because she was appearance conscious and coquettish, and frightened about losing a breast. Dédé doesn't know whether she had chemotherapy and radiation! The cancer had returned, on her chest wall. When Dédé has told the story, he leaves early to go to his room. He must be feeling guilty, and with good reason: Amélie was probably very insecure, and felt that her femininity was being threatened. Dédé had failed to reassure her, and to make her realise how unimportant losing a breast was for their relationship – that in his eyes it didn't mean she'd be disfigured or mutilated. Because he doesn't even know whether she had chemo and radiation, my conviction is reinforced that the poor woman met with a sad fate and that he failed to stand by her during her time of hardship. I wonder how many other women have to face the trauma of losing their lover along with their breast.

Cindy: Good point!

In all instances, Dédé can never talk about a woman without mentioning whether she's beautiful or ugly.

Jane: Very French!

Madeleine: True, but they're not alone: the Italians, the Spanish – Mediterranean men in general – all react in the same way.

Even in the case of Sophia Loren, who was on a TV show – and who I found to be stunningly beautiful! – he felt obliged to say that her time had passed!

Jane: What a jerk!

During this whole conversation, Sylvie keeps quiet, remains self-effacing, submits and bends – it's a rather revolting scene.

Paris, 23 March 1995

I'm at Orly Sud Airport, waiting for my flight to Tunis. I feel so excited about being back with Amel, especially because at present, I'm feeling anguished and depressed, and I know that when I see her, my mood will change and I'll feel better. There's a chance that Alban has a small, cancerous tumour in his prostate, and these past few days I've had a very bad backache, so I'm suffering from quite a bit of anguish. I feel so lucky to have such wonderful friends around the world: Marie Claire, who I saw a few days ago and who I find so reassuring and well balanced, in spite of all the misfortunes she's had to go through, and now, my 'soul sister', Amel.

This time here in Paris, I also meet with Merri and Jean-Pierre, who have also invited Genevieve, who's a clinical psychiatrist, and Julien, who's a lawyer, to come along. I find Genevieve extremely interesting. She first studied medicine, then psychiatry, and started working to rehabilitate drug addicts – a highly challenging job, she says, because very few addicts manage to kick the habit, the reason being that with drugs come the promise of fulfilment, a sense of the absolute and no affective attachment: an otherwise unachievable response to the emptiness of the addicts' world – or so they think.

Genevieve has now opened her own clinic, and treats a lot of women who are undergoing treatment for breast cancer. They're between 40 and 45, and the worst thing for them is losing their femininity. For most of them, it's worse than the disease – and worse than death! Some of them refuse to have a mastectomy, because they can't accept being mutilated in that way! One of them has emerged free of cancer, even though she refused the mutilating treatment; however, most women aren't as lucky.

Genevieve also thinks that breast cancer is on the rise, and believes that the increase is related to psychological problems. Almost all the women who've been hit with it have had a traumatic experience, a period of deep mourning or a time of profound grief; otherwise, they've lived through a very difficult, painful event, which, although it sometimes occurred many years earlier, they've linked to their disease. I wonder about this reasoning, even though I find it quite compelling. Don't most people have traumatic experiences in their life? Why don't they all develop cancer if the event is the cause? The same goes for pollution and toxic waste: even though most of us are exposed to bad environmental conditions, not all of us develop cancer or other diseases. Is it survival of the fittest? How come some people smoke like chimneys and never develop lung cancer despite the fact the connection between the two has been made very clearly?

Jane: I've heard the hypothesis that because the immune system is lowered as a result of stress, the timing of the moment of stress with the moment of exposure to a cancer-causing agent is very important. Does it make any sense? Your question about survival of the fittest could be a factor, because it's now being shown that genetic factors are very important. However, most women have already had their children, that is, passed on the gene, when cancer hits; therefore, the 'evolution' argument doesn't seem to work – it's all so complicated.

Alban: In reality, breast cancer is hitting younger and younger women – apparently, all cancers are tending to appear at a younger and younger age; therefore, cancer selection could play a part in evolution of the species. In socio-biology, a debate of the utmost importance is raised here. What's the option? Should we accept that the human body has to adapt to conditions through a selective process created by humans – various forms of pollution, and so on – and thereby be led to consider that what we call progress is a kind of absolute, which has its own extra and supra-human law governing the world, whereby the species has to adapt to the decisions of this quasi-divinity – and eventually disappear? Or should we choose collective conditions of existence to measure survival of the species as we know it today?

This survival would therefore become the measurement device for all the transformations that humanity could engender. With reference to the everyday, concrete choices involved in collective life, it's often probably more difficult to clearly distinguish between these two opposing options – the question is more to do with having a choice between two general orientations, and most of all to do with asking clearly about the significance of the first: the myth of progress.

I'm thinking of Alban a lot, and worrying that his body might've started manufacturing that nodule because of my disease, through which he became so upset and started to grieve. Could the nodule have developed so fast? I'm hurt to think it might be linked to my illness. I remember that his daughter Patsy told me that the benign nodule he has on his hypophysis gland started being manufactured when one of his daughters, Solange, died in tragic circumstances that he's never wanted to talk about, not even with me, because he was hurt so much as a result. I need to be with him at present. I dont like being separated from him at times like these, and am so much looking forward to our stay in Tunis; we both need it badly.

At my get-together with Merri, I find she isn't doing very well. She's suffering because one of her sisters, Pamela, is taking drugs, is suicidal, lives with her parents and is to have an operation to rectify her hip's decalcification – an operation that Merri thinks is unacceptable and will be useless! Merri is revolted and very upset at the way Pamela is being handled, within the medical system, within her family and within a society the members of which would rather operate than get her off drugs by detoxifying her.

Genevieve, the psychiatrist, is there listening to all this. She says that drug problems are linked to the victim's family. Children have to have parental rules and established limits. When these rules are absent, children become a law unto themselves whereby everything becomes permissible. It's distressing for them, and they can become destabilised if their family doesn't give them something else and provide them with some kind of balance.

I tell Monique that since I've lost my 'femininity' – the one I used to have, because I'm now trying to redefine myself in terms of my physical appearance – some men, such as Dédé and Jurius, haven't been looking at me the way they used to look at me. Monique responds, 'It must make you realise all sorts of things.' It's true that many social, cultural and esthetic values are thereby put into question. I also discuss the issue with Marie Claire, Françoise, Eva and other women, as well as with Alban. Because of the way people have reacted to me, I've been able to deepen the relationships that matter in my life and to drop the ones that don't. 'The envelope' – the surface of things – gets discarded as a result of the cruelty of some people, who think they know what's considered to be 'normal' or 'beautiful'. However, the experience can turn out to be a good one if and when you get to the heart of the matter, untie the knot and reveal the source of important meaning.

A bit later, on the plane

In Paris, I also speak with Alice. She misses her René: – poor man: he also died suddenly from cancer, which was discovered in his stomach too late; it'd already metastasised to his liver. He was a doctor, and worked in the nuclear sector, whereby he was exposed to radiation but was supposedly being 'closely monitored'. He was also in contact with asbestos, at Jussieu: one of many Parisian universities in which asbestos was discovered; a big scandal ensued because many people who worked at the uni were diagnosed as having cancer. Again, according to Alice, René was working 'under strict surveillance'. However, how can we know for sure that these so-called closely monitored conditions weren't dangerous after all? Alice also tells me that René liked his meat very well done on the charcoal grill, and that every morning he squeezed his own orange juice for breakfast. Orange peels are known to contain large amounts of pesticides that are linked to cancer. René didn't wash the oranges he squeezed. The pesticides probably got into the juice, even though he didn't eat the peelings. As for charred meat, their carcinogenic properties have been well documented.

Jane: My guess is that the nukes and asbestos got him before either the juice or the barbecue: what a job!

At present, Alice is doing research into women's cancers that are occurring in rural environments. She believes that many of the pesticides sprayed on fields can be directly linked to the spread of some cancers. She's applying for funding to finance the research she wants to conduct, in which she plans to use the vast amount of documentation she's compiled. So far, no one has come forward to finance her project; the reason being given is that it's a women's project as opposed to an environmental one. How disgusting!

Club Tahar Haddad, 24 March 1995

I'm in Tunis, at the Club Tahar Haddad, for the staging of *Wounding Words: A Woman's Journal in Tunisia* (Accad: 1996). More than 10 years have gone by since I wrote the text, during which I lived, cried and sang, and shared important moments of my life and of the other women's. I'm very moved to be back in this place, and to discover that these women, 'the daughters of the Club', 'the daughters of Tahar Haddad', as they call themselves, have experienced the text so deeply that they've decided to act it out on the stage. Iraj Zohari, an Iranian male theatre director who's living in exile in Germany, has done an excellent adaptation, interpretation and production. A lot of tension has been evident among the women during my past few visits, and I've been worried that some of the women would 'crack'. During the rehearsals I've attended, I noticed that Iraj tended to get upset and make hurtful remarks to the performers. Amel countered by making some remarks of her own, and soon everyone was unnerved and the tension continued to mount.

Jane: Wounding words, indeed!

On the plane between Rome and Beirut, 26 March 1995

What a pleasure it is to be with my dear Amel on this plane going to Beirut: she's wonderful, and so alive. She introduces me to her Italian family: Carla; Eric – her first love; Sandra; their parents and grandchildren; and Julio, Carla's son. Amel is so alive: she cries; she laughs; she lives! She moves me.

We're heading for Beirut, and my family members, who I'm anxious for Amel to meet. Mother is waiting for us. It's important for me that the two women meet. I'm touched when I think of this gift we're giving each other, these moments we're going to share. It's always very intense when I'm with Amel. The fact that she, along with Rachida, Renate, Hayat, Meriem, Iraj and the Club Tahar Haddad's director, Khadija Kamoun, have put together a dramatic adaptation of my novel *Blessures des mots: Journal de Tunisie* (Accad: 1993) is such a gift and an incredible revelation for me.

A couple of nights ago, when I'm sitting through the performance, I cry many times, especially when Amel recites some of the poems, during which she talks about her life, imprisonment, torture, hopes and dreams. I feel that the performance has a very strong impact; while I'm watching, I get goose pimples and shake all over. Also, when Hayat, Rachida, Renate and Meriem are reciting some of the lines, I can't believe I've written the same lines: they come out with so much strength and conviction. All the performers act very well.

Lately, I've been having a very bad backache and suffering from anguish. Today, however, I feel as if I've been delivered from both – and anyway, I feel deeply that I'm rid of cancer at present. However, I'm hurting for Alban; I hope that, in spite of his high PSA test, he'll be all right.

Amel has found us a wonderful little house located near

hers, in La Marsa: we're going to spend another of our honeymoons there! We're so fortunate she was able to find us this little paradise that overlooks the sea, has flowers and fruit trees in the garden, has furniture painted in the Tunisian style, and blue and white mosaic decorations.

Beirut, 31 March 1995

Amel and I arrive. At the airport, Amel cries, about having arrived in Beirut. Some passengers on the plane – a group of French people who'd come to visit Lebanon – look at her, and some of them express compassion for her in her suffering. They probably think, *Here's a Lebanese woman coming back home after years of absence, after the war!* Outside the airport, we find Faris, and he takes us to mother and Adelaide. Mother is in a wheelchair. Her meeting with Amel is very powerful and beautiful: two souls reach out to each other, join and communicate.

My back is still very sore. Yesterday, however, when Amel gives me a massage, the pain goes away, so I tell myself that if it were cancer, it wouldn't go away just like that. This morning, though, the pain is there again – perhaps the problem is the bed or the humidity.

Manicha: Backaches are said to come more from stress than from our modern way of life; this is why massages are helpful in untying muscle knots, and so on.

Wafa' has invited us over to celebrate Amel's birthday. She has a very beautiful place, in which she displays things that she and her husband, Andrew, have collected during their stays in many countries, such as India, Poland and Cyprus. I find that Wafa' is much more mature and poised than she was during my previous visit. She and Andrew have two adorable children, and for today's get-together, Wafa' has cooked a variety of delicious dishes. She's quite amazing: she's always so enthusiastic about life; she has a big appetite for living, which I've always admired; and she's somehow able to combine studying, raising children, inviting people around, cooking, collecting art objects, reading, writing and engaging in a thousand other activities.

Magda also arrives. She tells me a horrible story about a 23-year-old woman who died of a cancer that no one was able to do anything about – not even her father, who's a surgeon, an oncologist and a well-reputed cancer specialist. He felt completely hopeless as he watched his cherished daughter die! When I hear the story, I shiver. Amel thinks that people shouldn't be telling me these stories, but I'm glad I have them to include in this book and thereby let the world know of them. In this story, it's especially evident that doctors don't have all the answers, and that we have to be all the more vigilant about our health.

Magda tells me that our visit couldn't have happened at a better time in her life. She's reached a turning point, and she wants to change many things in her life. She says that Amel and I are an inspiration to her! When I talk to her, memories of my past, especially my adolescence, come flooding back, such as when we used to act in plays and operettas together. I used to be fascinated with her: her liveliness, her many flirtations, her openness and her free spirit. She was very different from the other Lebanese-Arab women who were around, perhaps because she came from such a cosmopolitan background: big families such as hers, of Italian or Greek origin – similar to Claire Gebeyli's – had had to leave Egypt when then president Nasser was nationalising everything. She used to inspire me. Now, the situation has become reversed – but I'm wondering how she could be inspired by my experience with illness; one day, I should ask her to explain.

Nazik and Mona are also present. They're among my

dearest friends in Beirut, and two of my top reasons for going back. This time, Mona seems fragile: she's had a second car accident, and I'm a bit worried about her. It's true that people drive crazily in Lebanon – as a motorist, you have to push, shove and act daringly, as if you're making your way through a crowd, whereby there are no rules other than the reaching of a consensus that the most daring driver has right of way. I'm surprised there aren't more accidents on the roads in Lebanon.

Manicha: Was it like that before the war?

It's always been like that – ever since the arrival of cars on the scene!

Yesterday evening, after I attend my reading–concert organised by Samir Khalaf at AUB – the American University in Beirut – Mona drives Amel and me to Claire Gebeyli's place, after which Claire takes us to a nice restaurant. This evening is very powerful, intense and beautiful, and includes women I admire very much and who belong to the chain of friends I have around the world who make my life so worthwhile. However, in the evening, I can't eat and drink as much any more.

Tonight, Amel and I sleep at my sister Adelaide's place, My brother Augustus is also here, staying in Beirut to be with mother. Amel and I can't fall asleep, and the next morning, I wake with a headache. I'd prefer to have only wine and cheese or salad with my friends, but how can I tell them that when eating and hospitality is so important a part of Lebanese conviviality, and I know they want to celebrate every moment, as well as my regained health, with us?

We've barely fallen asleep when we're woken again, this time by the phone ringing: Augustus's wife, Joy, is giving birth in Singapore. Augustus has been travelling, because he and Joy weren't expecting the baby to arrive before the end of April – but now their little boy is here, and they've named him Joël, after the biblical prophet.

Manicha: I understand that Augustus is an uncle of yours: why this lack of precision with reference to family links? One gets the impression that your appropriation of your family – 'my' brother, 'my' sister, 'my' cousin, 'my' … and so on – isn't one of your strengths, Evelyne! On the other hand, 'my friend' and 'my love' don't have the sense of this forced, congenital 'privatisation'! There: it's chosen, elected. Another comment: often, the names coming from all the corners of the globe, notably Arab and North American first names, aren't easily recognisable as feminine or masculine.

Madeleine: It seems to me that Augustus is one of Evelyne's brothers, not an uncle of hers.

The lack of precision was planned, and you've understood it well. As for the Arab or North American first names, they're easily recognisable for people who come from these countries or for the people who know the names … However, aren't we more and more becoming citizens of the world?

I like Mona Kouloub's attitude about her disease. She also had breast cancer and a mastectomy, about 10 years ago. She has a very positive attitude: she thinks there are worse diseases. Until she got breast cancer, she was in very good health. Her doctors removed her breast and gave her radiation, as well as radiation on her ovaries. I ask her whether a woman's libido ever comes back, because since my treatment, I've been feeling quite down in that area. She laughs and said it does, but gradually. She believes that if you're able to look beyond and to not dwell on the disease, you can feel very well later, be full of energy and engage in projects again. She reminds me of Caryl, my friend in Alabama, and

I'm glad to meet a woman such as her in Lebanon: someone who's willing to talk openly about her disease.

Jane: When I've read the 'medical' sections of your story, I always enjoy reading these sections about your recovery phases with your friends. I can feel you healing. However, I didn't realise that just when you were getting better, Alban's condition was threatening to worsen. What a tragic irony!

Cindy: I like these remarks when they connect with the main story and we're given ideas about the priority of friendship and its connection to healing.

A cancer cell, then, is made, not born. Cancer arises through a series of incremental changes to chromosomal DNA. Some of these DNA alterations can be inherited, but the vast majority are acquired during the lifetime of an individual when genes perfectly healthy at the time of conception become damaged. This process can happen through numerous pathways. Routine errors made during DNA replication are one. Sabotage by carcinogens is another. About 100,000 different genes are strung along our chromosomes. To contribute to cancer, at least some of these encounters between carcinogens and genes must involve the handful that help govern cell division. (Steingraber: 1997: 241)

Genes that are normally quiescent, for example, may become activated. Estrogen, in some cases, acts as a cancer promoter. As demonstrated in lab animals, so do many organochloride compounds. The good news is that these effects wane when such agents are removed from the body. (Steingraber: 1997: 243)

The trace presence of a cancer-promoting pesticide in drinking water, for example, may represent an absolute hazard to those whose breast, prostate, colon, or bladder tissue has already been initiated by some prior event (perhaps during childhood or because of occupation) or those rare few born with a mutated gene that predisposes them to cancer. Individuals whose genetic material has suffered less previous damage may more successfully ward off the effects of promoting agents – as would those lucky persons who happen to possess a set of metabolism genes that allows for especially efficient detoxification and excretion of promoting substances. (Steingraber: 1997: 244)

We are measuring more and more particulate matter and dust in the atmosphere; sulphur dioxide; nitrogen oxide; carbon monoxide, a killer at high concentrations; hydrocarbons; hydrogen sulphide; and ozone, which accumulates through pollution and becomes toxic in the lower atmosphere, even though it has a protective role when in the stratosphere, where it is becoming rarer; there is radioactive fall-out from bombs exploded in nuclear-testing programs, not to mention accidental fall-out such as was produced at Chernobyl on April 26th 1986, when, at 01h32 and 40 seconds, an explosion at that power station released iodine, strontium, cesium, plutonium – more than 50 million curies, or 200 times that of the bomb at Hiroshima. All of this has spread and can be measured over practically every breathe-able area, because at the end of the day, the atmosphere is nothing but a closed space around us, and a well-ventilated one, meaning that exchange is favored all over the planet.

It has been calculated that the equivalent of over 10 billion tons of coal are burnt annually, particularly by industries and motors of all kinds, not counting other chemical products that are even more unhealthy. Not all cities have the means to measure and analyze their atmosphere. It should be revealed that in 1996, not all cities had taken samples to measure which of the substances mentioned above are present, the reason being that they have yet to develop systematic programs to carry out these measurements. And yet air is the primary source of life, and our very existence depends on its quality. If this is the case, why are we ordering our economic priorities as if we didn't know this fundamental piece of information? Polluted air adds weight and even creates a cushion of contaminants above our heads that stifles everything below. The ocean absorbs these contaminants to saturation point, because we pollute faster than it can absorb. Antarctica, which occupies 20% of the world's ocean area, is absorbing two times less carbon dioxide than it used to, perhaps due to iron deficiencies, or to pollution, or to ultraviolet rays that prevent algae from growing. This cushion of unabsorbed gas tends to heat and to poison the surface below, and at some more sensitive places could lead to disturbances such as droughts, followed paradoxically by floods, and even tidal waves in some parts of the world. (Séralini: 1997: 52–3)

14

MY LOVE HAS CANCER
FACING UP

Treatment is administered by 'specialists' who, at best, know nothing of one another: the surgeon, the cobalt therapist, the chemotherapist. But does anyone imagine the anguish of the patient in this fragmented world, wondering whose speciality area is involved when this or that problem arises – that is, before he finally figures out that it's no one's area, because … no, no: there's no such thing, or, if this or that test has to be done, by whom, because each specialist believes, in good faith, that someone else is supposed to take care of it. Improvement must occur by way of a corps of generalists, not less specialized, as is the case at present, but better trained and capable of integrating overall patient care. This generalist will see to it that there is proper follow-up, giving the patient an anchoring point somewhere in the system, something that is impossible to achieve in the current situation. They will then realize that they are dealing with human beings, and some aberrations will no longer be enabled to occur. (Hyvrard: 1987: 192)

Beirut, 7 April 1995

I attend a meeting of Lebanese women who've had breast cancer: a meeting for women who wish to both help and be helped. I'm so glad to find that this type of group exists in Beirut, and that Lebanese women are speaking out poignantly and in ways that were previously unheard of.

At the meeting, one of the participants says, 'I have a great need to be loved, to be listened to. I have a metastasised breast cancer that I've been battling for three and a half years. Sometimes I get fed up and would like to die, but at other times I feel strong.' Another participant says, 'In Lebanon, the word 'cancer' is strongly taboo; consequently, patients need to speak, be reassured and be listened to. In Lebanon, there's a problem with telling the truth, and doctors don't tell their patients the truth. We Lebanese need to be in control, to speak, to listen, and to promote exchange of ideas and information among the sick and the healthy.' One of the people in charge says, 'We provide support. On Wednesdays we have an administrative meeting, and on Fridays we meet with patients. All of us are concerned about the problem of breast cancer.'

It was Dr Saadé who, acting on the request of one of his patients, started the group, a year and a half ago. The members call the group Faire Face: 'Facing Up'. They were inspired by the group Vivre Avec: 'Living with It', which is based in Lyon, in France.

The meeting leaves a tremendous impression on me: I never thought I'd see this type of group in Lebanon, and I'm very encouraged having participated in it. I know how important it was for me to be able to participate in a similar support group in the States when I was being treated. It helps a lot to be with other cancer patients – people who've gone through the same ordeal and who are able to express their anxiety and distress.

Bettina: When it comes to illness, we always think we're a special case, so when we encounter a similar case, we're better able to put things in perspective and find the strength we need in order to get better. Also, our guilt is reduced – when we get sick, we're torn between sensing injustice and feeling guilty.

The Beirut support-group meeting I attend is also a sad occasion, because, as we talk, one of the women, a co-founder of the group, is dying of cancer. The phone rings, and some of the people in charge have to leave to be with the poor soul.

Here in Beirut, I'm hearing a call, and feeling that people have an expectation of me – a need for my presence, for my work and my reflections about cancer; I therefore feel sad that I have to leave Lebanon. When I get back to Paris, I'll send the support group some books and information – the women are trying to set up a library of books about breast cancer and have very limited financial resources.

⧗

I have a strange dream, in which I'm in a hotel with Monique and Bruce, and Bruce is no longer interested in me because of my mutilation. I'm trying to reach Alban, and in doing so, I'm traversing a village by having to clamber over the roofs of houses that are all connected in a strange way. A bird comes into my hand and starts biting me. With a sharp, swift blow, I break its beak. Then I wake up.

When I attempt to analyse the dream, I note that the image of having my hand being bitten often recurs in my dreams – in one dream the offending animal is a dog, and in other dreams it's a bird. I interpret the biting animal to be the experience of chemo coming back: intravenous injection of poison in my hand, poison through which I'm supposed to be cured. In the dream, though, I don't accept the poison, and get rid of the offending animal every time. However, in this night's dream, the bird is also my desire to fly over the roofs to join Alban faster. I'm suffering inside my mutilated body, and being caused more pain because of people's reaction to my mutilation. Geographic obstacles are being placed between me and Alban, and I'm frustrated. My desire for freedom, symbolised by the bird, is more of a handicap than a help, so I break the bird's beak in order to get back my wings.

Cindy: I love these dream sequences and the analysis: they constitute the kind of poetic symbolism I relate to.

Manicha: How did Evelyne learn to decipher dreams – does it come from being a poet?

Perhaps! It's also like reading the 'grounds' in a coffee cup.

Madeleine: Elderly women in the Mediterranean regions, in North Africa especially, are real champions when it comes to interpreting dreams.

Rome, 8 April 1995

Amel and I are at Rome's airport, in transit on our way to Tunis. She's doing some duty-free shopping, and because I didn't have enough time to write when I was in Beirut, I'm now trying to remember a few notable events that occurred during my time in Lebanon. I'm always amazed at Amel's ability to adapt, to listen and to communicate – she's incredible.

⧗

I think about the trip that Amel and I make to the Ain Saadé mountain, with Théophile, Eloïse and Augustus, and about our kitchen dinner, for which we're joined by Cécile and Said. It's a very warm and relaxed atmosphere, thanks to

394

the love that Théophile and Eloïse express for each other and everyone else: a beautiful love that permeates their surroundings.

⌛

The next day, early in the morning, Théophile takes Amel and I to the south of the country. It's a luminous, glorious day, and we have a great time together. In Sidon, Théophile stops at a roadside restaurant so we can have some delicious *kanafi bjibin* – a special pastry filled with sweet cream-cheese and sprinkled with orange-blossom syrup; the restaurant is renowned for the delicacy. In Tyre, we have coffee, in a beautiful eatery located in the port.

While we're sitting at the eatery, I look at the men fishing. They're immobile, and no doubt thinking about their persecution by Israeli officials, who often forbid them to fish these waters, which are very close to Israel. I can feel the men's calm strength and their resistance to the persecution they endure every day. I associate the image of them with Théophile: his deep, Christ-like commitment to helping people, his charismatic message and his following in Christ's footsteps. It seems as if these fishers have always been here, since Christ's time.

At one moment, I feel sure that these men would've left everything to follow Christ if He'd appeared there in that instant. I feel Christ's presence – not from a faraway past, but as an immediate presence. Are these merely Orientalist images? Perhaps, but for me they reflect some unutterable reality. When our party has visited the ruins, we go to see the pastor of a church that's also remained as it was in Christ's time; Théophile often goes there on Sundays to preach, and my father used to preach there as well. The church has benches that have a rugged texture, like the wood of the Cross, and I feel that their being is inhabited by the Spirit. When Théophile preaches there, both Christians and Muslims, and even the members of so-called fanatical groups, come to listen to him. Today, the church's pastor – who according to Amel looks like the famous Arab singer Farid El-Atrash – gives Amel some candles, a gesture through which she's moved to tears.

Manicha: Why should you have to apologise for using an 'image' such as Christ and the fishers? These strong visions remain a reality!

Because ever since publication of Edward Saïd's book *Orientalism* (Said: 1979), it's been impossible to view these images uncriticically.

⧖

In the evening, back in Ain Saadé, Amel shows a film entitled Tanitez-moi, in which she's acting. Yves, one of Théophile's sons, who's in the film industry, likes it a lot. It's about the connection that exists between Carthage – present-day Tunisia – and Phoenicia – present-day Lebanon – through the countries' famous women, who are often political leaders.

⧖

The next day, we go to Théophile's church, in which he and I sing as we used to when we were adolescents and sang for an evangelist radio program that came out of Addis Ababa. Amel cries. It's very moving to see all the young people in Théophile's church singing, praising and connecting harmoniously through their faith. Many of them have been saved from the war's violence, or from drugs and death, and are on the road to physical and spiritual recovery. When we get home from the church, we have a delicious couscous that Amel has prepared. It's a beautiful weekend.

⧗

My back still hurts. I talk to Nabil Tawil, Augustus's famous cardiologist friend, who comes to see Augustus and to examine mother. He tells me to go to his hospital, located in Jbeil, at which he'll have my back X-rayed.

Because Amel and I have decided to go to Byblos, I go to the hospital while she's visiting the ruins. Fortunately, nothing troublesome is revealed in the X-rays. Dr Tawil is very friendly, and refuses to talk about fees. He tells me he was worried because the spot I showed him is sometimes the site of cancer metastasis. I feel reassured: even though everyone around me was saying they were sure it was nothing, and were praying for me, I had to have the 'scientific' confirmation from the doctor.

⧗

We also go on a beautiful trip to the Chouf, the Druze Lebanese mountains, with Mona. The mountains have remained wild and breathtaking. The area's roads and villages are clean and esthetically harmonious, and stand in stark contrast with other Lebanese spots that have been constructed with profit-making motives in mind rather than as the result of architectural ideas and lines that would be in tune with the landscape. We visit Afaf, one of Mona's great-cousins, in Ba'kline, the village of Mona's childhood. Afaf makes a great impression on us: she reminds me of Mona because she exudes the same serenity and harmony. We visit the palace of Beit Eddine, and eat in the village of Dar El Kamar – a gorgeous place, like the full moon to which it owes its name. It's an unforgettable visit.

Manicha: Your description reminds me of the orientation of the Iranian filmmaker Abbas Kiarostami, who's made films about the wisdom of peasants.

La Marsa, 17 April 1995

It's wonderful to be with my love in this house in La Marsa, across from Amel's.

I've just been reading two books about cancer: Léon Renard's *Le cancer apprivoisé: Cancer Tamed* (Renard: 1990) and David Watson's *Fear No Evil: A Personal Struggle with Cancer* (Watson: 1984). I find the latter title, a present from Juliana and Martin, depressing because it ends with the death of the person who's been suffering from cancer: a preacher for whom many people have been praying but whose cancer has already metastasised to his liver. People who haven't gone through cancer wouldn't understand that this is precisely the kind of book that someone who's just gone through the experience finds very difficult to read. Books that have a happy ending are what we feel like reading.

In the other book, *Cancer Tamed*, Renard relates some very interesting and important facts about what you can do to either avoid getting cancer or help cure it. However, I get annoyed with him because he emphasises personal effort and doesn't broaden the book's scope to include the political dimension. It's as if human beings were creating their own cancers and, if they really wanted to, could heal through their own efforts. The book does contain issues that are worth considering, though, such as how important it is to know and understand what it is inside yourself that's provoked the cancer: your unresolved past conflicts. It's important to understand these conflicts in order to bring them to closure.

Cindy: This idea is similar to what Deena Metzger says on her two cassette tapes *This Body: My Life 1* and *This Body: My Life 2* (Metzger: 1992), about the practice of creativity and healing.

But Deena Metzger says it in such a convincing way!

20 April 1995

Amel, Alban and I go to see Amel's doctor, Dr Hassen, the surgeon and oncologist who impressed me very much when I went to see him because I was feeling anguished that the Beirut doctor, Dr ES, had told me I should do another six months' worth of chemotherapy. Hassen says I have to watch the other breast carefully by having ultra-sound scans and annual mammograms in order to make sure everything's all right, because the kind of cancer I've had – lobular – often bilaterises.

He finds that Alban has a high PSA: the indicator that marks the likelihood that cancerous cells are present in the prostate. In 1992 and '93, Alban's PSA was 13; now, in 1995, it's moved up to 59. However, it shouldn't be more than 3. Hassen says that good treatments are available for prostate cancer, and that it's possible for the patient to be completely cured. He tells us he favours the method of injecting an anti-testosterone preparation in the stomach once a month over either surgery or radiation, which can have undesirable secondary effects. If the patient has the injections, the secondary effects are reversible once the cancerous cells have been gotten under control, and the treatment can then be terminated.

When the doctor starts talking about expediting a chemically induced castration as opposed to a surgical one, and says that Alban should also have a bone scan, pelvic ultrasound scans and a total medical check-up, I go into shock. The drug he mentions, which I'll call XTN, is what father was given at the end of his life. I can't believe we have to go through another ordeal. I know we all have our share of sorrows in life, but why Alban and I, and why now? We were so happy, and had such a fantastic sexual-love life. We were totally fulfilled and in harmony with each other.

If I were in Adelaide's kind of world, I'd think we had to be punished because we were too happy in leading a 'sinful life'. Alternatively, if I believed in the 'evil eye', I'd think someone had cast a spell on us because our happiness was flagrantly scandalous. However, I'm searching for the causes for this disease, this plague of our century, and I can't help but wonder why one of Alban's doctors, the endocrinologist, gave him testosterone when his PSA was already 13. Had he read Alban's medical records? Why wasn't he careful? The fact that Alban was prescribed testosterone is repetitious of my being prescribed estrogen. Both of us were prescribed a hormone to aid our bones despite the fact that other methods were available for dealing with osteoporosis. And I'm sure we aren't the 'exceptions to the rule': how many other people are contracting cancer without knowing it's caused by the drugs their doctor is prescribing them? Why aren't people forming groups around these issues, in order to take political action, and to change the practice of drug prescription indulged in by careless doctors and profit-making pharmaceutical companies?

Manicha: In France, we're still too respectful of – and dependant on – the powerful players who govern our lives: doctors, lawyers, architects and, of course, politicians! But it's changing!

Fortunately, Alban and I are able to talk about all this: we're so much in love. Through this trial, our love is being reinforced, and, if possible, being made even stronger.

Tunis, 21 April 1995

Amel, Alban and I go to a conference organised by a group called Communication and Personal Development. There, we meet Lucienne, who belongs to a communication institute in France through which support groups are organised for cancer patients. It's as a patient that Lucienne has experienced the group, and as a patient that, tonight, she gives her testimonial.

In 1992, Lucienne was striving to make a successful career in filmmaking. She was diagnosed as having advanced ovarian cancer. Her sister had died earlier of the same disease, whereby Lucienne was left quite alone. When she received the news of her own diagnosis, she decided the disease wasn't going to take her life as it had her sister's. She told herself that if it was perhaps the case that she got cancer as a result of how she'd behaved, she could perhaps change the state of her disease if she changed her behaviour. She attended a visualisation workshop. From the day she started doing visualisation, her whole chemotherapy changed and her entire attitude became more positive. She was cured.

She tells us about a man named Simonton, who discovered how mental attitudes and emotions can command the immune system, and who developed a method based on the discovery – a method through which she was given a great deal of hope. If the brain can communicate with the immune system, it's a matter of changing your belief in the treatment you're having: to get your body to better accept the treatment in question. To be able to practise visualisation, you have to be relaxed and find a scenario you can adapt to your own case. The idea is that you imagine that the chemo isn't poison but rather a positive substance that will help your body fight the bad cells. In Simonton's view, when you make this adjustment in your attitude to the treatment, your body is able to heal.

Lucienne also believes it's important to visualise life a few years down the track. When people get sick, they're receiving a message that they haven't been listening to their body, and that they must learn to understand their primary and secondary body messages. She admits that before she became ill, she could never have spoken in front of 30 people as she spoke tonight; she overcame her shyness because she wanted to help other people. She warns us not to remain in the realm of *le non-dit*: 'the unspoken', because keeping things to ourselves too much can have a bad effect on our body. If we accept that negative thoughts breed negative reactions, we must learn to unwind and speak out. Lucienne assures us that many methods are now available for achieving serenity.

After Lucienne gives her talk, the group members have a discussion. A Tunisian doctor speaks out as follows. 'Most illness is influenced by the thought process. Stress is a big factor in many diseases, of which cancer is but one. Doctors should be trained in this area; social workers aren't doing anything about improving the situation, so doctors should take the lead.'

Lucienne talks about these transformative techniques. If we wish to undergo the process, we must first understand which events have weighed most heavily in our past life, and what the events' impact has been over the years. When we have an outburst of anger, we should seek what it was that provoked the anger. The technique involves writing down the event and analysing all the thoughts that have sprung up out of the anger associated with it. We then ask ourselves the question 'Are these thoughts good or bad for me?' It should become apparent that one thought is masking another. This leads us to reformulate the thoughts and to sort out the positive thoughts from the truly healthy ones.

Lucienne says that unlike in the States, support groups

don't exist in France. She tells us that most of the techniques she's talking about were formulated by Americans.

With reference to cancer, the warning signals to watch for are symptoms such as a chronically sore throat and a stomach ache. Cancer-connected stress cancer manifests two years before the cancer actually develops and is detected, and cancer that develops in this way is often associated with the death of a loved one.

I raise the question of the relationship between cancer, hormones and the environment. Another Tunisian doctor, Dr Chtou, who practises alternative medicine, speaks up. He says the body should be left to age naturally, and that in general, the human body produces enough estrogen on its own. Decalcification occurs in both men and women, so he wonders why hormones are prescribed for women only.

Cindy: They aren't, as you've already shown, in Alban's case.

Yes, but for men, they aren't prescribed systematically.

Jane: Perhaps Dr Chtou doesn't recognise the studies in which it's been shown that although both males and females go through decalcification, women lose proportionately more bone mass: how else could you account for the preponderance of fractures and deformations among women, unless it's simply because women tend to outlive men and are therefore more subject to the forces of degeneration for a longer time?

Madeleine: When it comes to bone decalcification in women, perhaps we should also take childbearing into account. It's a simple equation: to give something, you have to take something away from somewhere else. For nine months, women create another being out of their own substance; this supreme creation is something that some men have never been able to accept.

Bettina: At menopause, specific hormones that protect women from undergoing decalcification are no longer secreted, whereas for men this isn't the case.

Tonight, as Dr Chtou is speaking, a woman in the audience almost cuts him off, saying that hormones aren't the issue being discussed at the conference. In fact, both Alban and I find the conference disappointing, and Alban articulates what we've both realised: that the meeting has been nothing more than an outright return to the auto-suggestion method. We believe that since Coué, a lot more has happened, and even if people are sceptical about Palo Alto, they should know that other reflections exist. I ponder over the fact that tonight, we've remained squarely in the 'blame the victim' corner. In that corner, everything is brought back to the individual, who must take charge of himself or herself, even though we know that the responsibility lies with our stress-laden society and our polluted environment.

25 April 1995

We have to go before a censorship committee in order to obtain a permit to stage *The Daughters of Tahar Haddad*, an adaptation of my novel *Wounding Words: A Woman's Journal in Tunisia* (Accad: 1996), for a theatre located in the middle of the Medina of Tunis. The committee is somewhat comically named The Communication and Information Committee – a title through which no one is fooled as to the committee's real purpose. I'm reminded of the name given to a branch of the American Cultural Center in Tunis and other countries: the centre is also called The Communication and Information Center, and various people in the countries often ironically refer to it as the CIA.

While I'm here in Tunis, I'm acting in the play. I introduce the women and voice my reasons for writing the novel, and at the beginning we all sing together. I also sing during each set change, and at the end, we all gather again on the stage to sing and dance. Today, we perform the play just for the censorship committee. No one else is allowed into the theatre, except one or two friends who help us do the lights and make-up.

Alban is also here, encouraging us. It's a surrealistic experience. The committee, which comprises seven middle-aged men, sits in the front row. The men sit stiffly until the middle of the play, even though some of the acting takes place behind their back, throughout the room, where the women recite some of the poems or I sing. However, towards the middle of the show, the committee men start to loosen up a bit. They turn their heads to see the performers around them, and begin to laugh and clap. They're now like fathers watching their daughters performing, and they're showing tender, fatherly compassion. At the end, they rise together as one, and clap. We can hardly believe we're seeing this response, especially because the play is so strongly feminist, and features women voicing their revolt against their environment and oppressive conditions. We wonder whether the committee men are simply being polite and will later forbid the play to be staged once we're no longer in front of them and they're supposed to give us the go-ahead. But no: after several weeks, we do get our permission, and one of the men even comes to one of the performances – as promised, with his daughter!

However, tonight, I'm very tense and don't sleep well. We've spoken about cancer with Alban. I dream I'm having to warn people about the dangers of environment-related cancer but that no one is wanting to listen. I'm having to climb on to a table and to scream very hard in order to attract their attention. I'm unable to express everything I want to. When I get down, I have to look at my mail. I remember there's a box I haven't opened for a long time. It contains lots of messages written on red pieces of paper: messages of support for the cancer victim – Alban in particular. The dream reflects my anxiety about Alban's cancer, the censorship committee, how the committee would react to the play and what decision it would take, a conference I have to give tomorrow, and all the mail that'll be awaiting me when I return from my trip. In previous dreams, the box has signified traumatic experiences I must work through and resolve, whereby lots of red, urgent messages are waiting to be addressed by me.

I must listen to my body's signals without losing my perspective on the political action that must accompany my personal therapy, even when people are unwilling to listen to me.

Dioxin is known to depress immunity, an outcome that may promote a variety of cancers. Sometimes it is associated with cancers that originate in the immune system, such as lymphoma. Dioxin also influences thyroid functioning, blood glucose levels, sexual development, and testosterone production. In rats, it interacts synergistically with PCBs to alter certain liver functions, and in monkeys it has been linked to the painful uterine disorder endometriosis. (Steingraber: 1997: 229)

Our bodies are living scrolls of sorts. What is written there – inside the fibers of our cells and chromosomes – is a record of our exposure to environmental contaminants. Like the rings of trees, our tissues are historical documents that can be read by those who know how to decipher the code. (Steingraber: 1997: 236)

Sampling urine, researchers have estimated that the bodies of most members of the US population contain detectable levels of the insecticide chlorpyrifos, a common ingredient in pet flea collars, lawn and garden pest control products, indoor foggers, and roach, ant, and wasp poisons ... In a 1996 study conducted in Mexico, researchers found that levels of DDT in living human tissues varied predictably across geographic space: residue levels in both abdominal fat and breast fat were highest in areas of intense agriculture and in tropical regions where DDT was used for malaria control. (Steingraber: 1997: 237)

During pregnancy, the placenta and other maternal defenses do not provide enough protection for future babies, who act like veritable sponges when it comes to carcinogens and environmental toxins, and they build their tissues with these pollutants. This should be enough to give pause to even the most cynical, and to pity those little toddlers who, for want of more conscientious adults, are being given this blemished world, with the promise of a future full of misery and illness, unless we do something to raise our standards. (Séralini: 1997: 170)

15

MALE HORMONES
LIBERTÉ, ÉGALITÉ, FRATERNITÉ!

With plastic surgery, i.e. breast implants, it is surprising to realize that the medical establishment does not consider amputation of breasts as a problem, ostensibly because they are now able to reconstruct them ... with silicone! It would be generous to suspect that this attitude should come as some relief to the mastectomized subject. What it really means, though, is that medicine has lost its mind. Technically super-powered, it has lost all sense of perspective, of life. Because there is a difference between human flesh and silicone that seems to have escaped the medical experts: the reconstituted breast (that's the official term for it) can no longer feel anything. (Hyvrard: 1987: 169)

It's clear that a woman who comes down with breast or uterine cancer has something to say about the condition of women. Does removal of her female organs resolve the problem? There is reason to doubt it. A few social reforms through which women would be enabled to live their life would be much more appropriate. When are we going to amputate the daily horror of sexism? (Hyvrard: 1987: 170)

On the plane between Tunis and Paris, 1 May 1995

Alban and I have just left these marvellous friends: Amel, Renate, Khalil, Meriem, Hayet and Rachida, and are on a plane in which most of the passengers are French, cold and distant. Some of the conversations we're hearing are racist and superficial. I'm having a hard time hearing such empty remarks, and leaving Tunisia and my dear friends. I'm crying about being separated from the warmth of a world I cherish and from friends I love dearly. I'm concerned about Alban's health, and hoping with all my heart we'll find the right treatment through which he'll be quickly healed. The way he's able to empathise with me is simply incredible: I love him so much.

I'm looking forward to going back to Tunis to perform in the play, if we get the authorisation we require from the censorship committee. I never would've imagined that people would be inspired to write a play such as that because they'd read my novel. I'm drying my tears: there's hope at the end of the road, I know.

Paris, 5 May 1995

Since I've been back in Paris, I've wanted to write but I haven't been feeling well enough to. I've had a headache, and been feeling nauseous and dizzy; the symptoms are partly physical and partly psychological. I've received the news about my dear Zohreh's ovarian cancer. I couldn't believe it, and on the night she was supposed to receive her chemo, I was sick, and remained sick for a total of 24 hours. I couldn't sleep a wink, thinking about her.

Alban and I have made all kinds of appointments with doctors for him, and are hoping that a workable healing program will result from their concerted efforts.

When I return to my apartment, I find several letters waiting for me. I include an extract from two of them as follows.

Caryl: ... *I liked your indignation in the face of silence. You've spoken out, and your words will contribute to the changes that must come. We must learn to talk back to our doctors; to refuse their treatments; to ask them questions every time they prescribe drugs to us. Your voice is so strong, Evelyne, and you enable me, as an American, to feel solidarity with the mutilated of this world ...*

Gilles: *... You speak to me about the death of this friend, and, what is even darker, of the 'decline' – your word – of your mother. We know, don't we, that death is in life? However, we don't even feel resigned to the realisation. On the other hand, it seems to me, and from your letter, that you're feeling better, and, in a word, that you're healed. It's very possible that the 'stress' you're talking about played a part in your illness – try not to replace it with another one ... My heart is with you.*

Jane: I heard a program the other day, on WILL Radio: an entomologist from the University of Illinois speaking about a not so distant time when they used DDT to eradicate everything that moved. He said that at one point, they almost closed the department of entomology because DDT had been so effective there were no more insects! In those days, insects were the number-one enemy of the large-scale farms. The university had created that department essentially to find ways to eradicate insects in order to increase agricultural productivity. At least this is what they thought they'd do, before they discovered the various mutating species that'd slowly become resistant to DDT. What's scary is that at the time, they didn't think at all about the effect on the environment, and on other species, including human beings. And this professor was admitting very openly to this blindness, this great scientific pride: to have wiped out the kingdom of insects! This is what you're paying for today: this blind scientific pride. Today, he said, they eliminate those pests by making them sterile.

Not very reassuring either, in my opinion. The green weapon hasn't finished causing disasters!

Cindy: And what about birds that depend on 'those pests' for their food?

6 May 1995

Two days ago, I wake in the middle of the night to hear mother calling me: 'Evelyne! Evelyne!' I rise suddenly from my bed to discover I've been dreaming. Today, Adelaide phones to let me know that mother isn't at all well. Mother has a lump in her stomach, and although it might be only a hernia, she'd be ill-advised to have surgery because of her age and physical condition. Mother feels she's slipping away, and wants to talk to me. When I have her on the phone, she says, 'I'm leaving to be with Jesus; if I've waited for so long, it's because I wanted to make sure everything was all right with you. You know you chose the best for your life –'

But then the line is cut. What did she mean by those words? I feel she's giving me her approval for the life I've chosen. Later, when I'm able to phone back, Adelaide tells that mother is feeling better, and has told her she wants me and Théophile to sing at her funeral the hymn that father and she liked so much. I quote the hymn as follows.

> *Simply confide in Him*
> *And you will see He will fulfil His promises.*
> *In the train of His triumph and of His grace,*
> *He leads all His children victoriously,*
> *So simply confide in Him ...*

⧖

Leslie and Ruth come for lunch. Leslie has two friends who have breast cancer, and they're only 45 and 38! One of them, Marguerite, has told Leslie that her sex life has been completely obliterated as a result of the treatment, whereas before she'd been very active sexually. Now, her vagina is so narrow from the chemo that any penetration is painful if not impossible. She'll have to be operated on to enable her partner to penetrate her again. Her doctors haven't succeeded in making her vagina smooth and elastic, as it was before, by applying other treatments. No one warned Marguerite that the chemo could have these effects. *Just like me*, I think: no one warned me that penetrative sex would become painful, and that the only pleasures I'd be able to continue enjoying would be clitoral orgasm and erogenous caresses.

Manicha: Would you have refused the treatment if you'd known the consequences?

Good question: I intend to address it in the epilogue to this book. I'd perhaps have refused the treatment after I'd read several books and studies that I later got a hold of. In those texts, it's revealed that the breast-cancer mortality rate hasn't changed as a result of chemo and radiation, and it's suggested that when a cancer is aggressive, nothing can be done – see *Dr Susan Love's Hormone Book* (Love: 1997) and other books and articles I've listed in the References at the end of this book. Above all, I feel that if I'd read Susun Weed's book *Breast Cancer? Breast Health! The Wise Woman Way* (Weed: 1996), which unfortunately was published only last year *[1997]*, I'd probably have tried her plant recipes before I had chemo and radiation. I say 'perhaps' and 'probably' because when people are hit with a disease such as cancer, and have no previous experience of it, the shock can be so great that they prefer to trust the medical establishment – which, remember, they most probably have never had to confront – in order to understand the disease's mechanism.

9 May 1995

I've just finished reading Penelope Williams's *That Other Place: A Personal Account of Breast Cancer* (Williams: 1993).

Williams says some very interesting things, and I identify with many of her remarks, such as about the contradictions contained in the various treatments, risks, survival rates and so on. I include an extract from her book (Williams: 1993: 40–1) as follows.

Risk factors, like survival rates, are another area of conflicting information. What causes breast cancer to strike one woman and not the next? Again, depending on the book you read, the documentary you watch, the doctor you listen to, these factors range from too much repressed emotion to not enough carrots ... The biggest risk of all is just being a woman ... The final answer is that no one really knows where or why cancer strikes. The one positive aspect of this lottery is that you can't blame yourself when you win ... i.e. lose. Another area of confusion: success rates of treatment. Some studies suggest that treatment of breast cancer is more successful than it was 10 years ago. Others state that although the percentage of breast cancer survivors is the same as 10 years ago, the treatment is more successful because there are more people with breast cancer these days. This kind of analysis makes me crazy. Are we talking good news or bad news here? Hard to say.

Like Penelope Williams, I go crazy when I encounter this reasoning, and when I read the so-called scientific books and articles about the subject, I find no logic – but who ever said that science was logical?

When Williams is writing about how important your attitude is in being healed of the disease, I couldn't agree with her more. I again quote from her book (Williams: 1993: 186).

One must have tremendous courage to face the unvarnished truth of cancer. It is not another disease. It will only become so, as did tuberculosis, as did the plague, when a cure is found for it. Or better to say, a cure for them, since there are hundreds of different kinds of cancer. Then we can pack up our myths and imagery, then we can shake our heads in rueful amusement at the silliness of our attempts to deal with the disease. But not yet. Keep your arsenal well stocked; use whatever works, or whatever feels as if it is working. And when breast cancer is brought to its knees by a new antibiotic, a new genetic attitude or a mutant extract of seaweed, then we can throw away our metaphors or transfer them to the new disease waiting in the wings to scourge our world anew.

⧗

Today, I go to see Dr Marty at Hôpital Saint-Louis, to find out the possibilities for having a reconstruction. Dr Marty thinks I don't have enough extra flab in my stomach for her to be able to use it to make another breast. Also, because I haven't had children, my belly skin isn't stretched enough. She favours an implant made of either silicone or serum, the latter which is a salted liquid, much like the natural liquid we have in our body.

I tell her that in the States, I was advised to have the stomach flap instead of the artificial implant because my skin has been made less elastic as a result of the radiation, and because it'd thereby be more difficult for the reconstructionist to create a pocket under the skin in order to hold an implant in. She doesn't agree, and thinks my skin is supple enough to be stretched out. She says she'd have to also operate on the other breast to make it a bit smaller so it matched the other one. I'd have to stay in hospital for 10 days and pay a daily rate of 4500 francs, all expenses included – about $US900.

After three months, I'd go back into hospital for three or four days in order to have a nipple reconstruction. The first operation lasts for between two and three hours, and I'd have a general anesthetic; then, I'd have 15 to 20 days of convalescence. As is the case with any operation, the two main risks involved are hemorrhaging and contraction of infection. Dr Marty doesn't at all favour the 'flap trap' for me. I remember that in the hospital in the States, I had a stay of fewer than 32 hours for my mastectomy, a more serious operation, and now realise that here in France, breast-cancer patients are kept in for about a week for a similar operation and for 10 days for their breast reconstruction – and that the cost is about a third of what it is in the States.

Dr Marty is a young doctor who has a pleasant personality. She talks about all this as if it were the most natural process in the world. Alban and I find the century we're living in to be astonishing in terms of manipulation of the body via hormones and the scalpel. I wonder whether I'll ever decide to undergo this reconstruction of my lost breast.

Paris, 10 May 1995

I feel completely depressed about the prosthesis I've just bought: compared with the one I got in the States, it's just as heavy – perhaps heavier because it's larger; just as cumbersome; exorbitantly priced; and, with its little flowers and all, insultingly packaged.

Madeleine: Mightn't it simply be an awkward way to soften something painful? 'Say it with flowers,' is part of our day-to-day way of dealing with things.

Bettina: But those prostheses really are much too heavy.

It's all about making money out of people's misfortune. I'd hoped they were making lighter, less expensive and more esthetic ones in France; however, this isn't the case, except that the price is about a third less, and the pocketed bras you can get with them are more attractive – all in lace – and fit me better.

Jane: Typically French: sexy, even in misery! Good on them, I say!

Madeleine: Often, when we women wear clothing and underwear that are refined and delicate, we feel better about ourselves, much more than we would if we 'let ourselves go' or dressed in dull, shapeless things – especially those of us who've become disgusted with our own body.

⧗

Today, to add to my depressed state, I have a bad experience at the bank. I go to sign the papers to get a loan in order to purchase additional rooms for my Paris apartment. The papers include questions about my health; whether I've had a serious operation over the past few years; and whether I've received chemotherapy and radiation. In my usual honest, frank and naive way, I answer yes to all the questions. No sooner have I left the bank than I realise how stupid I've been, and when I talk to French people – from my friends and acquaintances to my neighbours – they reinforce my uneasiness, and tell me I shouldn't have answered such personal questions that no one has the right to ask.

I feel completely demoralised. I remember Kathleen's friend who was refused a loan because of her cancer, and think I'll probably be denied one as well. I feel I'm caught in a completely unfair situation: I want to acknowledge my cancer; let people know I've been hit with this plague of our century; warn them about the dangers; and not hide my condition; however, if I do, I risk being ostracised and penalised. It's this civilisation that gives you cancer and then penalises you for having done so. I don't want to lie: I want to be honest and frank in my life. However, I'm finding it very difficult to maintain my high ideals in this world that has neither light nor vision; that's withdrawn into itself; and that has a selfishness eating it, like a cancer.

Paris, 12 May 1995

I'm at Villejuif, at the Institut Gustave Roussy, with Alban, to see Dr LS, who was recommended by Dr Hassen in Tunis. I never thought we'd have to come back here for my sweet Alban. Two years ago, cancer was a faraway disease that hit only other people. Since we've been confronted with father's cancer, mine, my friends' and now Alban's, I feel I've been plunged into the disease, and that I'm surrounded by all kinds of cancers that are continuing to hit people who are very dear to me – sometimes the dearest, most beloved people in my life. Is it chance? I don't think so. I truly believe we're living in a time in which cancer will go on increasing. It could be said that the disease has become almost commonplace if each and every case of it weren't so devastating.

Manicha: It's about time we asked why and how we can face it all together.

Having had my experience at the bank, I'm extremely depressed. I sleep very poorly: I think about what I can do if I don't get the loan, but can think of no other option. In the morning, I go back to the bank and ask whether I can alter the statement I made yesterday. The officer tells me I can because they haven't yet sent the papers for approval. *Good*, I think, and change my declaration. The officer tells me the previous one has been cancelled and that they'll send this one for approval. After I've done this, I feel lighter. I can't help but think I'd never have been able to do the same in the States: there, no bank or insurance company would've allowed me to retract a statement through which I felt that my rights and freedom were being jeopardised. France is really the country that I love to live in, and that I feel is the best for many reasons, not the least of which is the fact that the spirit of freedom is kept alive there and thrives in all areas of life.

Bettina: I find that summation surprising!

Jane: I don't think many Americans who know France and the French would agree with you: most think that the French are bureaucratic maniacs; however, perhaps they're unaware of the advantages of France's welfare system. Your comments about being able to retract the statement you made to the bank is also pertinent here. In a sense, the bank officer who allowed you to do it is showing solidarity with you in making it possible for you to beat the very bureaucracy he or she is working for, that is, the bank. In the States, a clerk would be more likely to start giving you morality lessons about telling lies or cheating the system, no matter how immoral it is to deny someone a loan on the grounds that he or she might be seriously ill and could at some point become unable to repay the loan.

14 May 1995

I've been dreaming a lot about the treatment that Alban will have to have: I'm sure my subconscious is busy dealing with my worries. In one dream, a nurse is telling me, 'I believe the best thing would be to give him an injection to stop the process immediately.' I tell her I agree. As for Alban, in the dream, it seems he's accepting anything that might happen along the way. When he has to have the injection, he's placed on a bed that's being lifted up by a machine attached to the ceiling; this, in fact, is radiation being administered to his feet. The doctors don't make me leave the room, and I say to Alban, 'It isn't like in the States, where they used to make you leave the room when I was about to receive the radiation,' to which Alban replies, 'It's France: here, everyone must suffer along with everyone else!'

Jane: *Liberté! Egalité! Fraternité!*

It's a funny dream, in which my anxieties about Alban and what he must choose are revealed. 'My dear, sweet, wonderful love' – from the Jacques Brel song: *'Mon doux, mon tendre, mon merveilleux amour'* – who can crack a joke even in my dreams. Why do we have to go through so much suffering this year? The dream also reflects my experience at the bank and the loan I've applied for.

⧗

At the Institut Gustave Roussy, Dr LS reads Alban's medical records very thoroughly. In 1992 and 1993, Alban's PSA was already 13: too high, because the normal reading is 3; by 1995, it'd climbed to 59! The cancer seems to be a localised one, but we can be sure only if Alban has a total check-up, including a bone scan, an abdominal scan and an ecography. According to the pathology report from the biopsies, Alban has a 'Gleason' of 7, which is quite high, because this indicator is the one through which the potential for cellular evolution is supposed to be revealed, although these results are inconclusive. In the report, hormonally sensitive cells are also indicated: a positive sign for Alban to take the hormone-therapy option. Dr LS tells us he's against local surgery, because bad side effects can result from it; like Dr Hassen, he's for hormonotherapy.

16 May 1995

Today, Alban and I go to Hôpital Bichat in order to have him undergo a bone scan. I get very scared, because at one point, both the technicians and Dr SP, who analyses the tests, ask that one image be redone: the image of Alban's back – his weak spot, on which he often gets pain. Accompanying him and watching the process, I think I've seen two tumours on the image: two phosphorescent, larger dots. I fear the worst.

We wait for Dr SP to talk with us – luckily, here in France, a doctor always comes and talks with you right after you've had the tests, in order to give you a first assessment; then, the results are sent to other doctors for a second or third reading, and confirmation of the first one. Fortunately, Dr SP tells us that the troublesome-looking dots are micro-calcifications and osteoarthritis. It isn't a wonderful diagnosis, but compared with the prospect of their being cancer, it's a thousand times more favourable. I feel like throwing my arms around Dr SP for joy, to thank him; instead, I throw them around my sweet Alban when we're leaving the hospital. Maybe I'm too sensitive and I feel everything too strongly – but I can't imagine my life without Alban.

We've had too many misfortunes this year: first, my cancer, and then Alban's, and we've had to deal with father's death from the disease. I'm sure I'm overly anxious, my nerves are on edge and I'm having unpredictable mood swings because all the trauma from these events is working in my subconscious. My sweet Alban soothes and reassures me. How does he manage to remain so serene in the midst of his discovering he has cancer and that he'll have to undergo an unpredictable treatment for this intractable disease? We talk, analyse all we're going through, laugh and joke, and, in the middle of our misery, manage to make love.

In my mail, I receive the *ARC – Research into Cancer –* journal. The statistics it contains are frightening. One in three French people will develop one form or another of cancer in his or her lifetime – as they will in the States – and the numbers are continuing to rise. One in 10 women will contract breast cancer – the figure is greater in the States.

Each year, 25,000 new cases of breast cancer are diagnosed, and about 9000 people die from the disease – the proportion of deaths is higher than it is in the States, a fact I ponder over. The death toll from lung cancer, which can easily be controlled, remains high. Each year in France, tobacco-related illness is the cause of 60,000 deaths, is responsible for the premature death of one in two smokers, and is responsible for their losing about 20 years off their life.

23 May 1995

Yesterday, we see Dr NM at Hôpital Bichat. Fortunately, Alban's tumour has been caught in time, and there's no metastasis. He'll have to have 'only' *hormonotherapy*. Like the other doctors we've seen, Dr NM is against surgery; he says that given Alban's age, it wouldn't be reasonable to subject him to it. The risks involved in surgery would be that Alban would suffer from incontinence and be irreversibly impotent. The doctor says that although radiotherapy on the prostate can be effective, it's very tiring. It can have serious side effects on the patient's bladder, and the disease isn't always cured as a result.

Dr NM is also for a hormonal treatment for Alban. He explains that too many male hormones are stimulating Alban's prostate. The treatment, by way of injection of a drug, would be administered in Alban's stomach every two months, to slow down the production of testosterone. The treatment's disadvantage and downside would be that Alban would have problems achieving erection; however, the doctor says that the erectile function can completely return to normal once the patient has concluded the treatment.

We ask Dr NM about the DNA content, which is aneuploid. The day before, I read that the prognosis for a diploid content is better than that for an aneuploid one. When I read my own pathology reports, I discovered two different readings, the first of which was 'Diploid' and the second of which was 'Aneuploid'. I was confused and depressed as a result of seeing this discrepancy, and wondered how there could be such flagrant contradictions, and what the implications were with reference to my care.

Dr NM tells us that Alban's readings aren't very conclusive: they don't signify as much as it was previously thought they signified in terms of predicting how the disease would evolve. It's like the PSA test: revolutionary when it was first discovered, but now its popularity has waned. If the DNA test were so revolutionary, it'd be being done systematically; in practice, however, it isn't as effective in determining the disease's evolution as was once thought.

At present, I'm having trouble coping with what's happening with Alban, and all my anxious memories are being dredged up. Françoise notices my state, and tells me she understands. Alban takes things so calmly; I love him for it, but can't help thinking that when I was ill, he might've kept his anxiety so well hidden that it's now coming out in the form of cancer. However, I don't believe that cancers are mainly psychological in origin, so I tend to reject the idea.

Jane: The fact that the thought even occurs to you must mean that somewhere in your mind, you can't totally discount the psychological factor. This reminds me of how I feel about some religious precepts. I don't, for example, believe in original sin and the notion of guilt in simply being human, or in the idea that Jesus died on the Cross in order to 'save' us from our guilt. However, because I was raised to have that belief, somewhere inside me I'm always ready to accept that I'm guilty about something.

Manicha: Evelyne is an epicurean: she finds much enjoyment in sensuous pleasures, and manages to integrate her strength and her weakness in this self-destructing world.

Ⴠ

Yesterday, Adelaide phones about mother. They have to move to another house, and Adelaide isn't only worried about moving mother; she herself isn't feeling well these days. She sounds quite depressed, and I so much wish I could be taking care of mother myself. I tell her she should try to get more help, because there's money for it. I tell her I'll try to get to Lebanon in order to be with her.

Augustus has sent me John McDougall's book about eating habits, entitled *The McDougall Program: 12 Days to Dynamic Health*. I quote from the book (McDougall: 1991: 360, 383) as follows.

Recent concern has been raised because of the findings that women who take progesterone for years have four times the risk of breast cancer as women who took none.

Estrogens slow bone loss, but at a price. Risk of cancer of the uterus is increased by 5 to 14 times over that for women not taking estrogens and may be quadrupled with the combination of estrogens and progesterones.

I wonder how doctors can continue prescribing these hormones when they must be aware of these blatant statistics.

The possible relationship between carcinogens in breast milk and breast cancer (or cancer in offspring) has not been systematically investigated. A study of more than eight hundred nursing mothers in North Carolina has uncovered three patterns that make this question an urgent one. Researchers found that the concentration of organochlorine chemicals in breast milk increased with the age of the mother, increased with the amount of sport fish consumed, and decreased dramatically over the course of lactation and with the number of children nursed. The first trend indicates that our bodies are still amassing fat-soluble contaminants faster than we can eliminate them. The second attests to the ongoing contamination of our rivers, streams, and lakes. The third fact is the most ominous one. Organochlorine contaminants are not easily expunged from our tissues. Their sharp decline in concentration over the course of breast-feeding, therefore, represents the movement of accumulated toxins from mother to child. It signifies that during the intimate act of nursing, a burden of public poisons – insect killers, electrical insulating fluids, industrial solvents, and incinerator residues – is shifted from one generation into the tiny bodies of the next. (Steingraber: 1997: 238)

Mad-cow disease is one thing, but there is also the media hype over this affair ... At times, we would rather fear ghosts than real murderers ... How many proven cases have there been that the disease has been transmitted to people? An infinitely small number: a dozen at most. And, as we have seen, there have been tens of thousands of deaths directly ascribed to the harmful effects of pesticides. (Séralini: 1997: 98)

It is a scandal to turn all this into a top-priority issue, while ignoring the hazards linked to the presence of carcinogens in meat that originate in fertilizers and pesticides, or other pollutants that livestock graze on, or while ignoring the risks involved in the highly detrimental preservatives that they continue to inject into cheap ham and lunch meats that are so often fed to young children. This is a dirty trick being played upon our society, while cancers that are obviously food related are gaining ground before our eyes, causing millions more deaths than mad-cow disease. (Séralini: 1997: 99)

16

ALL AROUND, YET AGAIN
IS THERE AN END?

I am now in the concentration camp, and my share of
'parental' inheritance is in the process of gassing me. But I
am inside the camp, and those doing the gassing are on the
outside. On the inside, I have a measure of individual freedom, however limited it might be. I have the freedom to
choose whether or not to scream when the blows begin to
fall, or to give my consent to this mistreatment. I can choose,
as they gas me, whether to shout 'Heil Hitler' or 'Killers!' I am
free to acknowledge the perversity of the society that made
me what I am, and to suffer from that recognition. I could also
resign myself, and say yes and amen to my murder. This will
to distance myself from my family's past, to the degree that it
causes me to suffer, is what makes me free. I have been
demolished and destroyed, castrated, assaulted, poisoned
and killed, but it is precisely within this individual freedom of
mine that I can distinguish myself from a head of cattle sent
to slaughter; that is where even I can attain some degree of
human dignity. (Zorn: 1979: 251)

On the plane between Tunis and Paris, 5 June 1995

Here in Tunis, I have an intense stay while I'm performing
in *Les filles de Tahar Haddad*: *The Daughters of Tahar Haddad*,

the stage play adapted from my novel *Wounding Words: A Woman's Journal in Tunisia* (Accad: 1996), for which we finally received the necessary permit. I go to Tunis with Ruth, who's filming the play, and with whom, thanks to the trip, I get much closer than I've ever been. I feel that Ruth is fragile and vulnerable, despite the fact she seems strong and assured. I didn't know that her father died of pancreatic cancer at age 52, while Ruth was still quite young.

I know that Amel also lost her father to cancer, when she was in her twenties. If I hadn't gone through cancer myself, I wouldn't be as affected when I hear the story of these two losses. In fact, Amel – and perhaps Ruth as well – has already told me about her father. However, that first time, I didn't react as strongly. Now, though, I feel differently about the loss, especially when Amel shows us the house her father built just before he died, the house that still bears her name, carved on the wall of the entrance door, even though the house is no longer her family's. Her father had to sell it when he became ill: he didn't have enough money to finish building it or to cover its upkeep!

⧗

A lot of tension is evident among the women performing my play, and I can't come up with a way to smooth things out in order to get them talking again. However, the play is a success. The Club Tahar Haddad's performance space is fully booked for the five shows, and by the last night, we'd managed to achieve a measure of professionalism. For the amateurs that we all were – except for Meriem – the show isn't so bad after all. Ruth is there filming, and her presence behind the camera is like the extra eye we need to reveal all of our mistakes. I wonder whether we'll stage the play again as we'd all like to, in Tunis, Paris, Beirut and even the United States.

Paris, 8 June 1995

I'm going through another spell of anxiety. I'm sore under my arm and on the right side of my abdomen, and I'm also having dizzy spells. These symptoms feel too much like those warning signs I've been told about, and I'm scared. Sometimes I tell myself, *That's it: the cancer's come back all through my body. I don't want to die – not yet, not with all the things I still have to do.* But then I remind myself that worrying only makes things worse, for both my body and my morale; I should have a more positive attitude. However, it's hard to be positive when the pains are so real.

It's pretty clear why I'm having all these depressing thoughts, what with all the stories I've been hearing recently: Zohreh and her sudden ovarian cancer; Caryle Kyle, a professor in the English department, who's about our age and who died recently, unable to be saved from a recurrence of cancer in her spine; sweet Séverine, with her recurrence; and all the other people who've been hit. No wonder I'm getting scared every time I have the slightest ache or pain.

Manicha: It could also be the case that the so-called depressive state is simply your true perception of what existence really is: not much; neither good nor bad; not progressive; a flat line. The idea of 'progression' is completely ideological. Humanity has to maintain this illusion in order to get out of bed in the morning and walk around! Why can't we accept, from time to time, that we can be 'non-positive' and exactly as we are and who we are, that is, nothing: we come from nothing, and we go to nothing. Once we've humbly admitted this truth to ourselves, we can accept that we're in this floating state – of nothingness? – and we realise that we must give ourselves an illusion – work, family, love: any kind of aim, big or small, to get up and walk around. Isn't 'depression' the true condition of human beings? At least this is how I've lived it.

Jane: Yours is a very European view – you're not at all the 'get up and go' American.

I make myself some *hab al baraka*: literally, 'blessing seed', but also an expression that Lebanese people also use in order to wish someone good luck, as Cindy rightfully reminds me. I've been given the grain in Beirut, by Maria, the woman who cleans Adelaide's house. Before I left, Maria brought me a whole bag of it and assured me that if I had some of it every day, my cancer would never return. It's a dark grain, a bit like sesame seeds but black, and North African people sometimes sprinkle it on bread dough. Maria has told me to boil it in water and drink the juice, and to then press the cooked seeds with olive oil and place the concoction wherever I'm feeling pain. In her village, she knows a woman who cured herself of a cancer recurrence as a result of taking *hab al baraka*. I've since found out that it's an old medicine that's long been prescribed all over the Mediterranean basin, and that its medicinal properties are even cited in the Qur'an (Koran).

I'm also taking mistletoe – *Viscum Album* – at night. Extracted drops of it can be purchased in French pharmacies, and mine was prescribed by Dr Joyer, the doctor who Patsy's acupuncturist recommended.

I'm practising relaxation using some meditation cassettes I brought with me from the States. Also, I'm thinking about contacting Amel's kinesiologist, who she introduced me to while we were in Tunis and who lives in Paris.

Somehow, my anxiety is being eased as a result of all these self-help measures. Next week, I have to have blood tests for a check-up. I'm glad I have to have them: I need to be reassured.

14 June 1995

I meet Michèle Brun, a militant for women's rights, who created and produces the journal *Dialogues de Femmes: Women's*

Dialogues. She knows a French female doctor, Dr Adjani, who's a breast oncologist practising in El Manar, in Tunis. Dr Adjani has told Michèle that many of the women she treats would rather die than be treated for their breast cancer. They tell her they're tired of living, and that they'd welcome being rested in death. They've chosen what they consider to be a final place of peace and rest over struggling through everyday life having lost a breast and been through a debilitating treatment that would've left them even more diminished in their daily life and with their family. I think of Adelaide, who's told me similar things, and I'm hurt, because these women have lived a life of such pain and quiet desperation that they'd rather die than suffer from it any more.

Paris, 16 June 1995

I go to the kinesiologist Amel has suggested. However, I don't know whether I'll go back: the exercises the practitioner has given me to do aren't very exhilarating. They're meant to be done in order to integrate the body with the spirit and the emotions. The practitioner has told me to 'do them well intellectually', because the two sides of my personality, the yin and yang, react well; however, I wonder whether my body truly follows the 'doing well'. I resolve to write to Amel to ask her about all this, because if I don't do the exercises correctly, I'm wondering whether it's worth it for me to go back to the kinesiologist and have a treatment for which I have to pay quite a bit of money that isn't even partially reimbursed by my insurance company.

Jane: This short paragraph is interesting: you've raised the question of non-reimbursable forms of health treatment, that is, most so-called marginal medicine. You've demonstrated what for some people must be a terrible dilemma: having to choose between a questionable treatment the cost of which is reimbursable and a milder treatment that's costly in the long term because you're 'put out of pocket'.

Bettina: It's worth highlighting this dilemma.

Madeleine: Some people might find this 'marginal medicine' more acceptable, but its effectiveness remains to be proven.

20 June 1995

I go to see Dr Joyer, the female doctor who practises both traditional and alternative medicine. She lives close to Monique's place, and is extremely warm and friendly. She's just attended a conference about cancer and found it highly revealing. I'll list just a few points she noted: (1) That cancer is provoked by a psycho-affective shock experienced in isolation; (2) That the left breast is linked to shocks related to the 'family nest'; (3) That there's no such thing as metastasis: a cancer that comes back is usually another cancer linked to *devalorisation* of the body, which is often caused by previous cancer treatments or other shocks provoked by the first cancer; (4) That it's important to understand all this in order to not repeat the experiences that hurt in the past and provoked the cancer: we must resolve past conflicts in order to eliminate the source of disease.

Manicha: And what about the effects of the environment and of the way we live? I believe that for some of us, these are the first causes; they're triggered by one weakness or another that's linked to our living conditions.

I agree with you, Manicha.

Dr Joyer examines me where I hurt, on the right side of my stomach. She thinks the pain is being caused by gas, and prescribes a natural medicine called Carbolevure, which is made of charcoal and yeast. For my bone loss, she prescribes a *phosphonate* called Didronel, as well as calcium with vitamin D, which help fix calcium in the bones.

Madeleine: It's the treatment that's been prescribed by any good generalist, in Paris at least, for more than 20 years now. I've been on it for a long time now, but I've never been able to fix the calcium.

I analyse what Dr Joyer has told me, and find it corresponds to the set of circumstances in my life whereby cancer might've been provoked in my left breast: father's illness; Milo's death; the great solitude in which I live here in France. I realise that until I contracted this disease, I never knew I had so many people who loved me and were concerned about me in France. For the first time since I've been ill, I've been feeling surrounded by friends and as if I'm no longer in exile. And now, I'm tending to *devalorise* my body because of the mutilating treatment I've had. I must resolve to work on this process and to overcome the feeling of dislike I have for my body; also, I should tell Alban not to react negatively towards his body and towards the treatment he's receiving that's causing him to be depressed. Dr Joyer believes it'd be good if both of us worked on this aspect and perhaps went to see the doctor who developed the theories. Unfortunately, though, that doctor lives quite a long way from Paris.

It's good that Alban and I can talk about all this and exorcise our pain, anger and frustration. I must learn to stop carrying the weight of the world on my shoulders, and must learn to unwind and live with less stress. Fifty is a difficult age, and if I can get over the hurdle without being damaged too much, I'll be able to view the journey as being an exploit. I've already lost a breast, and the damage must stop here. I wish I could be like my Swiss great cousin

Nelly, who was visiting mother the last time I went to Beirut with Amel. She's so serene, and her face always has such a sweet smile on it. She exudes happiness despite the fact that she's older and has experienced many losses.

27 June 1995

Augustus is here in Paris for a few days. We go to the Marché de la Poésie, and for a gift, I give him Andrée Chedid's novel *L'enfant multiple*: *The Multiple Child* (Chedid: 1995). Set during the time of the civil war in Lebanon, it's the story of a beautiful child who has multiple identities. I know that Augustus will enjoy reading it, and this afternoon, I'm glad that Andrée personally signs his copy, at the Marché bookstore, at which she's signing purchasers' copies of the book. At the store, she greets us warmly, and doesn't want me to pay for my copy; however, I like to buy books written by writers I admire, and even more so when the writer is a friend.

The Multiple Child has special significance for me because in it, Andrée deals with the literal scars of war as the body is affected by the conflict, as well as with attempts at covering up the scarring through use of artificial limbs. The 'multiple child' is Omar-Jo, born of an Egyptian Muslim father and a Lebanese Christian mother. Although Omar-Jo has lost an arm during the war in Lebanon, he wears his amputation, a bruised stump, with pride. When he goes to Paris to seek refuge, he's shown a selection of artificial limbs to choose from to replace his missing arm and so he'll thereby become 'able' again. However, he refuses the offer. I quote from the novel (Chedid: 1995: 217–18) as follows.

> With all his body, with all his being, Omar-Jo had summarily rejected the apparatus, the artificial limb that would have been joined to his mutilated but still living flesh. The child had gotten used to his stump little by little. Even the sutures, dissolved now

in the closed wound, were part of it. He'd forget the member momentarily, so that he could continue to exist and to function better. Yet, at the same time, it must always live in him as the representation of an amputation, of a permanent cry. You couldn't trade that arm for another nor betray its image. Its absence was a reminder of all absences, of all deaths, of all sorrows.

In this passage, Andrée is expressing what I've been feeling about having my breast amputated, the questions I've been asking about reconstruction and implants, and the relationship I have with my mutilated country.

Augustus tells me that Myrna, a friend from my younger days in Beirut, is struggling with a lymphoma, but that no one should know about the problem. Myrna is only a few years younger than I. I remember the times we went to the beach together in Beirut, when we were in our twenties – we had so much fun together. I'm hurt to think she has to undergo a difficult treatment: she's still relatively young. Again I ask myself what's now become a recurrent theme: *Why? Why?* Let no one tell me that the environment isn't implicated in all these cancers that are hitting people I never imagined would be suffering so young in their life.

Jane: I wonder why the issue is shrouded in so much secrecy. Are people ashamed? Are they afraid they'll be ostracised?

Madeleine: It's fear, to be sure; however, it's also a feeling of propriety. In France, haven't we got into the habit of saying, about someone who's died of cancer, that he or she 'died after a protracted illness'?

Paris, 28 June 1995

I'm disturbed by a TV film about an American blues singer who had a double mastectomy. Her heroic attitude comes through loud and clear, as do trivialisation of breast cancer

433

and absence of even a mention of the epidemic's environmental causes. The singer, a beautiful, harmonious woman, a 'believer' and a holder of traditional values, proudly wears her two implants, which are shown to be esthetically more pleasing than her natural breasts. Her fiancé vows to become a believer if she's healed. She overcomes the disease because she maintains her courage and her faith. Throughout her story, American values are reinforced: values to do with the American way of life, triumph over a desperate situation and success against all the odds.

Jane: When there's all this sentimentality in a story, attention is deflected from the real problem.

3 July 1995

Today, I have my third check-up with Dr Esper. Everything's all right: what a relief! I thank the doctor for risking not giving me another chemotherapy treatment. Humble, and happy not to have been mistaken, he barely smiles. I'll continue to be followed up by him, even though I'm shortly returning to the States to resume my teaching.

⧖

Now that the worst is over, how should I end this book? Well, it has no end, and neither does this disease. Until a real cure is found for every kind of cancer, how can I or anyone else rejoice? I've decided to share with you, my readers, a few more 'flashes' from my journal, as follows.

Beirut, 22 July 1995

I'm in Ras-Beirut, at the Nasr café, Pigeon Rock. I have taken a long walk, and now I'm enjoying a cold beer while

I'm writing. The sea, in front of me, is raging, like the unfathomable violence of this country.

Yesterday, Eloïse and I go to pick up Théophile at the airport. A guy in uniform hits our car from the back. Eloïse ignores the accident. We're stuck in traffic. The guy starts insulting Eloïse. She talks back to him and insults him. I'm worried, because the man's probably armed. Eloïse tells me it'd be worse to let herself be intimidated, and that she should've insulted him right from the start. I admire her for her courage and for the fact that she supported Théophile throughout the war. However, I don't like the fact that people here have to push and shove their way through traffic and queues, and I'm disturbed by the aggressiveness that some people express.

⧗

This time last year, I was having radiation treatment. Although it was a very difficult period in my life, I discovered many new friends in the States, and some friends I'd never really gotten to know until then. I didn't expect to have the kind of support I received.

Manicha: Every rose has its thorn: you make the best of each situation.

⧗

Two days ago, I attend the wedding of one of my nephews. It takes place in Théopolis, in the church in the mountains beneath which father is buried. Across from the church, we can see the house that father and his brother built, in which we spent our summers and father thought he'd spend his old age. It was almost destroyed as a result of the war, and remains standing because its hewn-stone walls are so strong. Father died before he was able to enjoy the fruits of his labour: his book and his houses. He suffered too much in the end, but was at least happy and in love with mother.

Manicha: It's good to underline the fact that this love was 'sustainable', just as we nowadays talk about 'sustainable' development and 'sustainable' peace.

⏳

I'm here in Ras-Beirut, the place of my childhood and adolescence. I'm sitting in the same spot in which Jay and I sipped a beer, almost 25 years ago, when the war hadn't yet started and we didn't know it'd take place. We also didn't know we'd split up one day. So many things have happened since then: how quickly time goes by.

I'm in Beirut with my sweet Anaïs. Twice a week, she has to give injections to Adelaide, who's suffering from a terrible backache as a result of which she's been laid up in bed.

Jane: *[I first wrote 'nailed up in bed', which is a translation from the French expression.]* For Adelaide, from the way you've described her, it probably would've been better to keep the first expression, which recalls the Crucifixion! Too bad English doesn't have an expression that's similar to the French one.

Mother is declining, but she's holding on despite wanting to leave this earth. I find life terribly cruel.

Manicha: Life isn't cruel; it simply *is*. The desire to leave this earth is natural: if people feel tired, or if they want to rejoin their loved ones. This is a right, and an honorable wish.

⏳

Last night, Alban phones. He's feeling awful because his brothers and sisters have decided to put his mother into a nursing home: a decision he's always been against. There's a silence. I ask him whether he's crying, and he replies, 'I never cry!' My sweet love: so attentive; so sensitive; so present. I'm often struck by the minimal amount of attention that most men give other people, and by how different Alban is in this way.

Paris, 6 August 1995

In 12 days' time, I'll be back in the States. Although I'm looking forward to returning there, I'm a bit apprehensive because I must learn to maintain my distance and not let myself get stressed out any more. How will I deal with my memories of my disease, and with all the sick people around me?

I phone Séverine, whose intestinal cancer has come back. She, Charles and Laura are leaving for Colorado. She's just spent three and a half weeks in hospital, and Alain visited her there every day. She's scared about dying, afraid to leave her daughter, and afraid of the risks her daughter has of contracting the disease. She's convinced there's 'something in the air' that's causing all the cancers around them. She's written an article for her city's newspaper in which she denounces the cancer-causing factors in the environment. I'm convinced that assessment of the problem is sound, and I'd like to see the article. Alban thinks that people at Séverine's university should mobilise and request that more research into the subject be undertaken. Séverine tells me not to worry about her and to instead think of myself – my sweet little sister: how I love her!

There's also Zohreh, who I know I'll find weakened by her treatment. And Myrna, who has Hodgkin's disease. At first, Augustus warned me that Myrna didn't want anyone to know she had the disease, but when I talked to Myrna myself, she said it was her husband who didn't want cancer mentioned: the word made him 'flip'. However, Myrna seemed calm. She's having chemotherapy – eight sessions of it – and will have to have radiation treatment if her cancer isn't completely eliminated as a result of the chemo. Also, she's taking cortisone, and as a result, and much to her displeasure, has gained 14 pounds. I told her I also gained weight due to the chemo, but that I subsequently slimmed down again. She told me she started losing her hair and so has had it cut very short. Poor, sweet Myrna, who's always been hyper-sensitive! When I told Narsay, a mutual friend, about Myrna's disease, he told me it's the very tender, extra-sensitive people who contract it!

And my poor, sweet Alban: he's being castrated as a result of the anti-testosterone injections he's receiving every two months. He can't get an erection any more. I hope the little tumours in his prostate are going away, and that he'll quickly be healed so he can cease having this treatment, through which his energy is being sapped and his ability to have sexual pleasure is being negated.

11 August 1995

I dream that Séverine and Charles have had another daughter and son, in addition to Laura. I'm telling Séverine, 'It's incredible how you've managed to make children despite your disease.' The dream reflects my desire to see life triumph over death, and to see my little sister triumph over her recurrence.

Alban is distraught because his mother isn't doing at all well in the nursing home. And Adelaide tells me that mother isn't doing well either. This week, Adelaide is finding her to be too isolated and quite depressed. Sometimes the condition of older people is heartbreaking.

Manicha: This must be the same feeling we had as kids, when we were told to go and have a nap while we were in the middle of playing – except that older people have no strength: they're being led; they show not an ounce of resistance; they're ready to let go any minute. They know the end is near. For people who don't believe in God, what attracts them is the calm, the eternal rest.

⧗

Before I depart, I have dinner with Noureddine and Madeleine Aba. I know that Noureddine's days are numbered, because he's had so many operations and been very close to death many times this year. I interview him, and fill two cassettes with his talking about subjects such as his life, his writing, his political engagement, Algeria and Palestine. Actually, what's come out most strongly in the interview is his relationship with Madeleine: he views it as being his life's greatest achievement. I find it moving to hear him talk about Madeleine so lovingly.

Yesterday, Alban and I go to see the film *L'Année Juliette*. It's very funny, beautiful and dramatic, all at once. The director and actors depict the role that dreams play in the life of the imagination, and all that the dreams help bring out, in an unusual, forceful and interesting way that's also filled with humour. We laugh a lot.

Urbana, 24 August 1995

Being back in Urbana is hard: I feel surrounded by sick people. Petite-Fleur's disease has been diagnosed as being Poliarthritis Nodosa; she's just been hospitalised in order to undergo some intensive, high-dose treatment. Zohreh, my dear, sweet friend, has just received the first half of her final chemo treatment: Taxol, which is very strong. And Séverine will have to go to Chicago in order to have a bone-marrow transplant; she wants to try and survive, so she doesn't have a choice.

⧗

One day, I have a bad cough and pain on the side I received the treatment on. I make an appointment with Dr Land to make sure everything's all right and that I don't have to worry about the cough. Fortunately, I have a good class today, so I feel better.

I wonder why all kinds of conferences about cancer are being scheduled that have names such as The Challenge of Cancer Treatment. Being treated for cancer isn't a challenge; it's torture, a horror – that's what they should call the conference.

Alban phones to tell me his mother has died. From his voice, I can tell he's devastated and angry. I wish I could be with him at moments such as these. And from what Adelaide tells me, mother is very morose and depressed. I wish there were something I could do for mother, such as bring her here to be with me, but she wouldn't survive the trip. And I know that Alban wishes he could've done something for his mother. We're all so helpless, sometimes.

26 August 1995

Dr Land gives me an antibiotic for my cough and tells me that if it hasn't gone within two days, I'm to go back to him for a chest X-ray. He's very communicative. I tell him about my experience during my follow-up in France. I feel that my cough has lessened since I've been taking the antibiotic. But how anxious I'm constantly feeling!

I like the book I'm reading at present: Sharon Batt's *Patient No More: The Politics of Breast Cancer* (Batt: 1994). Batt reveals that we aren't hearing enough about the fact that the horrible disease of breast cancer is hitting so many women each year because women haven't mobilised to take political action and raise people's consciousness the way men have done with reference to AIDS. I couldn't agree with her more!

I'm reading about Petite-Fleur's disease. It's frightening: the patient has a chance of surviving for only five years, especially if he or she isn't treated soon enough. Why didn't Petite-Fleur's doctors do the biopsies of her leg sores sooner? She's feeling alone and abandoned; at only 30, she's already seeing her dreams and future hopes vanishing. This woman has real courage!

2 September 1995

In preparation for a worst-case scenario, Séverine visits me bearing a list of names and instructions with reference to care for her daughter Laura: next week, my sweet little sister is to go to Chicago to be treated for her bone-marrow transplant. It's a dangerous process, in which the patient's bone-marrow cells are taken from him or her and are frozen in order to have extremely high doses of chemotherapy, which should kill all the cancer cells, administered to them. In the process, the good cells, along with the bone marrow, are also destroyed, and if it weren't for the frozen cells, which are then re-injected in the body to enable the cells and bone marrow to regenerate, the person would die. I'm frightened, and I shiver, when I think Séverine has to go through this dangerous and painful process. I hug her, and can't hold back my tears. Should I let go of my tears and sorrow, my fear of not seeing her again, when she needs all the encouragement she can get? But I can't help it, and I have a heavy heart as I watch her leave my house. Fortunately, I'm going to Samira's place this evening, and we'll be able to talk and cry together. We're supporting each other, and I'm so glad to have her in town.

6 September 1995

This afternoon, one of my students, Amy, comes to see me. Over the summer, her mother had breast cancer, and had a mastectomy and chemotherapy. My poor student bursts into tears as she's telling me about the ordeal. She tells me she took care of her mother over the summer. Her grandmother had the same disease when she was Amy's mother's age, so Amy is afraid for herself. Her mother is my age, and it's just been discovered that she has a brain tumour. She's a cellist. I'm at a loss to know how to console Amy.

Another of my students, Britt, has a sister whose breast cancer has metastasised to her bones and who's in great pain. It's incredible, how many cancers are manifesting! I tell both Amy and Britt that women should speak out, denounce what's happening, mobilise to take political action, raise awareness of the issue and influence public opinion. What a world we're living in: a civilisation of terror!

Later, I see Amy at one of the university's athletics centres. She's with a friend, and they're looking for the swimming pool. She seems more cheerful. I tell her I've just been thinking about her and the conversation we had that afternoon. I show her my scar because I think I might thereby help neutralise her fear of mutilation. She thanks me, and goes off to the pool with her friend.

12 September 1995

In the corridors of Foreign Languages Building, I see Giri, an Indian colleague who's teaching in the Comparative Literature department and who was one of the first people I met when I arrived at the University of Illinois, almost 25 years ago. He's now bald, receiving chemotherapy for inoperable lung cancer. He says, 'They're giving me a substance that comes from Brazilian trees.' I understand the substance is Taxol, the same substance used in the chemo that Zohreh and Séverine are having. Giri looks well in spite of his treatment, and seems cheerful. It occurs to me that this building is turning into a cancer ward!

I'm reading Rosalind MacPhee's *Picasso's Woman: A Breast Cancer Story* (MacPhee: 1994), which is about the author's experience with breast cancer. It's very well written, and MacPhee raises a lot of important questions in it that I can identify with. I include three extracts from the book (MacPhee: 1994: 145, 145, 162) as follows.

I understood that it took time to adjust to a diagnosis like cancer. But I was torn between a desire to just get on with my life and a need to understand the disease. I had no desire to see myself as a victim, and that was the way much of what I read made me feel. I want to grow stronger and put the experience behind me. Yet I needed to know the enemy; I needed to know how to fight back. Finding out about the breast cancer had led me to know my own mortality in a way I never had before. Cancer might have killed me. It might still – unless I learned how to live with it.

In my research so far, I had come up with more questions than answers. Countless times I had read that breast cancer is considered the most unpredictable of all cancers. There are known causes for many other types of cancer, but not this disease. The best anyone seemed to have come up with was that either an inherited factor or a carcinogen creates a mutation in a normal gene, then something else comes along and causes a second mutation. When this second mutation occurs, you possess the gene for cancer. But it was all guesswork.

A third study found that pesticide levels were higher in the fat tissue of women who had breast cancer … I had spent my childhood in the Okanagan Valley at a time when DDT was revered as a wonder chemical. We used to play under fruit trees that were dripping with it. This same paper mentioned that breast cancer in Israel dropped 30% per cent following an aggressive program to phase out organochlorine pesticides ... I read that breast cancers are 6 to 5 times higher in countries with nuclear waste sites ... When Jimmy Carter was president of the US more than a thousand people were awarded damages from the government for cancers caused by the nuclear testing in Nevada. The award was reversed by a higher court, which decided that the government was not responsible for what had happened. The previous year I had read a book called *Refuge* by American writer Terry Tempest Williams. How many had she said it was? Seven to nine women in her family with breast cancer – and no cancer history before all those above-ground atomic tests in Nevada, where she lived as a child. It really gave new meaning to the expression 'depending on which way the wind blows.'

Cindy: It is indeed a beautiful book; I have a tape with the author reading it; however, it's sad, because her mother dies.

6 October 1995

Today, I receive a bill from the Share clinic, for the physical therapy I had for my swollen and painful arm. The 'damage' is $140 for the first 30 minutes of introductory evaluation plus $31.50 for a fifteen-minute session, making a total of $171.50. In Paris, for that amount, I could've had a whole month – once a week, for 30 minutes each time – of incredible massages and lymphatic drainage with my sweet Bettina, and in Paris, any physiotherapist would charge me the same amount. Here in Urbana, however, the two women therapists who treated me didn't seem to know what they were doing. The first one was quite sensitive and interested in helping women, such as her mother and me, who've had a mastectomy, but she knew nothing about my lymphatic system; the other therapist pressed on my arm so much while she was massaging it that after I'd had the treatment, I was in more pain than I'd been in before I had it.

Madeleine: I'm startled that these 'scrubbers from the Turkish baths' can qualify as physical therapists: I wonder what kind of training they have in order to be licensed?

In Paris, I was told that the practitioner has to do this type of massage very gently and delicately, to push the lymphatic liquid back into its place without irritating the arm. When I went to the second therapist, she covered my chest with one of those open-front shirts that nurses give patients to cover themselves up when the patient is asked to get undressed. In this book, I've already mentioned I thought I looked like a concentration-camp inmate in the photos that had to be taken for my radiation therapy. In those photos, I'm wearing an open-front shirt. Clinics must have to pay a fortune to have thousands of these shirts washed and sterilised every day – a task that's probably routine in the States. I seriously question how necessary it is to use them and whether the expense involved in laundering them is justifiable, considering that medical institutions are doing so much to reduce expenses. What's the point of making patients wear these covers? And I have to wonder whether the therapist in question can see what she's doing and where she's massaging me under my 'veil'.

Madeleine: She doesn't see anything – that's obvious: American prudishness, once again!

I'm reminded of a TV program in which the presenter was trying to teach women how to touch their breasts in order to discover whether a lump is present: every time a breast was shown, the image of it was purposefully blurred. I find this type of censorship utterly ridiculous. In France, patients get undressed without having a curtain around them and without wearing a special outfit, whether the doctor or therapist is male or female. At any rate, I was angry about both the physical-therapy treatment I received and the cost involved in having it, and decided to phone the clinic to lodge a complaint. The practitioners weren't sympathetic about either my grievances or the pain that resulted from having the treatment. I decided to cancel the subsequent sessions that'd been scheduled.

Madeleine: For French people, Americans are a real puzzle: half the time they have an unbridled, 'anything goes' attitude, and at other times they're grotesquely prude.

Petite-Fleur is feeling desperate about her two city clinics' monstrous bills, which she's unable to pay. Formerly, the officers at the university medical centre who sent her to the clinics had told her she wouldn't have to pay, which is why she'd agreed to go along. She has very little money to pay for basic living expenses, let alone for the expensive treatment she's been having. I must find a way to help her. I'm angry to think that some antibiotics she was given a few years ago for an infection of her genital system might've caused the disease she now has.

When Petite-Fleur was all alone in the hospital last summer, her doctors sent some psychiatrists to see her because she was refusing to take the medicine they were trying to force on her. The first psychiatrist, an Indian man, asked her who the president of the republic was. Petite-Fleur answered, 'Hilary Clinton'. He then asked her whether she intended to kill herself, but then apologised for asking these questions and said he'd get fired if he didn't ask them. Poor Petite-Fleur was being treated as if she were deranged, and as if it weren't normal for her to be terribly depressed and desperate when she'd been diagnosed as having a terrible and devastating disease.

※

For my birthday, my dear Zohreh takes me out to a restaurant. I'm very touched by the gesture, and I look at her and think, *Why does she have to go through this difficult treatment? Her parents are old, and didn't have to suffer with cancer when they were our age. Why? Why?* I find it all so unfair. Zohreh is one of the most generous, loving, sweet people I know, and one of the best professors we have at the university. Why does she have to suffer so much?

11 October 1995

I've just discovered I'm my department's lowest-paid full professor. I'm angry that I'm the one who 'gets the guernsey', because compared with most of my colleagues, I've published more; I direct more PhD theses; I'm more visible both nationally and internationally; and my reputation is greater. I know that in this society, the currency that's used for judging everyone is money, so I believe that my real worth isn't being appreciated.

I feel an incredible rage rising in me. I remember the time I had had to ask for a promotion that wasn't coming as soon as it should've been; how the psychotherapist I went to see during that depressing time in my life told me to assert myself, and said that 'wheels that don't squeak don't get oiled'; and how I obtained my promotion thanks to the psychotherapist's advice. I'll have to design an action plan in order to reveal my anger and obtain what's my rightfully mine. I hate this system, in which people are forced to act so aggressively; it's not my style, and I'd much rather be appreciated for what I'm worth without having to get angry and stake my claim. However, I have no choice: It isn't fair that I do all this work and remain underpaid.

I'm doing physical-education exercises, in which I force my body to lift weights, swim, walk, cycle and stretch in order to dominate my fear of mad cells, recurrence, individual pains and strange symptoms. When I'm exercising at IMPE, I look at my body and remember how it was *before*, when it was intact and un-mutilated. I feel heavy with the weight of the years.

17 October 1995

Today, I meet Cassandra, a colleague who works in another department, is about my age and had breast cancer almost at the same time I did. Hers was also a lobular carcinoma and, like mine, appeared as a mass in her breast. However, the treatment she had was very different from mine. She had a hard time finding someone to read her mammography, so had to endure a delay in having her biopsy. When a different surgeon from mine finally operated on her, she woke up to be told that the cancer might've already reached her bones, in which case she'd have very few years to live. She was told this devastating news in a brutal way, and was then left alone in a state of shock. She received six months of chemotherapy – Adriamycin and Cytoxin, like I had – whereby she lost all her hair and eyelashes, and both her eyebrows. She's now taking tamoxiphen and participating in a study. She's unhappy about having gained 20 pounds. She had breast reconstruction immediately, and is very pleased with the results, especially because she likes to go swimming and would feel very self-conscious if she had only one breast.

Cassandra tells me she thinks the disease will kill her one day. I tell her not to say it, because I've been told that lobular cancer is less dangerous than other types of cancer. She tells me a horror story about the oncologist who treated her – the one I first saw, who charged me the exorbitant rates that I complained about. On a weekend, while he was making an opening in her chest in order to get the chemotherapy in through a catheter, he pierced her lung and then sent her home, even though she was complaining she had pains and symptoms through which he should've gotten a clue that he'd misplaced the catheter. Cassandra could've died as a result of this ordeal. I find this oncologist's carelessness very upsetting, to say the least, and am happy I had a wonderful nurse, Eve, who was so efficient.

Having talked with Cassandra, I feel somehow depressed, because I don't feel she wants to take charge of her life. She accepts too much of what she's being told, without questioning it or revolting. When I say we should organise by first finding other women who've suffered as we have, and then talking about our worries and mobilising to take political action, she responds by saying she'd be happy to meet them but not to talk about cancer with them. I believe she has to put her cancer experience behind her. And I think to myself, *What would we women talk about, then?*

Cindy: I understand both her feelings and yours. She wanted relief from thinking about cancer so much that she didn't want to become politically involved, whereas for you, political action is part of your healing.

24 October 1995

Anxieties and anxieties;
diseases all around;
fear of getting sick again.
I'm fed up with this country:
the whole world is polluted and sick.

There's no place to go,
except in one's mauve shelter –
secure and warm inside.
I must take refuge there:
'Protect yourself; retreat into your bubble,'

urges my Amel;

The time will come when I'll no longer be scared
of this disease,
of each pain, of each physical problem,
of each weakness, of each doubt.
Let this time come!
I don't dare name my fears any more,
afraid their name may become reality.
I yearn for a horizon clear and light,
where the fear that grabs me deep inside
will have vanished!

⏳

I go to see Séverine, who's back from having her bone-marrow transplant, in Chicago. I've prepared her some meals: cooked, re-cooked and frozen – she has to be extremely careful about germs. She's wearing a mask. I'm so happy to see her, having been so afraid I'd lose her. I'm hoping so much that she's been definitively cured as a result of this treatment, and that she'll be able to fulfil her deepest wish: to see her daughter Laura through college. She tells me that the procedure she's just gone through is the most horrible experience she's ever had – and my poor little sister has had her fair share of torture! She says she'd never go through it again, it was so excruciatingly painful.

She and Charles sent the following letter to all their friends who helped them during their Calvary.

Dear friends,

We hope you'll forgive us for writing this form letter, but we didn't think we could get to every one of you otherwise. Séverine's bone-marrow transplant this past September–October was very frightening for all of us, but we're writing to say that she's doing better than expected, and that we're all finding a special pleasure and meaning in being home together with all of us active again. Being sick wasn't easy for Séverine. Some of you told her how brave you thought she was, but her own recollection of the treatment is much less heroic: more like concentrating on putting one foot in front of the other. And crying over how unfair this world had become … Séverine's refrain is 'I'm amazed I have any friends left, that they don't all get tired of me and my crises. But if that happened, I'd understand, because I sometimes get tired of it all myself.' … Thank you all for the tons of cards and letters you sent to the hospital: they all arrived a bit soggy and blurred – after being sprayed with disinfectant – but the messages were crisp and clear, and your encouragement, hope and laughter came when they were needed. And thanks for the phone calls, even if sometimes it might have sounded like Séverine was out of it …

19 November 1995

Zohreh gives me a copy of Greenpeace's report about the effects of chlorine on the environment, especially its effects on breast cancer and the statistical rise in the disease (*A Greenpeace Report*: 1993). Finding out the links is very frightening. In the report, it's stated that chlorine must be eliminated from the atmosphere right now, and that even if it is, it won't be soon enough to prevent the catastrophic consequences for the generations yet to come.

Cindy: Isn't chlorine also in the water we drink?

Paris, 14 January 1996

Why am I so depressed that our president, Mitterand, has died? Probably because he died of prostate cancer as did father, and because Alban is suffering from the same frightening disease. Also, I feel that with this death of our leader, a whole historical period of my life is receding.

I'm worrying about Alban, because he's been undertaking too many projects. He doesn't have the energy he used to have, and tires easily. He's adorable – always playing seduction games with me; we joke and laugh. Today, though, I'm sad, because I'm again leaving to return to the States in order to resume my teaching.

Over the past few weeks, France has been experiencing lots of strikes, so we've often been having to walk to places such as doctors' offices and hospitals. All these strikes are an expression that people are profoundly unsettled and unhappy about their both living conditions and life in general. On TV, I hear a French person ask, 'What are we going to offer our children?' However, I wonder how, having all these strikes, we'll be better able to solve the country's huge economic, social, environmental and other problems: why add more chaos to the existing chaotic mess? It doesn't make much sense.

Today, a taxi driver says to me, 'It's the end of the world.' I think, but don't say to him, that I believe it's the end of *a* world: the world as we know it. Will we be able to create another world in which our values are different?

Manicha: If you're talking about the big strike in December 1995, it's clear you didn't care much for it. However, both Parisians and visitors were astonished at how friendly with one another the local people had suddenly become — they were remarking that they hadn't seen that kind of solidarity since the '50s. As a result of the public-transport strikes, people started to pool their cars. Among the non-strikers in the private sector, there was no sign of anger being vented at the public-sector strikers. As for how necessary the strike was in the first place, that's the way it's always been: a show of force is the only way to get crises resolved, alas. And even if the strike served only to demonstrate that our society is fragile; that any little thing can destabilise it; that people – the strikers – are still capable of shaking up the establishment, I'd say it's a good thing: hurray for strikes, Evelyne!

Bettina: For once I agree with you, Manicha.

Madeleine: So do I – although the right to strike is a right that people mustn't abuse, because there are times when an already weak economy can be ruined as a result of strike action.

Over the past two decades, nearly two dozen studies have emerged that link chlorination of drinking water to bladder and rectal cancers and, in some cases, to cancers of the kidney, stomach, brain, and pancreas. These investigations include case-control and cohort studies in addition to eco-logic studies. The collective evidence on water chlorination, affirms Kenneth Cantor, 'supports concern over an elevated carcinogenic risk ... Chlorine gas is a noxious poison. However, the problem with chlorinated drinking water does not lie with chlorine itself. Rather, in a manner reminiscent of the way that air pollutants combine in the atmosphere to create new chemical species, the problem begins when elemental chlorine spontaneously reacts with organic con-taminants already present in water. Their organochlorine offspring are known as disinfection by-products. Hundreds exist, and several are classified as probable human car-cinogens. Trihalomethanes, a small subgroup of volatile disinfection by-products, are currently receiving the most scientific and regulatory attention. Chloroform is the most common one. As with waterborne volatile compounds, our

route of exposure to trihalomethanes is threefold: ingestion, inhalation, and absorption.' (Steingraber: 1997: 202)

In the EPA's chart of drinking-water standards, along the row
labeled 'Total Trihalomethanes' and under the column titled
'Potential Health Effects' is a single word: *cancer*. Many studies all telescope into this one word. The early investigations
were ecological in design and compared cancer rates in
communities with and without chlorinated water. Conducted
in Ohio, Louisiana, Wisconsin, Iowa, Norway, and Finland,
these studies consistently found associations between water
chlorination and cancers of the bladder and rectum.
(Steingraber: 1997: 203)

In 1910, a New Jersey court examiner declared that chlorination left 'no deleterious substances in the water.' He was
wrong. Nevertheless, it is clear that the disinfection of drinking water with chlorine has prevented widespread contagion
and death, even as it has also contributed to the burden of
human cancers. I do not advocate a ban on the chlorination
of drinking water. But neither do I believe we should blithely
continue old disinfection practices as though our bodies and
our water supplies still existed in the world of ninety years
ago. I say this as an ecologist with a personal relationship to
bladder cancer. In 1910, chloroform was not considered a
deleterious substance. When its toxicity was later recog-
nized, its use as a surgical anesthetic was phased out. We
need not be forced to drink it now as the price for contagion-
free water. (Steingraber: 1997: 206)

About one-third of Americans draw their water from aquifers.
The rest drink from rivers, lakes, and streams. Of course,
ecologically speaking, everyone drinks from aquifers: all running surface water was at one time groundwater, aquifers
being the mothers of rivers. As Rachel Carson pointed out,

contamination of groundwater is, therefore, contamination of water everywhere. (Steingraber: 1997: 210)

Cultivating an ability to imagine these vast basins beneath us is an imperative need. What is required is a kind of mental divining rod that would connect this subterranean world to the images we see every day: a kettle boiling on the stove, a sprinkler bowing over the garden, a bathtub filling up. Our drinking water should not contain the fear of cancer. The presence of carcinogens in groundwater, no matter how faint, means we have paid too high a price for accepting the unimaginative way things are. (Steingraber: 1997: 211)

Every minute, less time than it will take you to read this page, the equivalent of six football fields of rainforest is being irretrievably destroyed, ... and this kind of forest shelters 90% of known species living on Earth today. This is important not only for medications and other substances processed from these species for our daily use ... The forest, and the whole plant kingdom, in addition to regulating our climate and retaining water, supply us, along with algae, with two substances vital for our very existence: living matter and the oxygen we breathe. (Séralini: 1997: 192)

We have undoubtedly consumed, polluted and degraded the earth's natural resources more in the past fifty years than throughout the previous ten thousand centuries. Misery has grown with the population boom at different points on the globe. During this time, as a result of the production–consumption rates in the northern hemisphere, this region has earned its access to progress, even for people in initially 'underprivileged' income brackets: a slim minority on the globe has benefited from the scientific conquest of anti-bacterial hygiene, and from the improvements in health care in general. It started in the early part of this century, and resulted, with a time lag according to the region, in an increased life expectancy for rich countries (81.8 for women and 73.6 for men by 1994, for example, in France). One could, therefore, using a narrow set of reasoning, and taking into account these criteria for success, wish to extend these methods, this *modus operandi*. However, for the past few decades, chemical health has been regressing everywhere in the world, so that the life expectancy of today's children and young people is being placed in jeopardy, as the world's reserves of natural resources are being depleted, and there are no signs at all of regeneration. (Séralini: 1997: 219–20)

17

RECURRENCES

MOVE ON: THE EARTH WILL TAKE YOUR SHAPE

Throughout the year it took for treatment, I engaged in in-depth conversations with each of the caregivers, from the stretcher bearer to the head physician. Each time, I came up against a brick wall. Given this situation, I was compelled to reflect on the causes of this failure to communicate. By the end of a year of frustration, I decided to write this book, so that what they were unable to hear from registration number LM007 within the confines of the hospital, where the doctor is all and the patient nil, they will hear within the cultural space of a book in which a group is given a voice, a group that until now could be heard only in the most fragmented and scattered way. (Hyvrard: 1987: 177)

Urbana, 22 January 1996

Back here in the States, I find out that two on-campus research centres have rejected my application to them for funding to write this book about cancer. When I phone the relevant people who work at them in order to ask why they've rejected the application, they tell me that cancer

457

isn't my field of expertise. It's clear that they don't recognise the scientific import of publishing a personal testimony about cancer: only doctors and researchers are qualified to write about the subject.

Frankly, if I hadn't already had some positive reactions and encouragement to pursue the project, I'd probably be feeling really dejected and drop the subject altogether. If there's anything I should abandon, it's this institution, and I should instead devote myself to writing. Juanita, in her usual sarcastic way, says, 'What do you expect? You slap the system in the face, and then expect it to reward you with funding!' My dear friend is right, and that's what I like about her: the way she has of seeing a situation for what it is and communicating her 20–20 vision. She isn't afraid to talk straight to me, whereas on my own, I'm too naive to recognise the facts as they are.

Later that semester, I reapplied through another channel: the Program for the Study of Cultural Values and Ethics, from which I received a semester's worth of support to write the book. I'm very thankful to the people in the program, and at this point I'd like to acknowledge how important the program is on our campus. Through the program, our faculty members and students are enabled to develop other ways of analysing contemporary world problems and issues.

Last night, I sleep very poorly, having that day spoken with my friend Zohreh, who's scared her cancer might've come back, and who's having all kinds of tests. She's been over-extending herself recently, by taking on too many activities even though she's barely out of intensive therapy. I wake up in the middle of the night, feeling pain all over my body. I ask myself, *What if the cancer's come back?* The cancer survivor is grabbed, unremittingly, by this real terror, and it's a vicious circle, especially at night time.

Last night, then, I have a hard time getting back to sleep. I'm mulling over the issue of the university's lack of encouragement for me to express my creativity. It seems so wrong-headed, because my novels are among the books I've written whereby my international reputation has been established. I always make a point of encouraging my students to be creative, because I believe they have to be in order to develop intellectually as well as emotionally. However, will being creative get them anywhere in a system in which this aspect of scholarly endeavour seems to be discredited? This night, I feel very torn by all these questions and conflicts, and I end up taking a tranquilliser.

2 February 1996

Tomorrow, my dear Zohreh is to have a *laparoscopy* – exploratory surgery – in order to make sure her cancer hasn't come back. I'm absolutely beside myself with worry, and visibly trembling. My dear little sister, Séverine, phones to tell me she has 'good vibrations' that everything will be all right. We agree that we need to talk and reassure each other, and that only people who've gone through this hell could understand the turmoil and anxiety we experience whenever one of us enters a period of uncertainty. We stick together to keep this horrible disease at bay. Something tells me, too, that everything will be all right for my sweet Zohreh.

10 February 1996

Last Saturday, Séverine, Rick and I visit Zohreh in hospital. It's one of those absolutely freezing-cold days. I drive, and my car almost stalls a few times, the day is so cold. We meet Zohreh's companion Jim and son Camran, and her mother Anouk, and all wait for the results.

We talk, and Jim offers me a cup of coffee. Rick recalls that

459

for Zohreh's first operation, he arrived late with Camran. Jim tells us he was alone when he received the terrible news that Zohreh had a tumour that was so big – the size of a grapefruit – the doctors were giving her only five years to live; later, however, the prognosis was modified, because the lymph nodes weren't involved and neither was metastasis. I think about how big my tumour was: between 10 and 12 centimetres, and about the five-year prognosis that Dr ES in Beirut gave Adelaide for me. What is it with these fast-growing tumours?

On the Saturday evening, when Zohreh is back home and I take her some soup I know she likes, she reminds me that Jim was also alone in the waiting room when my surgeon, Dr Yoto, came out of the operating room to tell him it hadn't been possible to do a lumpectomy and a mastectomy has had to be performed. Jim was alone in the waiting room because Juanita, wanting to distract Alban and ease his anguish, had taken Alban away to eat, having convinced him that the operation would probably take much longer to perform.

Here, in Zohreh's hospital, we're all there waiting when her surgeon, Dr Stafford, comes out of the operating room. She's in her forties but looks twenty-something. She tells us that everything's gone well, and that she's found no cancer. She's cut a few adhesions and taken several biopsies, which she'll send to a lab to be analysed. The results will be ready in a week's time. She's videoed the whole procedure using a new recorder, and she gives Camran the video. Rick asks her whether it wouldn't be worthwhile sending the biopsies for a second reading at the Carslaw clinic; however, she doesn't think it's necessary. Séverine is nevertheless glad that Rick asked the question.

We then go to see Zohreh. She's just woken up, and now she's all smiles – and doesn't she have one of the loveliest smiles I've ever seen? We're all very relieved.

When she's home later that evening, I take her the soup I know she likes. I'm very tired, and aware that I have to get up early the next morning in order to drive to Chicago's O'Hare Airport to meet Alban, who'll be returning from Paris. However, I need to see Zohreh tonight, and there's indeed something restorative about going to her house and talking to her. We reminisce at great length about our life, our past, our illness and the three turning points we have in common: exile, divorce and cancer.

⧗

This week, we have both good and bad news: all Zohreh's biopsies were negative, but Séverine is afraid her cancer might've come back. In her blood tests, her blood has been revealed to have a very high ACA – tumour marker. Although she still has to have other tests, she's petrified about having to tell her daughter the news if the cancer has in fact come back.

The next day, the bad news is confirmed: a 2 centimetre tumour has come back at exactly the same place at which the preceding tumour was located, the place from which the surgeon has already cut part of Séverine's small and large intestine, and bladder. She now has to have other tests to find out whether there's any other metastasis. Charles wishes she'd try other therapies, but she's afraid she'll lose the quality of life she's barely regained since the last round of the disease, in exchange for a painful prolongation of her life – because it's now clear to her that she's terminally ill. She's already suffered so, so much, my poor little sister. Will silent, heroic victims such as she remain invisible forever? Why does their situation go unnoticed by the broader public? Why is the torture they endure, often for nothing, surrounded by so much silence?

I can't bear to see her go through this again. When I ask

her exactly what her doctors have said, she tells me they think she knows too much for her own good! She laughs, but I'm revolted by what she's implying! Doctors can be so condescending sometimes; how are we to trust them when they make statements such as this? I keep these thoughts from Séverine, because she needs to keep communicating with the doctors with whom she's been able to establish a line of communication. She adds that despite everything, she and the doctors at least respect each other.

Cindy: I'm also angry when I read these doctors' remarks!

Alex: Keep emphasising how arrogant doctors are: it's very important!

> *My little sister Séverine,*
> *how I suffer with you.*
> *How I'd like to find the means*
> *to transform your illness into flowers and gardens;*
> *take our tears and change them into bouquets;*
> *take the flame so beautiful, so pure in you;*
> *illuminate the world with your fragile strength,*
> *with which you say, without the shadow of a doubt,*
> *'The venom consuming me didn't come from within;*
> *the earth, infested with man's destructive products,*
> *sends back, in a hideous reflection,*
> *the horror of a merciless image.'*

14 February 1996

I receive the report from my Paris doctor, Dr Esper, along with my test results. Everything's all right, except for three micro-calcifications within an *opacity* – an opaque area – in the other breast, which are 'to be watched'. I'm a bit scared when I read this, and yesterday I can't stop touching my breast: I'm obsessed with the idea of a recurrence. It's also the two-year anniversary of the discovery of my cancer, so I guess I'm somewhat more anxious than usual. Fortunately, my Alban is here, and I feel reassured when I cuddle up to him.

I truly understand why this disease is so terrible: because we live in perpetual fear of it. My friend Elizabeth comes to see me in my office. She's just learnt about Séverine, and is in shock. She's another person who lives in fear of pain, opacities and micro-calcifications. Her sister-in-law, Sarah, is dying with cancer that's metastasised from her breast to her bones. Today, we share our sorrow, despair and worries.

Séverine's doctors have told her they don't think it'd be appropriate to operate again, but have given her the following three options: (1) Operate; (2) Wait, and operate only if it becomes urgent to do so; (3) Start another round of chemotherapy ... And these are options? It's as if she were back at square one again! Hasn't she only just recovered from the bone-marrow transplant she had in December? Hasn't she just barely triumphed over two months of the most wretched sickness a person can have? It's simply disgusting to think she has to go through it all again!

21 February 1996

I'm reading a book that Séverine has lent me, about all the toxic products that are infesting us and poisoning the planet. Over the past 30 years, cancer has climbed by 40 per cent. People of my generation, the so-called Baby Boomers, will be much more affected than will people of Alban's generation, and if no cure is found, Alban's grandchildren will suffer even more – and no one is sounding the alarm?

Cindy: You've just been quoting books in which alarms are being sounded – the problem is that governments don't listen: the research is here, but the action that has to be taken is missing.

26 February 1996

This morning, I phone Séverine. She's in tears: over the past three weeks, her CA 125 – which marks the level of ovarian and some other cancers in the body – has doubled! According to the doctor who treated her at the hospital in Loyola, Chicago, while she was having the bone-marrow transplant, she should undergo all kinds of other treatment. However, she's refusing to be a guinea pig any longer. Crying, she says, 'Let me die in peace: I know my body. I want a decent quality of life for the time I have left to live. I want to go to France to see my family, as planned. My daughter would never forgive me if we didn't go. But I'm worried I'll get sick there and that I won't have the support system I've established here.' She breaks my heart; it's so unfair. I don't know what to say, so I stupidly blurt out, so as not to remain dumbfounded, 'There are miracles, you know – do you believe in them?'

She replies, 'No: I don't believe in miracles. I prefer to prepare myself for death well, rather than to live with the illusion I'll be healed.'

I have to admit she's right; nevertheless, hers is an unenviable dilemma.

Alban: If God existed, He'd have to be judged for His crimes against humanity!

And what about the devil: does he exist?

Jane: Did you notice they're both males?

⌛

I re-read Judith Brouste's *L'Etat d'alerte* (Brouste: 1994), which I've decided to include in the syllabus for one of my classes. This second time round, I'm getting more out of the book; in fact, because of her disease, the narrator starts seeking a profound truth she can be satisfied with. She moves away from the sado-masochistic relationships she's been seeking, which are reminiscent of her cancer treatment. She has us believe she finds love and faith. However, her words are very ambiguous: in the end, you don't understand whom or what she's addressing her italicised remarks to – but perhaps the ambiguity is intentional. I quote from the book (Brouste: 1994: 124) as follows.

> You arrive right after the time of before my illness, when I had abandoned what I was from the deepest part of myself, what is being transformed but never changes. I can no longer bear the tumultuous struggle against myself. Since then, we have been going forth, even at night, in this world that is no longer ours. We are going forth, as if everything around us were heading toward decay. As if a secret past were resurfacing in the present.

20 March 1996

Since I've been diagnosed as having cancer, I've started to more acutely notice the people who truly achieve things in life although they remain virtually anonymous, as opposed to the people who constantly boast but don't achieve much at all. It's fortunate that the former type of person exists on this earth: they make being alive worthwhile.

My neighbour Rod is exemplary in this way: he practically lives to help people. He's divested himself, as much as possible, of all his material possessions, and lives in a simple life simplicity that we can only admire. I'm feeling less sympathetic about the academics surrounding me: they seem to succeed better in the system by way of making more money and getting invited to all kinds of prestigious places. And despite having great prestige in their field, many of them are managing to keep complaining to me. However, I'm no longer touched by their recriminations within the life they've carved for themselves; instead, I look at what Rod and Alban have been able to achieve both humbly and silently, and without the self-aggrandisement I'm constantly hearing from other people.

Théophile is a person who lives the true message of the Gospel. And among the women I admire, there's Marianne Ferber, who's been able to move to high positions in academia, within her field, and even to administrative positions, without losing sight of the truly important issues or taking herself too seriously, while remaining humble and attentive to people. And there's Andrée Chedid, who remains humble even having had a long and highly successful writing career, receiving many awards and achieving so much. She's a person who truly practises what she writes about, and I include my own translation of the following passage from her book *Fraternité de la parole* (Chedid: 1976: 32–3).

> *The Journey*
> *From obstacles to terraces,*
> *from branches to darkness,*
> *the journey is merciless.*
> *Go hand in hand*
> *with so many others:*
> *Their fire, your fire,*
> *will be allied.*
> *Move on:*
> *the earth will take your shape.*
> *It abolishes only your mirrors!*
> *In spite of our enclosures, our Babels, our ravages,*
> *somewhere the word converges and unites us.*

I think I've become more selective as a result of my illness. These beautiful people are the role-models I now look up to, the people I'd like to emulate – will I ever measure up?

8 April 1996

Lately, I've been having many dreams, about mother. In one, I'm adopting a little girl, who's between six and nine years old, in Lebanon. In the dream, she's chubby, wears glasses and has Walkman headphones on her ears. Adelaide is chatting with her parents: a couple who, in real life, I met while I was visiting in Lebanon. In the dream, they were forced to get married because the wife got pregnant, and now they no longer have the financial means to meet the expenses incurred in raising the little girl. Adelaïde tells them I'm willing to take the child on the condition she bears my name: it's important to me that she has my name. Mother and Adelaide are happy about my decision, and are telling the couple, 'We told you she'd take her.' However, I'm thinking *How am I going to raise this child, who won't want to listen to me because she's always wearing a Walkman, and who won't want to communicate? How will I manage? I notice that Juanita is having quite a few problems with her daughter Laxsmi, even though Laxsmi is extraordinarily intelligent and charming – but how will I manage, and what should I do?*

Manicha: I know of one case in which after the civil war in Lebanon, a married couple in Paris adopted a Lebanese baby. Soon after, the man died of a heart attack. The woman now lives alone with the little girl, who's grown into a charming little person – raven-black hair, and very lively. Life is stronger than our anxiety – it's beyond our comprehension.

Another night, I have another dream. I'm in my Paris apartment, and lots of people are wanting me to put them up, among them mother and Adelaide. I'm asking mother, 'How am I going to find room for everyone?' But mother is reassuring me: 'We've already found our place; we've settled in.' Lots of beds are stacked up, on two or more levels. Later, in real life, I narrate my dreams over the phone to mother. She says, 'How nice: what beautiful dreams!' Later on, Adelaide tells me that after my phone call, she found mother still holding the receiver, smiling and talking to me: she thought I was still on the other end talking to her! My sweet mother: I hope she'll still be alive this summer, when I go to Lebanon. Adelaide tells me she's sleeping most of the time and barely waking up for one or two hours a day. Adelaide also says she's often talking to father in bed as if he were sleeping next to her!

Cindy: It's good to relate your dreams, and to make the connection between lived reality and the other side, through your mother.

⧗

Zohreh has lent me the latest issue of *Time* magazine (*Time*: April 1996), which is all about prostate cancer. This type of cancer is a real epidemic: one in five men are expected to contract it, and soon there'll be as many deaths every year from it as there are from breast cancer – about 50,000 deaths! Most of the treatments result in some level of impotence and incontinence.

Bettina: That's something that should be emphasised out there!

For this problem, hormone-therapy works for only a specific period of time; after that, the cancerous cells manage to circumscribe the treatment. These articles have a really chilling effect on me! Not much progress has been made in eliminating this plague; no absolutely reliable tests have been devised for detecting how aggressive the cancer is; and no progress has been made in the therapies available. It's a terrible disease, and men are only now starting to talk about it.

The person on the cover of the issue of *Time* is General Norman Schwartzkopf, who commanded the United States' troops during the Gulf War of the early 1990s, and in the magazine, he's represented as being a leader in the war against prostate cancer! Here we go again: war vocabulary and images for dealing with cancer! I read that the general's tumour was completely excised, through the procedure that's most reliable if there's no metastasis, but that the operation is also risky because the cancer is located in a very delicate place that's connected to the man's other internal organs.

Manicha: A powerful comparison: the 'surgical strikes' undertaken against Baghdad by Schwartzkopf during Operation Desert Storm were as 'harmless' for the surrounding area as real surgery is for prostate-cancer victims – hundreds of thousands of Iraqis were burnt alive, and other casualties were suffered, during that televised war.

⧗

Today, I have a reassuring phone call from Miriam. She tells me that her eye operation to remove skin cancer on her eyelid went very well. It was a small, rather mild type of cancer, and she wasn't disfigured as a result of the surgery. What a relief! I was so worried, because when she was first diagnosed she sounded as if she were in such a panic!

⧗

I'm reading Karen Berger and John Bostwick's *A Woman's Decision: Breast Cancer Treatment and Reconstruction* (Berger and Bostwick: 1994). It's been lent to me by Dr de Camara, who I went to consult about having reconstruction. I wish I'd read the book before I was treated and given the options I thought I'd have to take. It would've been helpful if I'd had all the information provided in the book and been able to see, by looking at its photos of reconstructed breasts, that the result is actually less frightening and more aesthetically acceptable than anything I'd seen up to then.

Manicha: The better informed we are, the more levelheaded we are in making our decisions.

15 April 1996

Today, Séverine comes for lunch, and is understandably depressed. She has pain in her bladder; she knows her days are numbered; she needs solitude, and not everyone understands that. There are some people she's avoiding and whose phone calls she's not returning. Alban tells her about a Chinese doctor, Dr Ting, he saw this weekend, for a problem he has with his hand, and tells her that the doctor helped him a lot. Dr Ting practises both traditional and alternative medicine, is very mild mannered, made a great impression on Alban and helped him ease the pain in his hand. Alban thinks Séverine should try to get in touch with Dr Ting.

Séverine breaks the news to me that Resa's cancer has come back. Resa is only 42, and was free of her first cancer for more than 10 years. I never thought she'd have to be hurt and go through that hell again. She has no insurance here in the States because she was originally treated in France. What'll she do?

I'm also depressed, because Israel is bombing the south of Lebanon. There are 300,000 refugees who don't know where to go. The Israelis are calling the offensive a 'clean-up operation' that they're directing at Hizbollah; however, if that's the case, why are they attacking civilians? They've killed almost 100 women and children who'd taken refuge in a United Nations compound. This blight is like a cancer coming back into Lebanon, my dear country.

Manicha: That says something about the level of respect Israel has for the UN: their flouting of the international resolutions with reference to their withdrawing from the territories they started occupying in 1967, and their setting up of two states: theirs, and one for the Palestinians.

Today, I'm shouting in my head, *Stop the world: I want to get off!* It's just too hard to live in times such as these. I realise what a toll the war in Lebanon has taken on my life. I couldn't bear having a recurrence, just as I can't bear to hear of cancer recurrences among my friends.

Both total warfare and some of these all-out, aggressive cancer therapies serve only to shift the problem from the source to the symptoms. Both situations are preventable, and both are an expression of failure to resolve imbalances while there's still time. Cancer and wars of mass destruction are the hallmarks of this century, and of a world that's bursting at the seams with contradictions and conflict that continues to spiral.

Jane: This paragraph contains one of your strongest ideas: that war and cancer are but symptoms of a deeper ill, something that exists on a much larger scale than does an isolated war or an individual person's cancer debacle. Media representatives and even so-called specialists in the field often fail to see the bigger picture: that's left to the philosophers and prophets, who spend their time crying out in the desert and are rarely taken seriously.

O'Hare Airport, 15 May 1996

My life seems to always be unfolding in airports, planes, trains, ships, meeting places, and arrival and departure destinations. Not so long ago, I was going to meet my parents, in Switzerland. It seems like yesterday that they were in relatively good shape – very young at heart, full of life and making plans for the future. Now, father is dead and mother is close to death.

Life goes by too quickly. Not so long ago, I'd just been hired at the University of Illinois. Zohreh was holding one of her young sons in her arms. Both of us were at the beginning of our career. Now, she's had three operations and undergone heavy chemotherapy treatment. The most recent operation was for horrible pains in her stomach that were being caused by skin adhesions strangling her intestines. The pains result from her *ovariectomy* but also from her stress and nervousness. Both of us must learn to relax and avoid stress; however, in the academic system, it's very difficult to do so.

We're having a very difficult winter: ice and sub-zero temperatures, and it seems we've had no springtime. I'm glad to be leaving for a while – and I'm anxious to be with Alban.

Jane: It's occurred to me that people here live their life as if they're in airports, always looking at their watches, like people who have a plane to catch. The artificiality of the modern airport as a structure, with all the so-called amenities and comforts – you could practically live in an airport these days – isn't unlike that of the shopping mall, which has replaced what used to be public gathering spots. I think the airport could serve as an interesting metaphor in your work in general, and not simply because you travel a lot.

Tunis, 26 May 1996

I'm understanding why the dramatic adaptation of my novel can't be performed in Tunis again: the women performers have too many sources of tension and dissenting voices among them. Everything's become so complicated – it's a wonder the play was ever produced in the first place. The first time around, the concept reached fruition on an impulse of the heart and in a surge of enthusiasm. Now, however, the heart is gone, wounded and erased as a result of all the quarrelling. The production had to stop.

⧖

We celebrate Azza's birthday, and her father, Ramses, comes to share the birthday cake. He speaks about illness as being an evil we program in ourselves. I find his remarks repulsive and infuriating. I tell him that I think the intention inherent in the remarks is to victimise the victim, and that I'm surprised to hear them coming from a former Marxist; however, I then realise I shouldn't be astonished, because reformed Marxists are similar to most converts but often worse because they've had to fight against the very thing they'd believed in so blindly: their articles of faith. Ramses says to me, 'Before, we suffered for the workers, the miners and so on; we got sick fighting for them, but it was useless, because there was nothing we could do anyway. Now, we try to transform things from within ourselves, from our own wounds; it's much more effective.'

I reply that we should do both: work *on* and *from* the inside in order to effect change for the better on the outside.

Manicha: For public intellectuals, the fact that the common folk never go fast enough for them is the source of their neverending frustration! The common folk are all rotten sell-outs, or asleep, or hopeless – can't you see a Sorbonne-style Pol Pot on the horizon? I say, 'Let's do what we can for ourselves and help whoever we can on the way, and it'll all come together in the end.

⌛

I'm thinking about Séverine, suffering so much and dying of the same ovarian cancer that killed her mother. I'm thinking about her daughter, screaming every time she hears anyone mention cancer or recurrences. I'm thinking about the letter that Séverine wrote to Eric Siegel and other positive thinkers – everyone who believes that miracles spring from the conscience and that they come about because we will them to by working spiritually on the conscience. My sweet Deirdre, who's come along on this trip with Cindy and me, puts the problem with this way of thinking very succinctly: 'It's easy to talk about healing ourselves from the inside when we haven't been sick, but it's a completely different story when a devastating disease hits us in our flesh.'

29 May 1996

I'm travelling on the train from Tunis to La Marsa with Cindy and our friend Deedee. Yesterday, we visit Manoubia, Meriem's cleaning lady, who lives in a popular district located between Gammarth and La Marsa. It's thanks to Deirdre, who made special contact with Manoubia, that we're able to go. It's a truly memorable experience, the height of our stay in Tunis.

Manoubia's story is fascinating. In the district, she bought a piece of land with some help from her father. She started building parts of her house slowly with the help of some neighbours, who also provided her with a power line because she wasn't yet connected to the electricity grid. She's so excited about having us over, even though she feels sick and is running a slight fever. She gets out all her jewellery to show us; burns incense; plays music on a 'boom-box', complete with flashing, psychedelic lights; displays her many cassettes; and shows us her collection of talismans, such as a desiccated chameleon the head of which she cut off to put in her door lock. She and Meriem dance together like sisters – a delight to watch. Deedee has brought her a big white towel from the States, and in return, Manoubia gives her an African-Arab dress. Deedee puts the dress on, and Meriem tucks a cushion inside the front of it, thereby giving Deedee a round belly, and everyone begins to ululate, Tunisian style. Everyone then makes a wish that Deedee conceive.

Manoubia is exuberant: she shows us her driver's license, and proudly displays the title deed for her piece of land. She tells us her brother, Eli, asked for half of it to build on but that she refused, on the grounds that she didn't get along with his wife. He said that if she didn't accept, he'd stop talking to her. Her answer to that threat was that he didn't really love her if the love was only for the things she could give him. As it turned out, sister and brother are no longer on speaking terms, and if Manoubia goes to visit Eli and his wife, they refuse to see her and pretend to be not at home.

This woman has a rare courage and strength. She tells us that the people of her district talk behind her back because she lives alone – they say she must be abnormal, a prostitute or a Jew! She was married for seven years but then divorced, and now prefers to live alone. She's making all kinds of future plans to enlarge her yard, get a shower and make all kinds of improvements. When she gets home from doing her cleaning work, she sews, listens to music and is happy to be alone. The only thing she's anxious about is that she'll die alone in the house and no one will notice. Her mother died when Manoubia was 15, and her father remarried. He backs her up and gives her all the support he can. She shows us his photo, and kisses it to express her deep love for him. She invites Deedee and her husband Art to come and stay with her next time they visit Tunisia.

I remember Umm Ashraf and some other women I visited in the popular districts of Cairo. Compared with Manoubia, they weren't as independent and were unable to assert themselves. Their condition seemed to be much more desperate, and compared with the environment Manoubia lives in, their environment was sordid.

Manicha: I don't get why she's like a Jewish woman – somehow a 'super' character – just because she lives alone: what's so negative about living alone?

It has to do with both being admired and being rejected, I think.

30 May 1996

Amel and I go to a kynesthesiology session: she's making me go back to the centre in order to untie the knots of my past. The first knot was tied in my mother's womb: my feeling of well-being as well as my fear of hurting my mother. Then, at age nine, there were the knots of the negative image I had of myself as being too plump and my desire to be different. At age 33, there were again two knots: my divorce and the war in Lebanon. And now, at age 50, there are another two: cancer and my fear of hurting people. According to Amel, what comes back over and over again is my fear of hurting people whereas I should be thinking more about myself. It's clear that if I'm to heal completely, I have to understand and untie these knots, these unresolved dramas of my past. I'm grateful to Amel for making me do this work and helping me locate these wounds.

Amel remarks how strange it is that my fear of hurting people keeps coming back. I believe that our session together also reflects my relationship with her. When I learn that she suffered very much when she heard I was ill, and that she felt as if the earth were moving under her feet, it pains me to think I hurt her that much. It's true I don't like to cause people pain, especially the people I love. No one likes to cause people pain, and no one should.

Jane: What conclusions have you drawn from this, then? Could this form of self-denial have been a cause of your illness? Was it the very fact that you didn't let out your anger at people when they probably deserved it? Was it that you preferred to absorb hurt rather than inflict it? If there's some sort of closed system of positive and negative energy – and it seems that Amel leans in that direction – you've absorbed more than your share of the latter. Could that be a cause of your illness? Once again, it seems that the victims are being victimised for not performing better. I think this is quite an interesting debate, and one that I'm sure few medical doctors want to participate in!

Thank you, Jane, for expressing the debate so beautifully!

Paris, 17 June 1996

Augustus's wife Joy and their son Joël are here in Paris with me, and Augustus is arriving tomorrow. I've managed to get closer to Joy, because we've had time alone together. She's told me things I never knew about her life: that her father bullied her mother, Gabrielle, so much, by taking a second wife and throwing Gabrielle out of the house, that Gabrielle lost her mind. Gabrielle is considered clinically insane, but Joy thinks her condition is the result of what she had to put up with – that she reacted as if she'd lost her mind but that she's in fact quite lucid. Joy was raised in a Chinese Methodist orphanage with two of her sisters. There, the girls were taught the Bible and about Christianity, but Joy thought the teachings were rather superficial.

One of Joy's sisters and her best friend left the orphanage to become prostitutes, a move that Joy didn't understand.

She believes that women can make money in Singapore through working in jobs other than prostitution. She's persuaded her sister to get out of the racket, and has even let her use her apartment. She wants to persuade the best friend to do the same, but says it won't be easy to do so. Joy cries, and tells me that her mother, Gabrielle, was forced to live in an asylum and on the street, with only a plastic bag containing all her belongings. She carried the bag everywhere, and during the final years of her life slept on the steps of the temple, her only refuge. She remembers her mother coming to the orphanage to see her and her sisters. She brought them meals of rice and chicken, and Joy remembers thinking it would've cost her mother a lot to buy such a wholesome meal. Gabrielle watched her three daughters eat, to make sure they had equal portions.

Manicha: The image that springs to mind is that famous shot of the young Chinese man with his plastic bag, standing in Tianenmen Square in June 1989, facing down the tanks and diverting them a few from their deadly task for a few minutes.

I tell Joy that I understand why Augustus is so concerned about helping orphans, and that I understand why he told me one day that if anything happened to him, he wanted us to take care of her. Joy starts crying again: she doesn't like remembering all these painful memories, and rarely talks about them.

Augustus tells her that I'll include her story in one of my books if she agrees to open up about it. This is what I'm doing at present, not only to keep that promise but to provide yet another example that the diseases women suffer are often social ones, including spousal abuse, prostitution and total rejection by society. Joy's case isn't an isolated one, and is painfully familiar: her father was completely irresponsible and abusive, and never cared for any of his children, including the children of a third wife whose existence Joy's family discovered only after the father died. Among the women of the world, home is where the hurt is.

In getting to know my sister-in-law Joy better, I've experienced a lot of happiness – there's something so warm and beautiful about her. Whereas I used to think she was rather cold, I now realise she was just shy underneath a guise of indifference. We've gotten much closer this time, and I love the way she's raising Joël: calmly and attentively. The little boy reflects this calmness and assurance: he looks very secure and at ease.

On the plane between Beirut and Paris, 25 June 1996

Théophile has told me not to put off my next trip to see mother for too long, and I know what he's implying. Therefore, when Ghassan Tuéni sends me a ticket to go to Lebanon to help organise a conference about Mediterranean poetry, I seize the opportunity to go there, even though I'm scheduled to return there in July in order to take care of mother. Théophile isn't one to be alarmist: if he thinks mother doesn't have much time left to live, it must be true.

Alban was hoping his doctor would tell him he could stop having the anti-testosterone treatment, because it's making him impotent; however, his doctor has said he shouldn't stop. His PSA has dropped to 0,3, which is good, and it's thereby been revealed that the cancerous cells are reacting to the treatment; there might still be some left, though: escaping and travelling around, ready to metastasise. There's no absolutely reliable test for them. This is why the disease is so frightening: it's invisible.

Can we call it lovemaking when only one of us achieves orgasm and the other is prevented from reaching those heights?

Jane: *[I first wrote 'getting on that plain'.]* This is actually quite a funny word play here. The noun you need isn't 'plain', which means only 'level areas of land', as in the Great Plains of the Midwest. Rather, you need 'plane', which in French means 'plan, niveau' and so on – a geometrical term. However, in the expression 'getting on that plane' in your sentence, one would more readily understand 'monter dans cet avion-là', and because your subtitle for this section is 'On the plane between Beirut and Paris', I have visions of what you and Alban were doing 'on the plane'. It made me laugh – sorry!

I'm reminded of Alban imagining Dr Esper in his office!

Although Alban tells me he gets a lot of pleasure out of giving me pleasure, I get frustrated because I can't satisfy him the way I used to: yet another of the many ways in which this disease is so unfair. It's just one more of the many forms of 'collateral damage' inflicted on us as a result of this unjust cancer war.

⧗

My trip to Lebanon is painful but essential. Mother is now nothing but skin and bones: she weighs only 48 kilos, and some of her bones are even showing through. Adelaide is being very sweet with her: she puts her in bed in the fetal position, so she's more comfortable. Adelaide changes mother's bed sheets and clothes several times a week, and sometimes twice a day, to make mother feel better. Mother has to be spoon-fed now, so I feed her in that way; I also sing, which makes her very happy. She's the one who used to love singing and whose voice I inherited; now, she can barely speak, let alone sing. I could tell that when she hears me, for her it's almost like she's singing herself again – her whole face beams with joy, despite the pain

480

she's suffering all over her body. So I sing and sing: religious and folk songs; Swiss and French songs, from Piaf to Brel; songs in English and Arabic – whatever comes to mind. For mother, I do my entire repertoire. I find singing so therapeutic!

Manicha: That's absolutely true – it must be physiological.

It's probably both a mind reaction and a body reaction.

⧗

The mountain house in which the conference is being organised, the Nadia Tuéni Foundation, in Beit Merri, is a real wonderland. Located in a pine forest, it overlooks Beirut and the Mediterranean Sea. Here, in these beautiful surroundings, far above the traffic pollution and noise, I can imagine how Nadia Tuéni was inspired to write her poignant poetry.

We've all been very moved to see that Ghassan Tuéni has been very faithful to the memory of this extraordinary Lebanese Francophone poet. I try to be faithful in my own way, by teaching her work in my classes back in the States. While I'm here in Lebanon, her text *Juin et les mécréantes*: *June and the Miscreants*, which Roger Assaf has adapted for the theatre, is being staged at the Beirut Theatre. In the text, the number four is a thematic emblem: four women; four different Lebanese identities; four religions representing Lebanon: the Druze, the Christian, the Muslim and the Jew; four voices; four ways; and four wounds, expressing the women's despair, suffering, joys and sorrow against the background of the outbreak of war. I include my translation of an extract from the text, in *Les œuvres poétiques complètes* (Tuéni: 1986: 125), as follows.

Can one keep the desert from leaving with one's body,
naked as a prayer?
O, sumptuous rottenness!
Each day is a resurrection,
with the earth's complicity.
All those unconcerned with the sun
make a liquid noise.
The nights,
here and there,
have the flight of birds in their eyes,
and I cry the time of a star:
the one who stole my death.

As always, it's a very moving experience just being here in Lebanon: centre of culture; crossroads for so many fascinating exchanges; a country that's suffered so much. I'm enjoying being with people I can communicate with at the deepest level.

On the plane between Beirut and Paris, 20 July 1996

It's a month later, and I've been back to Lebanon to be with mother and take care of her, and as I always do.

During this trip, I take many walks down memory lane. I walk around the campus of the Beirut University College – BUC, in Ras-Beirut. During my childhood and adolescence, these hills were still wild and covered with wildflowers; birds sang in them, and whenever it rained, little torrents of water flowed downhill. Now, the hills have been disfigured by luxurious concrete high-rises, many of which are unoccupied because few people can afford them. It's sad to see Beirut being transformed into a huge 'construction' monster.

Some young gay people come to see me, and several times we have coffee at the City Café, right below BUC. It's a very polluted and noisy spot, but I'm glad to visit it with the young people. One young man confesses he feels rejected because he's gay. A young woman tells me that in this society, the only outlet for sex is marriage. She's made to think she has to find someone to marry in order to be accepted, and she feels marginalised because she doesn't have anyone.

I tell my companions about my life, including how I lived and experienced life when I was an adolescent, details I share in my novel *L'Excisée: The Excised* (Accad: 1982). I tell them I believe that Christ came to liberate, not to chain people up with rules and dogmas. There's no reason they can't be accepted in the church just because they're gay: their rejection makes no sense to me. I feel that things haven't really changed since I was young; rather, the bleaker side of history seems to be repeating itself and spiralling out of control. The promises of modernisation haven't been kept, and the spectre of chaos and disease looms greater than ever.

⏳

Here on the plane, my writing is interrupted when I have a conversation with the passenger sitting next to me: Fatima, a woman from Saïda, located in the south of Lebanon. This is the first time she's flown, and her brothers in Canada sent her a ticket to cheer her up after her husband died, two years ago, of liver cancer at the age of 41. She has four children, the youngest of whom is three. Fatima's mother is taking care of her now, but. while she's talking to me about how much she misses her husband, she cries. They loved each other since they were children, and got along very well. She also lost her father to cancer, when she was quite young, and her mother raised the family by herself.

Fatima's husband was feeling well when the disease struck, out of the blue. Nothing could be done for him.

Fatima is now very conscious of the importance of food and the environment. She gives me the title of a book in Arabic, *Al-Ashfa' Bi 'Ayat Al Qur'an*, which is about healing by using herbs and includes verses cited in the Qur'an (Koran); she tells me that *hab al baraka*, the anti-cancer grains that Maria gave me to take, are cited in it. Alban has told me it's a medicinal plant that's described in many medical books.

Fatima explains that the grain has to be washed and then browned in a pan, and that it produces its own oil. In Saudi Arabia, oil is extracted from the grain and sold on the market. It can also be ground to make a paste. It can be used in all kinds of dishes, rubbed into the skin as an ointment and taken as a medicine. Fatima tells me that dates and garlic are supposed to be excellent antidotes for cancer, and that we should eat a clove of raw garlic at least once a day, and avoid eating meats other than fish; unfortunately, though, her husband didn't like fish. I tell her about cabbage, carrots and lemons. I'm deeply moved by this woman from the south of my country. At Paris's airport, we cry when we part company. I show her where to go to catch her plane for Canada, and wish her well.

Cancer is really everywhere. You can't sit down next to anyone, anywhere, who doesn't have a story to tell like Fatima's.

On the plane between Paris and Chicago, 30 August 1996

Alban and I see doctors for him because he's having headaches and feeling diminished as a result of the medical treatment he's undergoing. One doctor tells us it isn't possible to suppress a hormone as in Alban's treatment without suffering 'side' effects such as fatigue and ageing. Alban responds, 'It's hard to be deprived of sexuality the way I am!' The doctor suggests he take Prozac to 'improve his mood' – I can hardly believe it! – and that he take painkillers to alleviate his headaches.

Bettina: Utter nonsense!

I'm glad that Alban is able to speak his mind, but I realise we've reached a dead end with these doctors and their so-called solutions. What can we do? Where can we turn?

⧗

The day before, I go shopping. I see lots of bras that have little pockets to fill underneath the breasts, and thereby lift and push the breasts up. This type of bra is called the Wonder Bra, and apparently it's now fashionable to have round breasts pouring out of one. I notice there are no bras that have pockets for prostheses: the manufacturers are obviously unaware of the disease that's hitting 10 per cent of the population! I look at these bras I can no longer wear, and 'wonder'!

Jane: If you've ever watched the Academy Awards ceremony, you'll realise it seems to be a contest to see how much breast the female actor can get to bulge out her Wonder Bra without having the whole thing spill over it. It's a real engineering feat: a 'wonder'! My mother always laughs when she's watching the Golden Globe Awards ceremnoy: she says the only globes the viewer sees are the ones bulging out of the women's dresses.

It's also interesting to note that many of those breasts are in fact implants, for making the woman look more 'busty' than nature made her. I have two friends from my youth who had breast implants after they were married! Did they want to give their husbands something to play with, and to have something that'd make them 'look sexy' at work or on the street? And as if America has a 'street' any more! It's a mystery to me why anyone

485

would run the risk of implanting silicone in her body just to look like a Barbie doll.

⌛

I can hardly believe it – I knew it had to happen, but I kept hoping for a miracle: my little sister Séverine has died, at 8.30 yesterday morning. It's Zohreh who phones from Urbana to let me know. She leaves a message on my answering machine, telling me it would be healing for them to have me there in the States tomorrow for the various ceremonies that are to take place.

I'm glad to be busy packing: I have something concrete to focus on, but I can't help thinking about Séverine all the time anyway. Her death is going straight to my heart, and it's a deep, deep hurt. She wanted so much to live to see her daughter at least through secondary school, but she wasn't granted even that small wish! I'll miss her terribly. I can't help reiterating how unjust and arbitrary it all is.

On the plane, I write the following few lines to read out at one of the ceremonies.

Séverine, my little sister,
I see you showing your scars to Eva's camera,
with a touch of shyness,
joining me in complicity,
in our common revolt.
I see you when you first arrived in the French depart-
ment –
you were only twenty;
I was thirty –
already committed, speaking out against the injustices.
We connected immediately.
You left for Senegal,
one of our first exchange students.

How much hope in your eyes.
I saw you there, with Molly,
in the popular districts of Dakar:
misery, poverty, human warmth.
It was the theatre of these districts that interested you.
Incredible research you carried out,
left in cassettes;
never put down on paper,
as if afraid to betray the thoughts of
these creators/rebels.
(I see you smiling as I write this; I can hear you say,
'Evelyne, aren't you romanticising?')
I want to sing for you, Séverine.
I'm here in front of you,
my hands wounded by your suffering;
my heart heavy with our tears.
I want to sing, Séverine, so that hope will rise up;
so that your daughter will pick up the torch;
dry her tears;
understand that your struggle wasn't in vain.
I remember, and Zohreh remembers,
you were always present when we needed you.
Zohreh told me that every time she went for chemo,
she opened her eyes, and there you were.
One day, I'd had enough with radiation.
I called you;
you rushed to see me.
We both cried; laughed; cried
over our cancer fate.
O, my tender friend,
all the wounds we shared.
You are life's beauty,
hope for a better world.
Dawn's flowers open up
in the snows of your suffering.

You're reborn to ecstasy.
The white mountain kneels in front of you.
With you I climbed the highest peaks;
the barbed wires couldn't hurt us.
We contemplated a placid, shining sea,
so smooth on the horizon;
in the end, a scarlet sun was waiting.
Séverine, Séverine, bird of the south;
Séverine, Séverine, jewel of the sea:
she gave back life to the sea;
she built alone in the enclosure
a road engraved with images;
she came alone in the evening;
she opened all the hopes.

Chorus:
She was born for the stars,
for the breath that runs in her.
She was born for the voyage
of the earth, of the sky, of the sea.
She was broken, mutilated.
She was wounded; she was killed.
She went to the sea,
and the sea accepted her.

Beirut Airport, 30 December 1996

So much is happening all the time here in Lebanon. My heart is both heavy and light from all the wounds, which are slowly healing; reopening quickly with the slightest movement of wings, with any aggressiveness, with every harsh word, with each painful image, with each unassailable dogma, with all the reminiscences this country holds for me.

Mother is no longer here. She died in September, a few

days before her birthday; father also died during his birth-day month, March. I hope they're together now, united in their eternal love!

Noureddine Aba also died a few days after mother. He was certainly one of the most human and touching North African writers, poets and playwrights I had the pleasure to know. I remember when Milo gave me Noureddine's 90-page dramatic poem about Palestine; I was a student at Indiana University, and when I read it, I was so moved I cried and cried. I translated it in one stretch, and I know that Noureddine also wrote it in one stretch, after he'd viewed films of Palestinians being burnt with napalm by the Israëlis during the 1967 war. Jay illustrated it with very fine and highly elaborate pen and ink drawings.

At the time, I was very inexperienced and shy. Emile encour-aged me to go and meet Nourredine during a journey to Lebanon because I had a stopover in Paris. And that's how I developed a long friendship with Noureddine and his wife Madeleine. My translation of his dramatic poem was subse-quently published in a bilingual edition, entitled *Montjoie Palestine!, or Last Year in Jerusalem* (Accad: 1980). Noureddine and Madeleine came to the States several times to attend conferences and teach, and I visited them in Algeria.

In 1990 in Algiers, Nourredine used his own funds to cre-ate a literary foundation through which prizes would be awarded to Algerian writers who both remained faithful to their identity and demonstrated their tolerance and feeling of brotherhood with the larger world. Any Francophone researcher was also eligible for the prize. Within the chaotic context that prevails in Algeria today, Noureddine was attempting, through forming this brave initiative, to fight against the intolerance and violence that were threatening to tear apart the country he loved. He died heartbroken about the atrocities that were taking place in his land.

As a way of bidding him *adieu*, Madeleine sent to people who knew him and had written to her a few lines from *Le chant perdu au pays retrouvé* (Aba: 1978). In them, Noureddine expresses his deep faith and a message of hope, which Madeleine believes must absolutely be transmitted. I include my translation of the lines as follows.

> *... And so that everything might be said, I add*
> *that it is not the origins that make man*
> *but man who gives to the origins*
> *their value, their richness;*
> *that it is not the country that makes a man*
> *but man who gives to countries*
> *their prestige and their light and their spirit;*
> *that it is he, the quality of his love,*
> *the strength of his faith,*
> *that are its ligneous and indestructible stem,*
> *that gives birth to its branches,*
> *that carry hope*
> *of a single fraternity,*
> *in tune with the universe ...*
> *... Tomorrow, I will depart*
> *before the sun*
> *is high in the sky ...*

⌛

It's hard seeing mother's empty bed, and even harder seeing the painful expression on the face of Sana, the fiancée of one of my nephews, as she gazes at the empty bed. Father's place has already been empty for more than two years – back when I started my cancer.

We're all here in Lebanon: we, the five children of this wonderful couple who were my parents. We're making plans to complete all kinds of projects in order to start fulfilling our parents' dreams. We're talking as if we still have more than half our life to live, but I believe we have about a quarter of our life left if we're lucky!

Nevertheless, it's good to be making these plans, to be starting to building structures, in both the concrete and the spiritual sense of the word, and to be mobilising people to work and live within them. We hope we'll be able to come to the aid of the abused, the people whose life has been thrown into disorder as a result of the war and of an endless series of aggressions of all kinds. It's good we're all here, united in our desire to realise our parents' vision, in building much needed bridges of peace among the various communities in this part of the world. When I die, will my nieces and nephews be as careful about fulfilling my wishes? Can I count on them as father counted on me?

While I'm in Lebanon, I visit the women's prison in Ba'abdat, with Agnès and her daughter Anne. We bring the women Christmas presents, and Agnès has asked me to bring my guitar along to sing. The prison is right next to the hospital. It comprises four rooms, the area of each of which is between 20 and 30 square metres, and in which between 12 and 20 women live.

Today, all the women are lined up next to each other. Most of them are chain smoking, so it's almost impossible to breathe in the rooms, in which only a tiny dormer window, close to the ceiling, lets in barely a ray of light or any air: stifling rooms, and wounded humanity – most of the women come from society's most disadvantaged groups.

There are a few foreign women: a small group of Sri Lankans, who've been thrown in gaol for not having the proper residency papers. These group members aren't smoking, and I think how hard it probably is for them to be suffocating in this terrible atmosphere, unable to say anything or go outside for a breath of fresh air.

Agnès tells me the food is atrocious – it looks more like

491

vomit than food. The women who have a family get their food from their husband or children and often share it with the other prisoners. I think about these poor foreign women, who are often persecuted in their own country: they were hoping to earn a bit of money by being slave labourers in Lebanon, but have ended up in these prisons and been left to rot.

We distribute some presents and sweets, then sing and talk with the women. I'm struck by one woman: very beautiful; all dressed in black; and all hunched up in a corner, crying and refusing to talk; her beautiful white face, with its halo of shiny, jet-black hair, is all puffed up from the crying. The women around her try to console her, and feel sorry for her. They tell us she's been there for only a short time. According to them, she's innocent, and was nothing but a dancer in a cabaret. On the night she was stopped, the police raided the club, and she was thrown into gaol for no obvious reason. Her back hurts, because the police beat her up.

Towards the end of the visit, as we're leaving, the woman accepts our invitation to speak with her. I say to her, 'Soon, you'll be out: your brother has come to get you out. The women here have told me you're innocent: you didn't do anything bad.'

She responds, 'I did something bad.' I ask her what it was. She replies, 'I threw out this bastard who was trying to abuse me!'

She reminds me of Ferdaws, the character in Nawal El Saadawi's *Woman at Point Zero* (El Saadawi: 1983). I wonder, now, what's happened to her.

⧗

I'm thinking of Yvette's niece, Chantelle, who one day was kidnapped and strangled when she was going to school, in Philadelphia. Chantelle was a beautiful young teenager:

innocent; trusting; just opening up to life; brutally crushed in the prime of her youth. Yvette continues to cry rivers of tears, tears that'll never run dry.

⏳

I'm thinking of Séverine's burial ceremony. It seemed to defy all reason: I couldn't believe that Séverine was in that little box filled with her ashes. Two pastors talked about her beauty, her strength and her straightforwardness. Samira brought three red flowers, a kind of flower that kind Séverine liked. I asked Samira for one of them. We walked together towards the box, and deposited them on top of it. Séverine's daughter let a red balloon fly in the sky above us – it climbed happily … and disappeared. Like Yvette's, my tears became rivers, rivers that flowed into the sea of our common tears.

EPILOGUE

MEDICINE, DEATH, AND RECOVERY

I speak out in favor of a kind of medicine that will take biological advances and experimental results and apply them without delay, one that will resort to modalities as complex as the disease itself, capable of shifting as knowledge of the disease evolves, or in response to an individual case, modalities that can nevertheless still be scientifically evaluated with the proper methods, but that will also be humanely applied. There remains much to be done in this area. And yet today, it is considered somehow indecent to raise this issue at specialized conferences, both in France and elsewhere. On the contrary, the protocol involving the practice of drawing lots is becoming increasingly commonplace … It can be expected that over the coming decades, there will be a steady increase in cancers among the sixty-plus age bracket. We can also expect, unless we change our lifestyles, a considerable increase in suffering and costs. (Israël: 1998)

Within a same kind of cancer, breast or thyroid cancer for instance, there are found these same differences between cancers that are histologically distinct, which evolve so slowly that they are almost never fatal, while others hurdle headlong toward inexorable death within a few months, no matter what the treatment might be … Nearly all cancers are preceded by pre-cancerous lesions … Over the first five years following treatment, about 80% of recurrence or metastases become manifest, with the others appearing within five to twenty years later. Once this period has elapsed, no more metastases occur. One could therefore consider that patients who show no metastasis after the twentieth year beyond treatment are patients in whom none had existed at the time of the initial treatment either ... In some cancers, the spread occurs very early, when the tumor measures only a few millimeters in diameter. In contrast, other tumors can reach enormous proportions (7 or 8 cm in diameter) without producing metastasis. Human cancers are therefore different from experimental cancers, in which practically all tumors engender metastasis once a critical size has been reached. (Tubiana: 1998)

Women who do not recover from their breast cancer are not to be held personally responsible. The characteristics of the disease are alone to blame. The powerlessness of modern science is the foremost cause of therapeutic failures. The field of cancer is not wanting for medical practitioners, but for true medicine. No one as yet has found the ultimate weapon against cancer, and science is advancing at a slow pace. Unlike leukemia, cancer of the testicles or Hodgkin's disease, the cure rate for breast cancer has not improved for decades ... On the one hand, doctors never cease to reiterate, and rightly so, that every breast cancer is unique; and yet medicine is moving increasingly toward standardization of treatment. Awaiting further progress, we would do better to adapt medicine to women, instead of the reverse. (Gros: 1994)

Help for our cells can come from the outside, especially from what we absorb. For instance, cruciferous vegetables, Brussels sprouts, broccoli and of course cauliflower, all contain phenols and indoles, substances that can trigger enzyme chains for cell detoxification ... But we are placing our greatest hope on vitamin A and derivatives of retinoic acid, which are natural and synthetic substances known as retinoids ... Retinoids are capable of interfering in the cancer-producing process at several levels: by protecting those areas sensitive to carcinogenic DNA, called nucleophilic zones; by modulating cell proliferation, since the division of a cell altered by a mutagenic substance is what definitively sets the lesion of the DNA; by promoting cell differentiation, which amounts to forcing cells to die of old age, thus promoting tissue renewal; and lastly, retinoids can stimulate immune reactions ... Let us be reminded, however, that although epidemiological data suggest that retinoids play a protective role with regard to a number of mucous membrane cancers, there is also the risk of a possible negative effect in the case of prostate cancer ... Selenium, a mineral found in soil and water, though in uneven amounts, depending on the region, has also recently experienced a certain popularity, based especially on animal studies ... We are hoping that this substance will help diminish some widespread human cancers, too ... But a macrophage, for instance, is capable of the best and the worst. It can both detoxify an organism and engender certain carcinogens. Even good old vitamin C, with its lemon-like taste, has certain weaknesses: though it successfully inhibits formation of some nitrosamines, it can also promote the formation of other molecules of that nasty ilk. (Jasmin: 1989)

A friend of mine, a professor of public health, knowing that I was writing this book, said to me, 'Whatever else you talk about, be sure to tell your readers how to tell your doctor or provider if you decide to stop taking hormones.' She admitted that, for all of her professional success, she was afraid to tell her gynecologist that she wanted to go off hormones after ten years.

Her fear reflects a sad reality, both about doctors' attitudes toward patients and about the pressure on doctors to prescribe hormones. When a woman chooses not to follow her doctors' advice, the medical profession calls it a 'compliance problem.' ... It's an appalling attitude, but most women, whether they want to be or not, are intimidated by it ... Before you go, marshal all your questions and arguments. Write down your points. Bring a friend with you to the appointment for moral support if you need to ... It's often helpful to bring a tape recorder as well ... If your provider has an opinion, ask why, and what data he or she is basing it on. It's important to feel that your provider is a partner you can work with to find the right approach to fit your life and values. If it doesn't feel right, it probably isn't – and you should see someone else. Don't forget other options – a herbalist, a traditional Chinese doctor, a homeopath. Remember: This isn't a disease you're treating; it is a normal part of life. (Love: 1997)

On this Friday the 13th of November, 1998, I'm looking out the window of my sixteenth-floor apartment in the 18th *arrondissement* of Paris. Spread before my eyes is the Montmartre cemetery. By now, almost all the leaves from the chestnut trees have fallen: yellow, red, ochre, brown and purple. Soon there'll be nothing left to look at but the gravestones, arranged in a semi-circle and set within the roundness of the Paris landscape, which I rediscover each time with renewed pleasure.

The Paris sky has an extraordinary, ever changing light. Its clouds break apart and rearrange themselves, and it's both threatening and comforting, and reflects the hours and the seasons: it metamorphoses in tune with the rhythms of Nature. I feel good here. Of all the places I call home – Urbana, Beirut and Tunis – it's here that I can write best, perched above the white gravestones that are dotted with splashes of colour: flowers and yellow leaves, like pictures painted by the Impressionists who once lived and worked in this neighbourhood, surrounded by the trees of the amiably round Montmartre hillside. Death here is peaceful: I'm not frightened by it – or rather, I'm no longer afraid of it.

In this book, I haven't reflected much on the question of my own death, as my friend Gilles points out as follows.

Gilles: I have reservations with reference to your explanation of the environment, whether psychological or chemical, as being the cause. Yes, the environment plays a part, but cancer is as old as humankind itself, and dates back to long before the onset of pollution. The practitioners of Chinese medicine puzzled over it long ago, and weren't particularly traumatised as a result. It's the whole issue of having one civilisation in which people don't consider death to be an evil, and another civilisation, ours, in which people refuse to accept it. And if we don't accept it, it's often out of narcissism – our great perversion. On this point, I'll leave you to reflect on this one feature, which really struck me: you almost never speak of the threat of death, only of how your image is being affected.

Gilles is right, up to a point. When I found out I had cancer, I actually didn't think about death. I can't really say why; I just knew I'd make it through. Perhaps it has to do with how suddenly and unexpectedly it all happened. If the idea of death ever did occur to me, I drove it out of my mind. I felt too young to make my exit: I said to myself, *No, not yet: there are still so many things to accomplish!* I repeat this sentence to myself even now, because a person never gets over cancer completely. We learn to live with the fear of a relapse, of pain and of death. However, I can't come to terms with my death. I accepted it for my mother, because she was old and sick, and was yearning for deliverance. I was less accepting of my father's death, because when he was struck down by cancer, he was a man who was still vigorous and full of life, and wanted so much to live.

I most definitely didn't accept the death of Séverine, or of Florence or Nnennaya: they were much too young, and had yet to experience so many things. I found the unfairness of it all overwhelming, as I find the death from cancer of so many other people at an increasingly young age. It's this flagrant injustice that I've tried to denounce in this book.

Cancer is, of course, as old as the world. However, in the twentieth century, it took on monstrous proportions and its spread now seems unstoppable. If nothing is done, if effective treatment isn't discovered, a massive death toll will ensue. This prediction is contained and denounced in the strongest terms in much of the 'scientific' material I've read, and I'd like to add my voice to this collective denunciation.

However, other questions are asked, and Gilles poses them as follows.

Gilles: Allow me to clarify a few points. Why were the practitioners of Chinese medicine stumped by cancer? The answer is that at the time, the conditions in which they'd have been enabled to solve the problem weren't fulfilled. By 'conditions' I mean the conditions we'd call scientific but that didn't exist in and of themselves: the ones that depended on society as a whole and on the choices society made for itself. This was the case in Europe's Middle Ages, when people were powerless in the face of the great epidemics; likewise, both Ancient China and medieval Europe were marvellous civilisations, and both included formulation of total responses to the question of death – and at the same time, the very existence of these responses is the reason that any attempts to overcome diseases were either prevented or rendered useless, because the diseases were accepted at the outset.

In order to fight against cancer, a culture had to emerge in which death was deemed inadmissable and science was allocated its central and preponderant place. The two phenomena are linked: on the one hand, the feeling of power connected to science, and on the other, today's narcissism, arrogance and will to prevail over the human condition – in short, belief in progress. Clearly, we've yet to notice that there's no such thing as progress without loss. We've acquired democracy, but at the expense of civilisation. We can cure one cancer case out of two or three, but in doing so we poison the people as well as the environment with the substances that are meant to cure them. On that point you're absolutely right, and on another you're partially right. It's indeed undeniable that cancer is very often psychosomatic, which means the subject bears responsibility for both the sickness and the cure. However, people wouldn't be as sick if society were less so – sick from stress, as we call it: the result of that will to dominate the universe at all costs, through which, in turn, the technological frenzy that drives capitalism as we know it today is triggered.

Capitalism has come up against its limits, and the limits are the human body. In capitalist societies, everything is viewed as being a means of generating gain, especially what Nature has to offer, and that includes the body. The body is considered to be an instrument of work: the body of the worker; the body as locus of renewal of life and therefore as an instrument of consumption; the body as space into which the profit-making machine casts off its waste, as it casts off its waste into the rest of Nature, and the body therefore as a space that does not have its own existence, is empty and has no status other than that of a waste dump – oddly, a kind of 'no man's land'! And it's this very space that, as many people have said, 'can't take it any more'. The human body is *co-extensive* with Nature, and the body of Nature can similarly be spoken of as a whole. It isn't abusively anthropomorphic to think of Nature's body and the human body as extensions of each other, because when the two are taken together, their functions, regulations and balances are too similar to be ignored. In this book, as in the many other books I refer to in it, I've borne witness to the body's current protest against capitalism, against this blind mechanism through which we're all being driven towards disaster.

Gilles: The writer Susan Sontag is also the person who established a link between capitalism and cancer; however, no one seems to know she did, because the past of knowledge has been so eroded. People don't know that it was in fact Michelet who not only described the homology between society and sickness down through the centuries but who actually based a whole system on the connection. It could be said that Michelet is to Sontag what Pasteur, the creator of immunology, is to Koch, who discovered the tuberculosis bacillus.

⌛

Now I've completed my manuscript, I feel the need to cast a critical eye over what I've written, to rethink things in light of some of the important works I've read over recent months. The sheer number of books being published about the subject of cancer are proof we're in the presence of a societal crisis of major proportions, although some of the writers would debate the extent of the crisis. I'd like to bring to bear a few thoughts that these books have inspired in me, and to locate myself within the debates their authors raise, by quoting extracts from them that seem to be especially pertinent to the points I've been trying to make in my own book.

Several people who read my manuscript, as well as some of my women friends, told me to write about alternatives in order to give my readers, both men and women, some ideas about how to 'avoid' cancer, or how to fight it more effectively should they be stricken with the disease. In this epilogue, I try to comply with their request.

⌛

It's now five years since Dr VZ prescribed hormones for me.
Three months later, I was diagnosed as having cancer. It'll
soon be five years since I underwent surgery, on Friday the
13th of June, 1994. It's said that to an extent, five years
means recovery; however, I've read too many conflicting
reports to believe that.

Do I feel cured? You never feel truly recovered from this
illness; in fact, you have the lurking fear that down the road,
the very treatment that 'cured' you will itself engender
other cancers – something that actually happens rather frequently. Every time you have a pain, every time you cough,
every time you have the slightest feeling of unease, your
repressed fears are awakened – and yet, the more time passes, the more the memory of the ordeal fades and life once
again resumes, undaunted.

Our loved ones who are now deceased are ever with us
and present within us. Their memory springs forth at the
sight of a flower; the aroma of a dish; the sound of a melody;
when your eye meets an image; when you read a text; when
you experience the thrill of travel. I sometimes have the
impression that Séverine is going to burst into my Urbana
kitchen with her lovely smile and her unfailing frankness;
that she's going to explain to me what happened to her; that
we'll have long talks together, as we had in the past. Alex
Sorkin, my eye specialist who founded Champaign–Urbana's
support group for cancer victims, has died. It seems his heart
gave out while he was undergoing a surgical procedure; otherwise, as his mother hinted to me, he simply wasn't being
properly cared for. He should've been kept in hospital longer
rather than been sent him home in such great haste, especially because he was sent home on a weekend, when it's very
hard to reach doctors. I can almost hear Alex saying, 'You see,
Evelyne: the arrogance of doctors! Nothing's changed: they
simply left me to die.'

My dear friend Charlotte Bruner, whose personal and

professional support for me has been unstinting and invaluable, is now having to face a metastasis to her bones, which means her days are numbered. More than 20 years ago, she underwent a double mastectomy, and everyone thought she was cured. Last year, however, cancer reappeared in her lungs, so she underwent radiation and chemo. People thought, once again, that she was cured. And here she is today, suffering from bone cancer. She tells me that her current treatment is serving to only lessen the pain. At this moment, she's mostly concerned that she'll be leaving behind David, her life companion, who'll then be alone. Knowing how very close She and David are, I feel terrible for her. Fortunately, I was able to visit them last year, and I'll try to visit them again soon.

So many of my friends and acquaintances, too numerous to list here, are currently undergoing treatment, in many cases for a recurrence. Many of them wouldn't wish their names to be included here, so strong is the conspiracy of silence surrounding this illness; however, I think of them very often.

The post-treatment period is a time of re-adjustment that many of us find challenging. How am I coping? Whenever my heart starts beating too quickly, I recall the red-coloured Adriamycin, the 'heavy' chemo drug I was administered: I imagine it's penetrated some of my heart cells, of which it's destroying some, and that it's weakening a vital muscle in my heart. Whenever I have pain on the left side of my mutilated chest, I can see the reddish eyes of the radiation machine; I hear the grinding sound of the electron production; I fear for my brittle bones and my spinal marrow; and I worry about suffering fibromatous effects.

The constitution of reactional fibrosis involves the activation of fibroblasts that surround the tumor and start secreting, and of excess fibers that make up connective tissue ... All

> patients who, after undergoing postoperatory radiation therapy
> for breast cancer, find themselves with the 'fat arm' syndrome,
> have come to know the unfortunate effects linked to compres-
> sion of the vessels in the armpit due to fibrosis … Fibroblastic
> sarcoma can appear anywhere from ten to twenty years after
> radiation … Another problem is the rays themselves: they
> destroy irreversibly any segment of bone marrow within their
> range of application, thus destroying the capacity therein to
> produce new blood cells. (Israël: 1998: 140–1)

When my arm feels sore, I'm afraid it'll go on hurting indefinitely and I'll lose the use of my arm; I then worry about
my other arm: whether the cancer will spread bilaterally to
the other breast, as is so often the case, I'm told, with lobular cancer. When I think I might lose the use of one arm, my
fear of losing the other becomes all the more intense.
Because I'm scared of becoming permanently disabled, I
start thinking about having a preventive mastectomy of the
other breast.

I'm also afraid for Alban. I can't imagine living without
him. For the moment, his current treatment seems to be
working. However, as soon we're told his PSA count has
risen, as it has in the past, we start panicking, and fearing
that the cancer cells have escaped and are somewhere
engendering a metastasis; therefore, whenever he has a bit
of pain here or there, we get nervous.

I can' refrain from repeating that in our view, we were
both prescribed hormones somewhat rashly and that his
current doctors aren't taking his medical record enough into
account. Why, for example, aren't they doing analyses of his
endocrine system and of the role that prolactin might have
had in his health problems, including his cancer?

> There exist prolactin receptors in many a case of prostate
> tumors, hence an added possibility, rarely put into practice, of

exerting a useful effect by administering an antiprolactin ... A well-reasoned multiple hormone therapy ought to be attempted in cases of prostate cancer when traditional treatment proves inadequate. It could turn out to be quite useful, even though currently existing medical references released under the auspices of Social Security make no mention of it, thereby implicitly condemning it. (Israël: 1998: 167)

With reference to hormones, over the past five years, the situation has changed drastically. A mere five years ago, it was a rare and timid person who questioned estrogen use in treatments, and he or she was more often than not ridiculed; today, hardly anyone denies the dangers involved in it. However, in 1998, Maurice Tubiana, a cancer specialist well known in France, could continue to make the following statements, which I quote from his book *Le cancer hier, aujourd'hui, demain* (Tubiana: 1998: 76).

The use of estrogen, both during and after menopause, has been incriminated. Consumption rates of this hormone have been highest in the upper income brackets. When estrogen is administered over long periods of time without progesterone, the risk of breast cancer increases. Currently, we are using hormone combinations less rich in estrogen, associated with various types of hormones, estrogen and progesterone especially, and this combination therapy reduces the risk of breast and uterine cancers. Treatments now in use for menopause should therefore no longer be considered dangerous.

However, his optimism is already starting to look a bit outdated, as indicated by Lucien Israël in his book *Destin du cancer*, which I quote from as follows (Israël: 1998: 229).

Estrogens are also dangerous ... it happens that estrogens are growth factors for breast cancer ... the risk is increased by 40%, as well as an enhanced risk among women whose substantial bone mineralization after menopause is the result of prolonged exposure to natural or artificially administered estrogen ... The same goes for contraceptive pills, less innocent than we may have thought, especially in high-risk families. If a compromise must be sought, then it should be in the direction of weaker doses, administered only intermittently, with the help of derivatives that stimulate only very slightly, and in association with differentiating agents.

Israel continues as follows (Israël: 1998: 164).

Most gynecologists are convinced that at normal doses, progesterone has preventive effects against breast cancer. That could not be further from the truth. On the contrary, it has been proven experimentally, but also through epidemiological studies, that the constant and often inappropriate use of progesterone can stimulate and favor the growth of breast cancer.

At the time of writing this epilogue, *Dr Susan Love's Hormone Book* (Love: 1997) had just been published. Love is the American surgeon and widely reputed cancer specialist whose *Dr Susan Love's Breast Book* (Love: 1993) I read during my ordeal. In the more recently published book, she sends a warning to women, whereby she states clearly that menopause isn't a disease and that it's highly erroneous to speak of prescription of hormones during this period of a woman's life as being 'substitution' therapy. According to her, the body knows why it produces hormones and why it ceases to produce them; it has a well-regulated device for interior programming that isn't to be tinkered with. Her book is also an account of how far she's come in her understanding since she wrote her breast-cancer book. She finds it scandalous that doctors persist in prescribing hormones to women who've already had breast cancer, as indicated in the following two extracts from the book.

Women who have already had breast cancer may increase their risk of a recurrence of the original cancer or of a second breast cancer if they take hormones ... Some research is beginning to confirm the danger. Studies looking at the basic biology of estrogen and progesterone suggest that progestins actually help cancers to become more invasive ... To be dangerous, cancer cells have to be able to invade tissue outside of their normal territory. Progestins make it easier for cancers to invade and spread. So giving progestins to women with breast cancer may make the difference between an *in situ* cancer and a metastatic cancer. Another worrisome study followed four women who were taking both estrogen and progesterone after treatment for breast cancer. They all developed metastasis ... Limited as this study is, it does give one pause. (Love: 1997: 123)

... at one time doctors – recognizing the likelihood of a connection between hormone therapy and breast cancer – were reluctant to give hormones to women who had had the disease. Now, however, with all the marketing of hormone 'replacement' therapy, there's been a disturbing turnaround: since there's no solid proof of danger, many doctors have decided that it's fine. To me, that's appalling. Logic suggests that it's dangerous to give hormones to women whose disease is already related to hormones. There's no proof that hormones don't increase the risk of recurrence, and these are human lives we're dealing with. Maybe I'm being unfair. Perhaps the doctors are just unwilling to tell these women their prognosis. Lord knows, it isn't easy to confront a patient with the fact that her chance of living long enough to get osteoporosis or heart disease is far less than her chance of dying from her breast cancer. But even if that's the case, doctors owe it to these women to give them the best shot at a longer life. Maybe I've just been too close to it. I've seen too many of my own patients die before they should have died; I'd have been so grateful if some of them could have lived into their seventies or eighties, even if they did end up with broken hips or heart attacks. Most women with breast cancer agree with me. A recent survey of women with breast cancer found that they weren't willing to accept hormone therapy if it meant even a very small risk of recurrence. Doctors who are promoting the use of hormone therapy for women with breast cancer cite the fact that both estrogen and progestins are given to treat metastatic breast cancer. This is true, but the doses are much higher. And paradoxically, high doses kill cancer even though low doses may cause it. (Love: 1997: 124)

The issues are indeed complex, and as I've already stated, Dr Love, who's seen many patients die and who's herself reached the age of menopause, felt the need to distance herself for a while from direct involvement with the illness:

While I was writing this book and wiping off the perspiration from my hot flashes, I suddenly realized that I needed a break from my medical practice. I'd been caring for patients for almost twenty years; I needed to take a break to focus on caring for myself. As a result, I retired from seeing patients. I have many activities I'm still involved in, from research, teaching, lecturing and writing to going back to school to get my MBA. Maybe I'll go back to patient care at some point, maybe not. I hadn't really thought that this change had anything to do with approaching menopause until I heard Susun Weed on that panel. But doing this for myself has made an enormous difference in my level of stress. (Love: 1997: 217)

In this epilogue, I can't address the polemics involved in Love's taking a stand against hormones, against detection of breast cancer through systematic mammograms of young women, against preventive prescription of tamoxifen, and against other unwise practices; I've spoken briefly about the subject in one of the chapters of this book. It isn't at all surprising that doctors as courageous as Lucien Israël and Susan Love are often criticised by some of their colleagues as well as by representatives of the big pharmaceutical companies. These doctors irritate the companies by calling into question the discretionary way in which they take charge of the patient's body; their kind of criticism strikes at the heart of the companies' profits.

By contrast, criticism such as Maurice Tubiana's, aimed at doctors such as Love and Israël, doesn't have much to do with real scientific dialogue; rather, it comes down to being an ideological debate. The debate can be outlined as follows. On one side – Tubiana, for example – the members of the medical establishment, whose ideological relations with the 'establishment' of society at large are quite visible, tell people not to worry; that there's nothing new under the sun; that cancer has always existed; that 'we're watching over you'; and that it's best to be silent and sleep in peace. Medical practitioners, in their incarnation as members of the pharmaceutical–medical complex, take full charge of your body. On the other side are the critics, such as Love and Israël, who are dissatisfied with current practice and tell us that everything must be rethought, from our relationship with our body and to Nature to treatment of the illness. According to them, we've got it all wrong: the risks we'll contract cancer are spiralling out of control yet we're treating cancer in the most bureaucratic way.

Clearly, on Tubiana's side of the debate, the proponents' opposition is total: they're opposed with reference to their relationship with the patient's body as well as with reference to the relationship of society as a whole with the environment. When I was reading Tubiana, I was struck by how insensitive he seems to be about environmental issues and their link with cancer, even though many researchers have established that the link clearly exists:

And yet, these myths still continue to affect the collective unconscious, and even wider health policy matters. The most false among them is the myth that attributes the 'epidemic of cancer' to modern civilization and to pollution. In reality, after adjusting for age, the frequency of cancer has not increased for over a half century. If we exclude lung cancers, 90% of which are due to tobacco and whose rate among non-smokers has remained constant, the mortality rate due to cancer has actually decreased by 14% between 1950 and 1990. This myth is not only false but dangerous, for by focusing attention on civilization, society, and pollution, it diverts attention from the real issues and has a demobilizing effect upon those who seek to do something about their health. (Tubiana: 1998: 32)

Of course, we must improve on the ways we keep chemicals in check, but do so without sawing off the branch where we're sitting. We must also take care not to encourage irrational fears, for these can prove more dangerous than industrial pollution. (Tubiana: 1998: 41) ... it is because radioactivity is frightening that it is considered as an important cause of cancer, and not the reverse. (Tubiana: 1998: 42)

Tubiana has clearly chosen to wear blinkers. As is the case with abuse of other substances, doesn't tobacco – or rather tobacco addiction – have everything to do with modern civilisation? Aren't personal habits linked to living conditions, such as stress? In any case, what control do we have over what we consume, conditioned as we are to consume the products that big corporations thrust in our face? When Tubiana's summations are thoroughly read, some patently economic designs are in fact revealed: he is in favour of putting a stop to ecology-conscious measures; he casts all responsibility on the individual – who of course cannot assume it; and he wishes to either limit or reduce to zero the amount of funding being used to establish the link between cancer and the environment – in other words, he has an obscurantist perspective. In his book *Le cancer hier, aujourd'hui, demain*, under the title 'Cancerphobia', he make the following statements (Tubiana: 1998: 429).

During medical conferences on the prevention of cancer, specialists deplore the huge sums of money being wasted on the fight against such minimal risks, money that could be better spent elsewhere. In the United States, these expenditures totaled some 200 million dollars in 1996, twice the amount spent on health insurance in France, with rather uncertain benefits. Unwarranted fears have limited the use of effective chemicals and slowed down the expansion of nuclear energy for power production ... ecology has become a weapon in the struggle for power in Germany, Russia and even in France.

Critics of this attitude have no need for these ideologically based approximations; rather, they construct a solid grid of scientific data, which I've consistently referred to in this book, especially to Sandra Steingraber and Gilles-Eric Séralini. I quote from Israël's *Destin du cancer* (Israël: 1998) as follows.

Genotoxic carcinogens that damage DNA do so by means of oxidation reactions. They create mutations in a certain number of genes, activating oncogenes, inhibiting anti-oncogenes, modifying the genes involved in repair work, upsetting the balance between proliferation and apoptosis ... It would be impossible to cite all the genotoxic families of chemicals, but some are worth mentioning: organochlorines such as DDT and its metabolites, which involve estrogenic effects that impact directly upon mammary cells. The same goes for dioxin and its derivatives. Aromatic polycyclic hydrocarbons, pesticides, gasoline vapors, especially from diesel engines, benzopyrene contained in cigarette smoke, all these are potent carcinogens. These hydrocarbons are also found in alcohols, such as certain types of whiskey, in many kinds of paints and mineral oils and in solvents. (Israël: 1998: 52)

... But the list is much longer. Derivatives of benzene, dinitrotoluene, paraquat (a herbicide) and its derivatives, quinones and quinolones, nitrosamine, which is present in fermented foods, all of these are carcinogens, as are metals such as iron, copper, and cadmium. Add to the list arsenic, asbestos, mercury, and vanadium, while zinc has protective properties against oxidation, as does selenium ... Thus, city air, salted and smoked food products, vegetables exposed to herbicides and pesticides, but also roasted coffee and the charred part of charcoal-grilled meat and such, all contain carcinogens. (Israël: 1998: 53)

... The more a tissue has access to differentiation, the less it will be susceptible to cancer, which occurs in cells that divide. In this area, it seems that the female breast is protected by early pregnancy and relatively prolonged nursing of children. In Western societies, where first pregnancies are postponed later and later, where birth rates are on the decline, and where nursing is often abandoned altogether, breast cancer rates are on the rise, and this does not appear to be mere chance. Add to this the massive ingestion of mood-altering drugs and pesticides that find their way into the foods we eat. (Israël: 1998: 53)

In compiling his essential information, Israël has laid bare the how complex things are when it comes to issues such as cancer and the environment, the truth about the statistics for ageing, and deaths due to cancer. Because this important information is the key to understanding cancer, I prefer to cite him rather than attempt to paraphrase him. I invite you, my readers, to take a closer look at his work, some extracts from which I include as follows.

We have now seen, through this accumulation of possible causes, that we are literally immersed in a sea of carcinogens. There are causes yet to be discovered, and some are known but so rare as to not merit a mention, but what we know is quite enough. We breathe carcinogens, we ingest them and we even produce them ourselves through our metabolism and through the radioactivity of some of the atoms that make up our bodies. We receive radiation from the sun and the stars, from the earth as well; we explode atomic bombs or allow nuclear power stations to blow up, we subject ourselves to X-rays and scanners ... Though knowledge of these factors is still a long way off from driving us to modify our social behavior, or even to modify our individual behavior – apart from the decline in tobacco addiction – life expectancy is on the rise in developed countries ... and certain indicators suggest – though there are conflicting studies in this area – that mortality rates due to the most prevalent cancers are actually on the decline ... But what about the cancer rate itself? It is more difficult to assess. A study carried out recently in the United States among a population of young people established that for cancers overall, the number of cases increased by 13.7% between 1973 and 1993, with a 12% increase for lung cancers. Unfortunately, breast cancers are not mentioned in this study (Israël: 1998: 62)

... It should be pointed out that the figures quoted above have been contested. Other American teams with larger scope and more means at their disposal made different observations. A very recent article suggests that in 1994, death rates due to cancer in the United States were 6% higher than in 1970, even though they had declined by 1% since 1991 ... There is thought to have been a slight increase in mortality due to brain tumors and melanoma, a substantial increase in deaths due to lymphoma, and a leveling off or decrease for other cases. (Israël: 1998: 63)

Thanks to the work undertaken by Sandra Steingraber and other researchers, we now know that a direct link exists between environmental pollution on the one hand and brain tumours and melanoma on the other. If these facts are covered up, it amounts to lulling people into complacency. We also know that the breast-cancer rate is clearly on the rise all over the world. To illustrate this point, I include the following five extracts from Claude Jasmin's *Cancer: aide-toi, la science t'aidera* (Jasmin: 1989).

Because of how fast industrial techniques are moving ahead, we are liable to identify new carcinogens only once it is too late, or even at a future time when the substance is no longer in industrial use ... Did you know, for instance, that chrome can be a carcinogen? Chrome is the most widely used metal in the world, for its properties of resistance to shock and corrosion ... it raises the risk of lung cancer among workers exposed to this metal ... The furniture industry is affected by cancers of the respiratory system (larynx, lungs) and the digestive system, according to epidemiological studies ... And what is there still left to say to the French about tobacco, when one observes what a brisk business the SEITA is still doing? *[The SEITA is France's state-owned tobacco- and match-manufacturing monopoly]* ... light cigarettes are as

dangerous for the heart and circulation as unfiltered cigarettes. Awaiting improvement, the massacre goes on: with
650,000 cases worldwide per year, lung cancer has stolen
first place away from stomach cancer, which is rapidly declining among wealthy nations. In France, at least 20,000 deaths
per year are attributable to lung cancer, a fifth of all cancer
deaths, and it has been estimated that there are at least
30,000 new cases every year. (Jasmin: 1989: 72)

Without going into too much detail – all the statistics are
equally depressing – it should be mentioned that tobacco is
also a major cause of mouth, pharynx, larynx and esophagus
cancer, in association with its old partner in crime, alcohol. All
of which adds some 20,000 cancer cases per year in France
due directly to tobacco. Alas, there is still room on the slate.
Also to be added are bladder and most probably uterine cancer. What is even more surprising is that a recent study has
confirmed earlier suspicions: tobacco could represent the
prime cause of adult leukemia. And if we add to this bleak toll
that smokers probably kill as often as bad drivers do by causing people in their immediate environment to inhale smoke
second-hand, we might well ask why cigarette use is not as
regulated in France as it has started to be in the United
States. (Jasmin: 1989: 73)

Carcinogenic viruses are in fact variants of quite common
viruses that are almost never dangerous, just as the danger of
chemicals can be quite variable. They do not act alone, and for
a cancer to appear, there must be an early infection, a major
multiplication of the virus that will remain within the organism,
where it will be able to attack repeatedly, as is the case with
chemicals in the environment or radiation. (Jasmin: 1989: 107)

Of course, in the case of cancer, it is likely that only repeated exposure to a carcinogen is capable of provoking cell

515

lesions that open up the way to malignant transformations. (Jasmin: 1989: 115)

In France, we hold the world record for cancers of the esophagus, particularly in the Calvados region, where it accounts for 12% of male cancers, as compared to 3.1% in the Tarn region, for example. This cancer would seem to be linked to alcohol consumption … Very recently, over-consumption of beer has been considered as a cause of pancreatic cancer. Under strong suspicion is the nitrosamine present in beer (though also in some wines and liquors), thought to be responsible for the carcinogenic effect of alcohol in general and for potentializing the effects of tobacco. (Jasmin: 1989: 116)

I find Lucien Israël's books especially interesting: he has courage and opens up new perspectives. One of his books, *Le cancer aujourd'hui* (*Cancer Today*) (Israel: 1976), bears the following lovely dedication.

To my wife, who did not capitulate when faced with the cancer of Auschwitz.

Often accused by his colleagues of using medication too intensively, he calls to mind the distinction that Thomas Kuhn makes between normal science and scientific revolution:

Today there ought to be recruitment in all schools of Medicine of young people who are capable of changing their point of view, should it become necessary. The same is true, in fact, for all decision-making positions, in all human activities. (Israël: 1976: 217)

I needed only to do a little cross-checking, a few uneasy statements from common acquaintances, in order to learn that my declarations had been judged as bordering on obscenity. I was asked to do no more than re-establish confidence, comfort and blissful ignorance. They rebuked me for playing the role of preacher, which is the last function I would ever hope to perform, but also for showing signs, so they said, of a positively sadistic side, truly disturbing for a doctor ... I must say that the position taken by French doctors, for instance, is far more responsible, more collectively courageous, than that of American doctors, who, for what is not often the purest of motives, deliver the unmitigated 'truth' to their patients, who are then left to digest the news on their own ... Nearly all doctors on the other side of the Atlantic live under the constant threat of malpractice suits, which is, incidentally, a distressing and dangerous civilizational phenomenon. They find themselves obliged to justify each and every therapeutic decision, get the patient's consent, discuss all the options, all of which cannot be accomplished unless the starkest and most straightforward truth is shared by all. (Israël: 1976: 246)

Lucien Israël won't stand for the medical establishment's techno-babble, and writes with utter frankness about the dilemmas a doctor faces when he or she is dealing with the multi-faceted and complex phenomenon of cancer:

I have no clear-cut solution to offer. I would claim that none exists, in fact, and that any global solution is necessarily false or dangerous ... I aspire at times to live in a world where relationships would be carried out on an adult-to-adult basis, among people who know the meaning of life and death, who, though not immune from fear, would not become its prisoners. A world of Stoics ... I have the greatest admiration for practitioners in the area of children's cancer and leukemia, for I know what a painful ordeal they face with each young patient, that they lose something of their substance with each new case. And I have no personal experience of having to tell children the truth. (Israël: 1976: 254)

I believe it is no longer possible to practise medicine without basing one's own practice on a deeply personal, even ascetic questioning, each and every day, of medicine's end purpose. This means taking into account as much real data as possible, in all its diversity, without falling under the influence of advisors and ideologues who think everything is simple, who seek and find, in their little books, all the answers. (Israël: 1976: 255)

Israël's attitude is a great comfort to me, and it seems my current doctor, Esper, has a similar approach to medicine. I can picture him right now, with his attitude of calmness, attentiveness and humility, attuned to his patient. How, during my cancer treatment, I'd have loved to come under the care of a doctor such as him! I have the feeling that if I had, before he or she had ordered the procedure I underwent, he or she would've done all sorts of tests and analyses of the biopsy, and would've adapted the treatment to my specific cancer's histological properties. Although Israël probably wouldn't have spared me the heavy chemotherapy I underwent, he would've spread it over a longer period, and I'm guessing he would've concluded that in my case, radiation wasn't useful. Esper said nothing to me about radiation – I didn't dare ask his opinion; however, I noticed he didn't hesitate for one moment to contradict one of his fellow doctors who was planning to have me undergo six extra months of chemo. Also, he phoned me in response to a worrying letter I sent him: a response I didn't at all expect and that in my experience of doctors is quite out of the ordinary.

I also have a high opinion of Susan Love's approach, especially as she defines it in her most recent work over these past few years. Like Israël and Steingraber, she's often criticised by 'scientists' and pharmaceutical-company reps who don't much care for someone who deigns to throw a spanner in the works of their money-making machine. Love has now distanced herself from the practice of medicine; however, if she'd been available and practising within a reasonable distance from my home, and if my insurance and professional commitments had allowed for it, I wouldn't have hesitated to seek her out to care for me.

For me, equally compelling has been the fine and subtle links that cancer specialist Dominique Gros sets up between the breast, myth, cancer and the psyche. I include the following two extracts from his book *Les seins aux fleurs rouges* (Gros: 1994).

> Maximalism is a permanent ontological temptation among cancer specialists. When faced with a cancer, aggressiveness seems to rhyme with effectiveness. When dealing with the Devil, all available weaponry must be brought to bear: chemotherapy, mastectomy, radiation therapy, hormones, immunotherapy, and not to forget the whole range of parallel medicines. The attitude is one of 'at least we tried everything.' The woman no longer has her breast, her hair, her ovaries, but the doctors, the patient herself, and her family members, will be shielded from any eventual reproach, should a complete cure not result. (Gros: 1994: 311)

> How can one make the decision as to one's own mutilation? ... When the chances of recovery are equal between mastectomy and conserving the breast, the doctor's role consists of opting for a solution that best fits the individual woman, not to apply some computer-driven set of procedures ... In the name of community harmony, individualism is made taboo. The breast becomes an object, cancer a thing, the person a number. A dehumanized society cannot induce humane medical procedures. (Gros: 1994: 321)

Gros refutes the theory that breast cancer can have psychological causes, such as the one whereby breast cancer is linked to female melancholia. These theories, though groundless, serve only to place the burden of guilt on women. Taking a different tack, he lays the blame squarely on contemporary medical practitioners, and on the lag in the area of research, in which he says not much has been done to date and real medical advances are sorely lacking. Like Israël, he includes himself among the guilty medical doctors, and has the courage to be self-critical:

The campaign messages devoted to the fight against breast cancer are very guilt-provoking. What always emerges is that the breast is a pre-cancerous organ by definition, and that women who are stricken by the disease are those who were not cautious enough to consult a doctor in time … As if the chosen were invited to sit at his right hand, and the damned to his left … This either/or dialectic is unhealthy, wrong and reprehensible. (Gros: 1994: 298)

Doctors are being trained to persuade rather than to seek to understand. To persuade women that they have to have mammograms, mastectomies, chemotherapy … It will take courage and strength to humanize medicine. Laws are not enough when it comes to the weaknesses of human nature. When confronted with cancer, physicians and care-givers also have their fears and their pain. They seek to protect themselves. (Gros: 1994: 299)

Gros poses the following questions, which I've been asking consistently ever since the onset of my illness.

Cancer still arouses an age-old and haunting question: 'Why Evil, and why me?' The idea that illness is simply a matter of chance is too scary … The idea that there is no fundamental Order behind the creation of Life or of Cancer is unbearable, for it would imply a reign of absolute incoherence … What

remains once all other explanations as to the possible cause
for cancer have been exhausted is the thesis that the psyche
is to blame. (Gros: 1994: 300)

The feeling of being powerless within the medical establishment is what drove me, during my own illness, to consider
alternative treatments, as well as to consider the possibility
of cancer prevention. The latter is something that licensed
medical practitioners never even mentioned to me. I've often
asked myself, *Can a person actually 'avoid' cancer by having a
proper diet?*

Whatever it is that triggers cancer is much too complex
for anyone to be able to provide a simple answer to this
question. However, I've come to make a complete reassess-
ment of how and what I eat. I've always had a very healthy
diet, which includes lots of fruits and vegetables and not
much fat or meat, but I was never careful about either the
water I drank or the likelihood that the fruits and vegetables
I ate contained pesticide residues. I never paid attention to
where poultry meat was produced or whether the animals
were fed hormones. Today, I try to be informed about alternative methods and *phytotherapy*, and make an effort to buy
organically farmed products. I filter the water I drink; otherwise, I buy bottled water, if I'm certain where it's from.

I've read quite a few books to help me discover an alter-
native planet, among them Duraffourd, Lapraz and
Chemli's *La plante medicinale de la tradition a la science*;
Montignac's *La Methode Montignac: special femme*; Frahm's *A
Cancer Battle Plan*; Joyeux's *Prevenir les cancers du sein*;
Michio's *Prevenir le cancer par l'alimentation*; Steinman and
Epstein's *The Safe Shopper's Bible: A Consumer's Guide to
Nontoxic Household Products, Cosmetics, and Food*; Weed's
Breast Cancer? Breast Health! The Wise Woman Way; and
Weil's two books *Eight Weeks to Optimum Health* and
Spontaneous Healing.

All these authors highlight the importance of having a diet that's rich in fruits and vegetables – especially cabbage-family vegetables, when possible organically grown – as well as in fish rather than animal meats. They promote olive oil; garlic; spices such as turmeric, which is good for the liver and has antioxidant effects that are more potent than those of vitamins C or E, or beta carotene – all of which are nevertheless nutritionally excellent. The authors are in favour of eating all sorts of mushrooms – wild, shiitake, maitake and reishii – and in favour of taking ginseng, astragalus and echinecha, through all of which the immune system is strengthened.

Dr Andrew Weil remarks that in the 1960s, the members of medical establishment wanted to ignore cancer's environmental and dietary causes, but that in recent years this attitude has shifted. Having a good diet is a condition that's basic to having good health. However, some foods should be avoided at all costs, as Dr Weil explains in the following extract from his book *Eight Weeks to Optimum Health* (Weil: 1997).

Avoid carcinogenic foods. Black pepper, button mushrooms (the most commonly cultivated kind), peanuts and all peanut derivatives contain natural carcinogens, and we ought to consume as little of them as possible. Celery and alfalfa sprouts also contain natural toxins that attack the immune system. In addition, highly salted and smoked foods, as well as the brine widely used in Asia (on radishes and turnips, for instance) are carcinogenic when consumed on a regular basis. Grilled meat is as well, as are all animal products when they are cooked until the outside surface is charred. Also to be reduced or eliminated are processed meats, those with a reddish appearance due to nitrates used in processing. Any foods that contain artificial coloring or artificial sweeteners should be avoided. Fiber-rich foods should be in everyone's diet, to avoid cancers of the colon and rectum, breast cancer and probably other cancers that are sensitive to hormones.

That means more whole-wheat flour and less refined, white flour. Include lots of fresh fruits and vegetables in your daily diet. That way you get the preventive chemical benefits of sulphraphane and other indoles in broccoli, of lycopene in tomatoes, of limonene in lemons, ellagic acid in grapes and apples, carotenoids in all yellow fruits and vegetables as well as in leafy greens, of isoflavones in soy, and many other elements that are yet to be identified. And don't forget garlic and ginger. (Weil: 1997: 250)

Through having my illness, I've learnt once again that we should avoid stress and take the time to do the things we enjoy, but that when necessary, we should practise techniques for reducing stress, and re-centring of the self, such as through meditation, relaxation and various forms of physical exercise. In the academic sphere, it's difficult to find time for yourself, and I'm finding myself once again being taken up in the whirl of meeting work commitments and demands on my time, and responding to requests that I'm often finding hard to turn down. However, when I feel the tension mounting, I've learnt to stop, breathe deeply, eat slowly, chew conscientiously, laugh, and simply walk away from any tasks it's become too disheartening to complete.

My relationship with my body has undergone a complete change. In the past, my bodily functions were so automatic I never had to think about them. My body existed as a part of myself, in perfect symbiosis with my self, and I never gave it a thought. Now, however, everything is different. I'm obsessed with my body image, and it's as if my body has become something alien to my self. This book is permeated with the obsessive fear that my own body inspires in me. At the same time, though, I categorically refuse to give in to this fear that's been imposed on me from without, this constant source of uneasiness.

I might spend a lot of time wondering about my body, but

this book is also about the connection between the body – my body – and the world. Our body belongs to Nature and to society, and society belongs to Nature. As a result of the mutilations I underwent during my treatment, I'm forever being led back to the same question: *Where does this kind of aggressiveness come from?* It hasn't caused me to turn away from the world, to turn in on myself or to regress; rather, I've been led to attempt to understand my relationship and my body's relationship with Nature and society. Within myself, I seek to awaken, or re-awaken, an awareness of this relationship, which in the prevailing ideological climate, society at large seeks to interrupt and divert, with all its agents, doctors and other people, who keep repeating that cancer springs from the individual, whether in the person's genes or mind; that the individual is responsible; that neither society nor Nature has anything to do with the disease. It's this same awareness that people such as Tubiana seek to shatter by openly waging combat against the idea that there could be anything new in the area of cancer, and to demobilise people by assuring them that the members of the medical establishment have patients' best interests in mind, and know what they themselves are doing. This is how they construct individuals who've completely withdrawn into their own body and who remain preoccupied with their bodily functions, having decided that because of the health-care demands their own body places on them, they have to ignore their connection to the larger world and deny their existence as 'beings in the world', in society. The irony is that their denial is coming at a time when people are being all the more passive as subjects as a result of their persistent refusal to acknowledge the relationship; in other words, they're being reduced to the state of medico-pharmaceutical super-consumers.

Because I constantly ask myself all these questions about the body and how I relate to my own body, I'm naturally led to address the central issue that all women who've been mutilated must confront: reconstruction. The question inevitably comes up, so great is the social pressure to consider the option, starting with the medical practitioners themselves. An article about the subject has recently been written by Jacqueline Julien. The translated title of the article is 'Breast Implants After Cancer: And That's an Order! For Whom? For What?' In the article, Julien frames one of the facets of this question in terms that are very close to the ones I'd have used, and makes a connection I've often made throughout this book: that of cancer and war. I include six extracts from her article (*Nouvelles Questions Féministes*: November 1997: volume 18: number 3–4: pages 117–27) as follows.

Is there not a semiological contradiction in this term which, on the one hand, calls to mind programmed destruction – such as that of a city razed to the ground during a bombing campaign – and on the other, the notion of reparation, trivialized under the enigmatic lexical guise of 'reconstruction?' (121)

There are throngs who would cry: hide this non-breast from us, that it be out of our sight! Why is this? Because this non-breast, this absence, is the sign and the obvious indication of your illness, of the dis-order that you have been subjected to … And to show *that*, well, it is simply not done. This non-breast is non-sensical. To expose this non-breast seems to give cancer the better part of the deal, offers it grounds to exist, whereas removing the breast but 'replacing' it is supposed to take those grounds away. (122)

For there is something vital at stake, after all, when this damage is done: something hideously powerful has, once in our life, attacked our very life, and the loss of a breast is indeed a reminder of that attack on vitality … But I ask you: when a city has been razed to the ground, annihilated, and its inhabitants wish to rebuild it, do you really believe it is only a matter of making it look nice? No, they wish to rebuild it for the life they want to relive in that city. They 'reconstruct' for immediate, practical, economic reasons, not mere aesthetic ones, nor to simply set upright again some stage set that has been knocked over. (123)

I did not accept breast reconstruction, because I did not feel destroyed or mutilated. Wounded, threatened, yes, but in my life as a human being, not in my 'femininity', whereas some people might have wished to reduce me, via a pair of breasts. (124)

I did not accept your reconstruction, because what does reconstruct me is the ongoing, delightful and delicious physiological sensation of what I have managed to come through alive. What reconstructs me is precisely that new asymmetrical body image that bears witness to the trials I faced, that tells the story of the battle won. Which tells it as it was, clearsighted. (125)

Why, indeed, could we not come up with a new fashion line for the thousands of women – a sizeable niche market – just as was created for expectant mothers whose fashions have become increasingly flattering precisely because they were designed with pregnant women in mind? Women who have gone through breast cancer and mastectomy have the need, just as anyone who has been harmed (and I mean by the disease itself), to share, to seek complicity. They need other women, and they need those other women to see them, not with looks of false pity but with warmth and intelligence (which is called solidarity). (126)

Like Jacqueline Julien, I have strong feelings about the artificiality of reconstruction, and especially about the discourse that surrounds it. When a breast is reconstructed, a living breast – a breast that's capable of enjoyment – isn't rebuilt. In this discourse, the key words are 'prim' and 'prudish', and only appearances are addressed. However, unlike Jacqueline Julien, I still feel mutilated in my body, just as I did immediately after I had my operation: physically mutilated; off-balance; as embarrassed and uneasy as a person would be after he or she had lost a limb. This is why I occasionally pay a visit to a plastic surgeon. As yet, I haven't resolved the problem.

'And what about faith and prayer?' my friends and family members will inevitably ask. I've already broached this issue in the book. As I've stated, I have the deepest respect for people who use authentic faith and prayer. In many recent 'scientific' studies, a direct link has been established between the practice of praying and being healthy, and even being cured. When we pray, we can attain a feeling of immense serenity: something I observed in my parents and that I continue to observe among other members of my family who pray on a daily basis. I find faith repugnant only when it's stiffened into dogma, and its practitioners seek to proselytise and take a judgemental turn; them, it amounts to a form of intolerance. In short, people who practise this type of faith do more harm than good.

For me, prayer is a form of meditation; during times of trouble, it brings me peace. In one sense, it's a form of relaxation, like singing or cooking. Making meals for people I love also has a great soothing effect on me, as does singing, which is also very helpful in keeping sadness at bay and in celebrating all the happiness I have in my life. Through singing, I was and remain able to overcome all the anguish and anger I felt during and after the civil war in Lebanon, and whenever I've been confronted with the reality of how women are treated in my part of the world. Through composing songs, both music and lyrics, I've had a way to express my suffering and my impatience for change. And later, composing become an outlet during the most painful periods of my cancer treatment. My mother was someone for whom song and prayer came as naturally as breathing, and today I can testify to the positive effects they had on her throughout her life, and especially towards the end of it, when her serenity shone like the sun on everyone around her.

I also had my writing to help me overcome my anxiety and allay my fears. Through writing, I've attempted to understand what was happening to me and to the people around me, and how cancer is related to the world and the environment. Writing, singing, cooking, meditation, prayer, physical exercise, relaxation techniques, and even laughter: through all of them, I've kept myself from sinking ever further downwards during the very worst of times. As well as being a way of remembering, writing is a way of forgetting. In Jackie Stacey's book *Teratologies: A Cultural Study of Cancer* (Stacey: 1997: 242), she puts it this way:

Narration makes it possible to exit from pain but also ensures that it will not be forgotten. Perhaps it is a kind of memory that heals. Restorative writing.

REFERENCES

Aba, Noureddine. 1978. *Le chant perdu au pays retrouvé.* Paris: Cerf.

Aubry, France, Dr. 1998. *La belle cinquantaine.* Paris: Stock

Accad, Evelyne. 1993. *Blessures des mots: Journal de Tunisie.* Paris: Côté femmes. English edition: *Wounding Words: A Woman's Journal in Tunisia.* 1996. London: Heinemann. Theatrical adaptation: *Les filles de Tahar Haddad.* 1995. Tunis: Médina.

Accad, Evelyne. 1982. *L'Excisée.* Paris: L'Harmattan. 1994. English edition: *The Excised.* Washington: Three Continents Press.

Accad, Evelyne. 1980. *Montjoie Palestine! or Last Year in Jerusalem.* (Translation of Noureddine Aba's long dramatic poem). Paris: L'Harmattan.

Accad, Evelyne. 1990. *Sexuality and War: Literary Masks of the Middle East.* New York: New York University Press.

Angier, Natalie. 1997. 'In a Culture of Hysterectomies, Many Question Their Necessity', in *The New York Times*, Monday, 17 February, page 10.

Barry, Kathleen. 1984. *Female Sexual Slavery.* New York/ London: New York University Press.

Batt, Sharon. 1994. *Patient No More: The Politics of Breast Cancer.* London: Scarlet Press.

Berger, Karen and Bostwick, John III, MD. 1994. *A Woman's Decision: Breast Cancer Treatment & Reconstruction.* St Louis, Missouri: Quality Medical Publishing, Inc.

Brouste, Judith C. 1994. *L'Etat d'alerte.* Paris: Le Seuil.

1993. *Chlorine, Human Health, and the Environment: The Breast Cancer Warning.* A Greenpeace Report, Washington, DC.

Butler, Sandra and Rosenblum, Barbara. 1991. *Cancer in Two Voices.* San Francisco: Spinsters Books.

1997–98. *Cancer Smart.* A Scientific American Publication on Cancer. New York: Yorktown Heights.

Carson, Rachel. 1962. *Silent Spring*. Boston: Houghton Mifflin.

Chedid, André. 1976. *Fraternité de la parole*. Paris: Flammarion.

Chedid, André. 1989. *L'Enfant multiple*. Paris: Paris: Flammarion.

Chedid, André. 1995. (Translated by Judith Radke). *The Multiple Child*. San Francisco: Mercury House.

Coney, Sandra. 1994. *The Menopause Industry: How the Medical Establishment Exploits Women*. Alameda, California: Hunter House.

Cousins, Norman. 1981. *Anatomy of an Illness*. New York: Bantam Books.

Cushman, John. 1997. 'US Reshaping Cancer Strategy as Incidence in Children Rises', in *The New York Times*. Monday, 29 September, pages 1 and 13.

Cutler, Winifred Berg. 1988. *Hysterectomy: Before and After*. New York: Harper and Row.

Delbo, Charlotte. 1970–71. *Auschwitz et Après*: 1. *Aucun de nous ne reviendra*; 2. *Une connaissance inutile*; 3. *Mesure de nos jours*. Paris: Minuit.

Déoux, Suzanne and Pierre. 1993. *L'Ecologie c'est la santé*. Paris: Frison-Roche.

Devi, Mahasweta. 1988. (Translated by Gayatri Spivak). 'Breast-Giver', in *Other Worlds: Essays in Cultural Politics*. New York/London: Routledge.

Dillard, Annie. 1974. *Pilgrim at Tinker Creek*. New York: Harper & Row.

Dossey, Larry. 1996. *Prayer Is Good Medicine*. San Francisco: Harper.

Dubrana, Didier, Ikonicoff, Roman and Guillemot, Hélène. 1995. 'Nucléaire et cancer: L'Enquête qui dérange', in *Science et Vie* (number 939), pages 85–94.

Duraffourd, C., Lapraz, J. C., Docteurs, and Chemli, R., Prof. 1997. *La plante médicinale de la tradition à la science*. Paris: Grancher.

El Saadawi, Nawal. 1983. *Woman at Point Zero*.
(Translated by Sherif Hetata). London: Zed Press.

Evler, Ewa and Séguin, Jackie. 1994. 'Cancer du sein:
Parlons-en', in *marie claire* (October), pages 133–42.

Erler, Brigitte. 1987. *L'Aide qui tue*. Lausanne: D'en bas.

Evans, Nancy and Martin, Andrea. 1998. 'Breach of Ethics at
the *New England Journal of Medicine*', in *The Breast Cancer
Fund Report* (Spring), pages12–15.

Faith, Jeanne and Nygren, Annelie. 1995. 'Breast Cancer: A
Feminist View', in *Off Our Backs* (August–September).

Felner, Julie. 1997. 'Dr Susan Love Cuts through the Hype
on Women's Health', in *Ms* (July–August), pages 37–46.

Frahm, Anne E., and David J. 1992. *A Cancer Battle Plan*.
Colorado Springs: Pinon Press.

Francos, Ania. 1983. *Sauve-toi, Lola*. Paris: Bernard Barrault.

Freud, Sigmund. 1955. *The Interpretation of Dreams* (1900).
New York: Basic Books.

Garrett, Laurie. 1995. *The Coming Plague: Newly Emerging
Diseases in a World Out of Balance*. New York: Penguin
Books.

Gille, Elizabeth. 1994. *Le crabe sur la banquette arrière*. Paris:
Mercure de France.

Gladwell, Malcolm. 1997. 'The Estrogen Question: How
Wrong Is Dr Susan Love?', in *The New Yorker* (9 June),
pages 54–61.

Global Action Plan Initiated at World Breast Cancer
Conference. 1997. *WEDO News & Views*. (Women's
Environment & Development Organization, 355
Lexington Avenue, 3rd Floor, New York, NY 10017–6603).

Greer, Germaine. 1993. *The Change: Women, Ageing and the
Menopause*. New York: Ballantine.

Gros, Dominique, Dr. 1987. *Le sein dévoilé*. Paris: Stock.

Gros, Dominique, 1994. *Les seins aux fleurs rouges*. Paris: Stock.

Hall, Stephen S. 1997. 'Vaccinating against Cancer', in *The
Atlantic Monthly* (April), pages 66–84.

Heller, T., Bailey, L. and Patterson, S. (editors) 1992.
Preventing Cancers. Milton Keynes, Buckinghamshire:
Open University Press.

Hitchens, Christopher. 1996. *Le mythe de mère Térésa*. Paris:
Dagorno.

Hjelmstad, Lois Tschetter. 1993. *Fine Black Lines: Reflections
on Facing Cancer, Fear and Loneliness*. Denver, Colorado:
Mulberry Hill Press.

Hœrni, Bernard. 1994. *L'Archipel du cancer*.
Paris: Le Cherche Midi.

Hœrni, Bernard. 1991. *L'Autonomie en médecine: Nouvelles
relations entre personnes malades et personnes soignantes*.
Paris: Payot.

Hyvrard, Jeanne. 1987. *Le cercan*. Paris: Des femmes.

Illich, Ivan. 1975. *Medical Nemesis*. London: Calder & Boyars.

Irigaray, Luce. 1985. *This Sex Which Is Not One*,
(Translated by Catherine Porter with Carolyn Burke).
Ithaca/New York: Cornell University Press.

Israël, Lucien. 1989. *Cancer: les stratégies du futur*.
Paris: Espaces 34.

Israël, Lucien. 1998. *Destin du cancer*. Paris: Fayard.

Israël, Lucien. 1976. *Le cancer aujourd'hui*. Paris: Grasset.

Israël, Lucien. 1992. *Vivre avec un cancer*.
Paris: Ed. du Rocher.

Jasmin, Claude. 1989. *Cancer: aide-toi, la science t'aidera*.
Paris: Plon.

Jasmin, Claude, in collaboration with Saad Khoury. 1979.
Cancer: De grands spécialistes répondent. Paris: Hachette.

Jasmin, Claude. 1983. *Parce que je crois au lendemain*.
Paris: Robert Laffont.

Joyeux, Henri. 1997. 'Cancer du Sein: un fléau social', in *Le
Figaro* (31 December), page 2.

Joyeux, Henri. 1998. *Prévenir les cancers du sein*.
Paris: François-Xavier de Guibert.

Julien, Jacqueline. 1997. 'Prothèse du sein après un cancer:

une injonction. Pour qui? Pour quoi?', in *Nouvelles Questions Féministes* (volume 18, number 3–4, November), pages 117–27.

Jung, Carl G. 1964. *L'Homme et ses symboles*. Paris: Robert Laffont.

Képès, Suzanne and Thiriet, Michèle. 1987. *Women at Fifty*. New York: Schocken.

Kfir, Nira and Slevin, Maurice. 1991. *Challenging Cancer: From Chaos to Control*. London: Routledge.

Khoury-Ghata, Vénus. 1993. *Mon anthologie*. Beyrouth: Dar An-Nahar.

Kierkegaard, S. (Translated by F. and O. Prior). 1943. *Le Journal du séducteur*, in *Ou bien ... Ou bien ...* Paris: Gallimard.

Kolata, Gina. 1997. 'Ticking Bomb', in *Chicago Tribune: Womanews* (Sunday, 23 March), section 13, page 2.

Koocher, G. P. and O'Malley, J. E. 1981. *The Damocles Syndrome: Psychosocial Consequences of Surviving Childhood Cancer*. New York: McGraw-Hill.

Kott, J. 1992. *La vie en sursis*. Arles: Solin.

Kuhn, Elizabeth. 1995. 'Lymphedema – the dirty secret of the breast cancer establishment, or Uninformed Consent'. Paper presented at the 1995 NWSA. Norman, Oklahoma.

Kuhn, Thomas. 1983. *La structure des révolutions scientifiques*. Paris: Flammarion.

Kushi, Michio. 1984. *The Cancer Prevention Diet: The Nutritional Blueprint for the Relief and Prevention of Disease*. Wellingborough, Northamptonshire: Thorsons.

Kushner, R. 1982. *Why Me?*. Kensington: Kensington Press.

Lacan, Jacques. 1977. 'The Mirror Stage as Formative of the I as Revealed in Psychoanalytic Experience', in *Ecrits*. (Translated by Alan Sheridan). London: Tavistock.

Lambrichs, Louise L. 1995. *Le livre de Pierre: Psychisme et cancer*. Paris: La Différence.

'Le cancer du sein: Hantise de toutes les femmes', in
   Réveillez-vous (8 April), pages 3–13.
Love, Susan M. 1993. *Dr Susan Love's Breast Book*. New York:
   Addison-Wesley Publishing Co.
Love, Susan M. 1997. *Dr Susan Love's Hormone Book*. New
   York: Random House.
Love, Susan M. 1997. 'Sometimes Mother Nature Knows
   Best', in *The New York Times*, Thursday, 20 March, page 19.
Lorde, Audre. 1980. *The Cancer Journals*. San Francisco:Aunt
   Lute Books.
MacPhee, Rosalind. 1994. *Picasso's Woman: A Breast Cancer
   Story*. Vancouver: Douglas & McIntyre.
Mathieson, Cynthia. 1994. 'Women with Cancer and the
   Meaning of Body Talk', in *Canadian Women Studies*
   (Summer, volume 14, number 3), pages 52–5.
McDougall, John A., MD. 1991. *The McDougall Program: 12
   Days to Dynamic Health*. New York: Penguin.
Metzger, Deena. 1992. *This Body: My Life 1* and *This Body: My
   Life 2* (two cassette tapes about the practice of creativity
   and healing). Boulder, Colorado: A Sounds True
   Production.
Metzger, Deena. 1992. *Writing for Your Life*. New York:
   HarperSanFrancisco.
Mindell, Earl. 1995. 'Soy: Rx for Breast Cancer, Menopause,
   and More', in *Women's Health Letter* (February), pages 1–3.
Orenstein, Peggy. 1997. '35 and Mortal: A Breast Cancer
   Diary', in *The New York Times Magazine* (29 June), pages
   28–52.
Payer, Lynn. 1988. *Medicine and Culture*. New York: Penguin.
Piver, Steven M., MD and Wilder, Gene. 1996. *Gilda's
   Disease*. Amherst, New York: Prometheus Books.
Plotkin, David, MD. 1996. 'Good News and Bad News about
   Breast Cancer', in *The Atlantic Monthly* (June), pages 53–82.
Powers, Richard. 1998. *Gain*. New York: Farrar, Straus &
   Giroux.

Powers, Richard. 1988. *Prisoner's Dilemma*. New York: William Morrow.

Pracontal, Michel de. 1995. 'La vérité sur les pilules du bonheur', in *Le Nouvel Observateur* (2–8 February), pages. 6–14.

Price, Reynolds. 1994. *A Whole New Life*. New York: Atheneum.

Radner, Gilda. 1990. *It's Always Something*. New York: Avon Books.

Read, Dr Cathy. 1996. *Preventing Breast Cancer: The Politics of an Epidemic*. Harper Collins.

Renard, Léon. 1990. *Le cancer apprivoisé*. Geneva: Editions Vivez Soleil.

Roy, Claude. 1983. *Permis de séjour, 1977–1982*. Paris: Gallimard.

Said, Edward. 1993. *Culture and Imperialism*. New York: Alfred A. Knopf.

Said, Edward. 1979. *Orientalism*. London: Vintage Books.

Scarry, Elaine. 1985. *The Body in Pain: The Making and Unmaking of the World*. Oxford: Oxford University Press.

Schwartz, Laurent. 1998. *Métastases: Vérités sur le cancer*. Paris: Hachette.

Sedgwick, Eve Kosofsky. 1994. *Fat Art / Thin Art*. Durham/London: Duke University Press.

Séralini, Gilles-Eric. 1997. *Le sursis de l'espèce humaine*. Paris: Belfond.

Sheehy, Gail. 1992. *The Silent Passage: Menopause*. New York: Random House.

Siegel, Bernie. 1986. *Love, Medicine and Miracles*. New York: Harper and Row.

Siegel, Bernie. 1989. *Peace, Love and Healing*. New York: Harper and Row.

Simonton, O. Carl, Matthews-Simonton, Stephanie, and Creighton, James L. 1984. *Getting Well Again*. New York: Batam Books.

Simha, Yolaine. 1985. *Eva comme Eve en ville*. Paris: Tierce.

Simha, Yolaine. 1998. *Je vous ai vue dans la rue*. Paris: Le Lieu-dit.

Soljenitsyne, Alexandre. 1968. *Le pavillon des cancéreux*. Paris: Julliard.

Sontag, Susan. 1977. *Illness as Metaphor*. New York: Farrar, Straus and Giroux.

Sontag, Susan. 1991. *1933 – The way we live now / Susan Sontag*. [etchings by] Howard Hodgkin. New York: Noonday Press.

Stacey, Jackie. 1997. *Teratologies: A Cultural Study of Cancer*. London & New York: Routledge.

Steingraber, Sandra. 1997. *Living Downstream: An Ecologist Looks at Cancer and the Environment*. Addison-Wesley Publishing Company, Incorporated: A Merloyd Lawrence Book.

Steinman, David and Epstein, Samuel, MD. 1995. *The Safe Shopper's Bible: A Consumer's Guide to Nontoxic Household Products, Cosmetics, and Food*. Macmillan.

Tait, Ann. 1986. *The Mastectomy Experience*. Manchester: University of Manchester (Studies in Sexual Politics).

1993. 'The Breast Cancer Warning: Chlorine, Human Health, and the Environment', in *A Greenpeace Report*. Washington, DC.

1992. *The New Our Bodies, Ourselves in the '90s*. The Boston Women's Health Book Collective. New York: Touchstone.

1995. *Time*: 'Estrogen: Every Woman's Dilemma' (26 June), volume 145, number 26.

1996. *Time*: 'The Battle against Prostate Cancer' (1 April), volume 147, number 14.

1996. *Time*: 'What Your Doctor Can't Tell You (22 January), volume 147, number 4.

Tubiana, Maurice. 1991. *La lumière dans l'ombre*. Paris: Odile Jacob.

Tubiana, Maurice. 1998. *Le cancer hier, aujourd'hui, demain*. Paris: Odile Jacob.

Tuéni, Nadia. 1991. *July of My Remembrance*. Beirut: Editions Dar An-Nahar.

Tuéni, Nadia. 1984. *La terre arrêtée*. Paris: Belfond.

Tuéni, Nadia. 1986. *La prose: œuvres complètes*. Beyrouth: Editions Dar An-Nahar.

Tuéni, Nadia. 1986. *Les œuvres poétiques complètes*. Beyrouth: Editions Dar An-Nahar.

Tuéni, Ghassan. 1993. 'Vivre avec le cancer', in *Conférence Internationale de Médecine*, Beirut, 8 July.

Wallis, Claudia. 1995. 'The Estrogen Dilemma', in *Time* (26 June), pages 46–53.

Walsh, Patrick C., MD and Worthington, Janet Farrar. 1995. *The Prostate: A Guide for Men and the Women Who Love Them*. Baltimore/London: A Johns Hopkins Health Book.

1994. *Watch Tower: Wake Up!* 'Breast Cancer: The Obsessive Fear of All Women', (April), pages 2–25.

Watson, David. 1984. *Fear No Evil: A Personal Struggle with Cancer*. London/Toronto: Hodder and Stoughton.

Weed, Susun S. 1996. *Breast Cancer? Breast Health! The Wise Woman Way*. Woodstock, New York: Ash Tree Publishing.

Weed, Susun. 1992. *Menopausal Years: The Wise Woman Way*. Woodstock, New York: Ash Tree Publishing.

Weil, Andrew, MD. 1997. *Eight Weeks to Optimum Health*. New York: Knopf.

Weil, Andrew, MD. 1995. *Spontaneous Healing*. New York: Fawcett Columbine.

Wiesel, Elie. 1994. *Mémoires: tous les fleuves vont à la mer*. Paris: Seuil. (Translated in 1995). *Memoirs: All Rivers Run to the Sea*. New York: Knopf.

Williams, Megan. 1994. 'Breast Cancer and the Environment', in *Canadian Women Studies* (Summer, volume 14, number 3) pages 7–10.

Williams, Penelope. 1993. *That Other Place: A Personal Account of Breast Cancer*. Toronto/Oxford.

Wilson, Alexander. 1992. *The End of Nature*. London: Routledge.

Winterson, Jeanette. 1992. *Written on the Body*. London: Jonathan Cape.

1997. *Worldwide Inventory: Environmental Links to Breast Cancer Research: 1990–1997*. An Action for Cancer Campaign Report. New York: WEDO, Women's Environment & Development Organization.

Yared, Nazik Saba. (Translated from the Arabic by Stuart A. Hancos). 1997. *Improvisations on a Missing String*. Fayetteville: The University of Arkansas Press.

Zorn, Fritz. 1979. *Mars*. Paris: Gallimard/Folio.

Chinese Medicine for Women
Bronwyn Whitlocke

... a comprehensive guide ... for women seeking an alternative to Western treatments. – *The Republican*

ISBN: 1-875559-70-1

Shiatsu Therapy for Pregnancy
Bronwyn Whitlocke

An instructive manual for pregnant women, partners and birthing partners caring for pregnant women.

ISBN: 1-875559-81-7

Help! I'm Living with a ~~Man~~ Boy
Betty McLellan

With a mixture of sensitivity and humour McLellan puts forward some thoughtful strategies to help men understand the difference between mumbled promises of future help and solid action.

– The Sunday Times

ISBN: 1-875559-79-5

The Menopause Industry; A Guide to Medicine's 'Discovery' of the Mid-Life Woman
Sandra Coney

An antidote to the flood of information extolling the HRT … a must read for women of all ages.

– Jill Farrar, New Woman

ISBN: 1-875559-14-0
(Available from Spinifex in Australia and New Zealand only)

The Day Kadi Lost Part of Her Life
Text by Isabel Ramos Rioja
Photos by Kim Manresa
Shortlisted, The *Australian* Awards for Excellence in Educational Publishing.

The Day Kadi Lost Part of Her Life is the moving photostory of a four-year-old African girl named Kadi, who is subjected to female genital mutilation in accordance with the traditions of her community. Black and white photographs document the activities of the day in which she undergoes this operation and an explanatory text details exactly what FGM entails.

I believe … that universal education and information about human rights and health needs to be spread as widely as possible. This book, with its direct, profound message, is a significant step towards this goal. I can recommend this book to fellow health professionals as a compelling and informative account and also feel that its visual impact will appeal to a general audience.
– Dr Kate Duncan, *Australian Medicine*

ISBN: 1-875559-74-4

*If you would like to know more about Spinifex Press,
write for a free catalogue or visit our website:*

Spinifex Press
PO Box 212, North Melbourne,
Victoria 3051, Australia
http://www.spinifexpress.com.au